MOTHERING
MULTIPLES

BREASTFEEDING & CARING
FOR TWINS OR MORE!

KAREN KERKHOFF GROMADA

Third Revised Edition

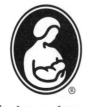

La Leche League International
Schaumburg, IL USA

Cover Photo: David C. Arendt
Book and Cover Design: Digital Concepts, LLC
Photo Credits on page 419

La Leche League International
957 N. Plum Grove Road
Schaumburg, IL 60173 USA
www.llli.org

For my parents, Ed and Peachee Kerkhoff, who continue to show me what parental love is all about; For my husband, Joe, whose love allows me to believe I can do anything I try; For my children (Elizabeth, Brandon, Tony, Joe, and Carolyn), who have taught me what is most important in life and who forgive me when I goof, but especially for my twins, Tony and Joe, without whose "help" this book would not have been possible nor would I have known it was necessary.

Contents

Introduction

If you are like most women, your emotions have seesawed since multiples were diagnosed! One minute the thought of multiples sounds exciting, and the next minute it seems frightening. Today you may resent getting more than you bargained for; tomorrow you may feel proud of your extra dividend(s). When you don't feel well, you may be overwhelmed with feelings of anxiety. At other moments, you feel in awe that your body can nourish two or more babies so well.

Questions may race through your mind. Will each baby be all right? Will they be born early? How will multiples change the plan for labor and delivery? Can I manage the needs of two, three, or four newborns when one seems a handful? What preparation should I make? What extra equipment will I need? Can I still breastfeed? How do I presume to know what you may be feeling? I have felt the surprise and numbness myself. I have experienced the ambivalence. And I have asked the questions. I am a mother of twins. I am also a La Leche League (LLL) Leader of a special group just for mothers who will be or who are currently breastfeeding and nurturing multiple-birth children.

For more than 25 years, this group has been meeting in Cincinnati to discuss the unique situation of breastfeeding and parenting multiple-birth children. All of the Leaders know what it is like to breastfeed and nurture multiples. Most of the women who attend are mothers of twins (MOT), but a number of mothers of triplets or quadruplets have also brought their babies to Series Meetings over the years. In the past, a lot of the Leaders' work was done by phone–with expectant mothers confined to bedrest, with mothers recuperating from birth, with mothers pumping for preterm babies, and with mothers too overwhelmed to coordinate getting two to four babies to meetings. Today, we also "meet" many mothers of multiples via the Internet.

Whether you currently are in contact with an LLL Leader by phone or email, attend "regular" LLL meetings, or even lead LLL meetings yourself, I hope you find this revision of MOTHERING MULTIPLES helpful. In addition to discussing some of the science of multiple pregnancy and birth, it is most importantly a compilation of years of mothers of multiples' experiences. There are frequent reminders that multiple babies are going to mean more adjustment and work for parents–no matter how they are fed.

Multiples do not plan to be born together. In spite of arriving as part of a set, each is a unique individual. Parents must constantly remember that. Having one another can never replace the need of each baby for your mothering. Since babies cannot be expected to compromise their needs, you and your husband or partner, as the mature members of the family, will have to give more. Because of this reality, several chapters in this book seem to focus on negative aspects of mothering multiples. When writing the first edition, I felt very frustrated by this.

Then it dawned on me. A mother does not need a book to help her enjoy the fantastic feeling of being at the center of two, three, four, or seven babies' universe. You don't need another mother to explain the joy of seeing all those little arms and legs waving wildly in greeting as you approach them. No advice is necessary when it comes to savoring the intangible pleasure of having four tiny eyes focused on your face as you breastfeed two simultaneously. Do I need to describe the awe you feel as you watch your babies sleep side by side? You certainly don't need me to explain why you feel so proud when your babies' pediatric care provider congratulates you on the babies' good weight gains–all on mother's milk! It is an incredible feeling to be given the privilege of eavesdropping on nature's most perfect "environment versus heredity" study, but I don't have to tell you that. Certainly, you will experience enormous personal growth as a direct result of coping with this intense situation without anyone having to inform you of it.

The positive aspects of mothering multiples are many and are to be experienced with joy. It is for the difficulties that assistance is required. When you are plagued with doubt or negative feelings, you may need a boost, a few suggestions, or a reminder that you are normal in a situation that is not normal. Fortunately, it is in overcoming any difficulties and coping with ambivalent feelings that the most positive personal growth can be achieved.

Remember that you are not alone. There are more than 25 years of other mothers of multiples cheering you on in this book. LLL Leaders who have breastfed multiples are available if you ever want to talk in person to someone who has "been there." La Leche League International (LLLI) maintains an updated listing of LLL Multiples Groups and Leaders and now hosts a "multiples" list on its Web site (www.llli.org/mother-to-mother forum). We are here for you, so please feel free to get in touch with one of us.

Good luck as you begin one of life's grandest adventures. And happy mothering–multiplied!

Karen Kerkhoff Gromada
September 2006

Acknowledgements

A special thank-you goes to Dee Keith, IBCLC, LLL Multiples co-Leader extraordinaire, and special friend. Thanks also to these wonderful women:

- Judy Torgus, Executive Editor, LLLI Publications Director, for her technical expertise and for her patience when this revision took longer and longer to complete.
- Nancy Bowers, RN, BSN, MPH, mother of twins and President of Marvelous Multiples childbirth program, for her expertise about multiple pregnancy, labor, and birth.
- The mothers of the Cincinnati LLL Multiples Group and those I've "met" on AP Multiples (Yahoo Groups) for the constant flow of multiples-tested parenting tips that demonstrate "good mothering through breastfeeding" and the value of mother-to-mother support.

I especially want to thank the mothers of multiples who contributed their personal stories and photographs for this edition. I hope they realize how their efforts will help other new mothers see that breastfeeding multiples is a realistic and wonderful way to feed babies–no matter how many arrive at one time!

MOTHERING
MULTIPLES
BREASTFEEDING & CARING
FOR TWINS OR MORE!

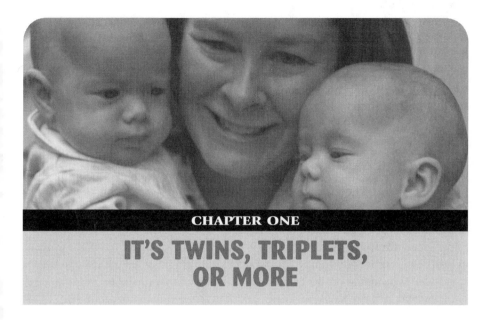

CHAPTER ONE

IT'S TWINS, TRIPLETS, OR MORE

Congratulations! You've hit the jackpot! You are carrying two, three, or more babies! Whether you simply "got lucky" or your odds for conceiving multiples were increased due to fertility-enhancing techniques, if you are like most parents of multiples, you never thought it would happen to you. Ready or not, here you are. You've now joined one of the fastest growing parent populations.

The number of multiple births in the United States (US) and most other developed nations rose significantly during the last decades, although the increase appears small when looking at the total number of births per year. For example, twins accounted for 3.2 of every 100 births in the US during 2004.* This represents a 42 percent increase since 1990 and a 70 percent increase in the annual twin birth rate since 1980. The increase in the number of higher-order multiple births, who also may be referred to as super multiples or "supertwins," is even more dramatic. Although the number of triplets, quadruplets, and quintuplets born each year account for only one-tenth of one percent of all live births in the US, the rate of supertwins increased from 37/100,000 to 193.5/100,000 births between 1980 and 1998 with an average yearly increase of 13 percent from 1990 to 1998. Since then there has been a slight decrease in the higher-order multiple birth rate to 176/100,000 live births—still far higher than the pre-1980 rate.

* The 2004 information is the latest year with complete information available from the US National Center for Health Statistics (NCHS) at publication.

Twin Types

The number of multiple births in the United States rose significantly during the last decades.

Multiples come in two types—identical (one egg) and fraternal (two or three or more eggs).

Identical, or monozygotic (MZ), twinning occurs during an early stage of cell division for a single fertilized egg (ovum). Once the fertilized egg cell begins to divide it is called a zygote. At some point in the process of dividing to form twice as many cells, the single zygote splits completely to form two separate zygotes—each containing the same genetic material since each originated from the same fertilized ovum. Because their genetic make-up is essentially the same, identical twins are always of the same gender. They share the same hair and eye colors, basic body build, ear shape, and so on. Unless someone knows them well, identical twins often are difficult to tell apart. Identical twins are born at about the same rate worldwide—approximately one in every 250 births. The incidence of MZ twinning appears to occur independently of a woman's age, ethnic group, or culture.

Fraternal twinning results from the fertilization of two (or more) separate eggs (ova) by two or more separate sperm, and it is referred to as dizygotic (DZ) twinning. Fraternal twins have as much or as little of their genetic material in common as any siblings who share the same two parents. They may look as alike or different as any two siblings in a family, and they may be of the same or opposite genders. Many factors influence the likelihood that a woman will conceive fraternal twins, including:

- Maternal family history of twins,
- Previous fraternal twin pregnancy,
- History of several prior pregnancies,
- Maternal age of 35 years or older at the time of conception,
- Use of fertility-enhancing procedures to conceive.

"Spontaneous" or "natural" fraternal twinning occurs most often in black ethnic groups and least often among Asian groups. An increase in the number of births for women over 35 years of age and fertility-enhancing procedures, also called assisted reproductive technologies (ART), are the main reasons for an increase in the number of fraternal multiple births in white ethnic groups, at least in the US. Fertility enhancement treatment especially influences the increase of higher-order multiple births; only 18 percent of higher-order multiples born in 2002 were conceived without some form of fertility treatment.

Multiples occurring due to fertility-enhancing techniques generally are fraternal because most of these techniques involve the administration of ovulatory induction (OI) medications, which lead to the maturation and release of multiple egg cells (ova) during a single menstrual cycle. (Depending on the procedure, fertilization may occur inside or outside of the woman's body.) However, it is possible for one or more induced fertilized ova to split during cell division and create an MZ pair, and a higher incidence of MZ twinning is seen after a woman uses OI drugs and ART.

All individuals within a higher-order multiple set will be identical (MZ) if after splitting once, one (or both) of the two "new" zygotes splits again (and possibly again). All members will be fraternal if three or more mature egg cells are released and fertilized within a single menstrual cycle. Higher-order multiple sets may include a combination of identical and fraternal members. For example, naturally occurring triplet sets can consist of an identical pair and a third fraternal member.

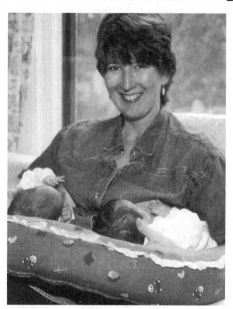

Breastfeeding benefits a mother as well as her babies.

Yes, It's Really Twins (or More)

An increase in the number of births for women over 35 years of age and fertility-enhancing procedures are the main reasons for an increase in the number of multiple births.

Until the last quarter of the twentieth century more than 25 percent of twin pregnancies went undiscovered until delivery. Today the birth of undiagnosed multiples is almost unheard of. When conception follows fertility-enhancement procedures, the possibility of multiples is always a consideration. Health care providers watch closely and test early for multiple pregnancy. Yet spontaneously occurring multiple pregnancies are also diagnosed earlier now. The development of simple but sensitive maternal blood (serum) tests, which are drawn in the first or second trimester of pregnancy, have helped. Blood may be tested for the hormone human chorionic gonadatropin (hCG) during the first trimester; the results of a maternal serum alpha α-fetoprotein (MSAFP) are more accurate when it is drawn between 16 to 18 weeks of pregnancy. Higher levels for either test are associated with an increased likelihood of multiples.

Ultrasound examination has had the greatest impact on multiple pregnancy diagnosis. Before the mid-1970s, x-ray was the only instrument able to definitely diagnose multiples and determine their positions in the uterus. Now a definitive diagnosis usually is made by ultrasound scanning—a method that creates moving "pictures" of the babies by bouncing sound waves off their body tissue in the uterus. (For more discussion of ultrasound, see Chapter 4, "What To Do If...")

When multiples are diagnosed early, you have more time to prepare for the birth and breastfeeding of two or more babies.

Early diagnosis gives you time to improve health habits that affect the babies' development. Also, once you know how many babies you are carrying, you will begin to form an attachment with each baby. When multiples are diagnosed early, you have more time to prepare for the special birth, and subsequent breastfeeding and care of two or more babies. And more preparation is needed—physically and emotionally.

Health Care with Multiples

A multiple pregnancy is monitored more closely, so it is important for you to have confidence in your health care provider(s) and in the health care setting where you will give birth. You need to be completely honest with health care providers** about every aspect of the pregnancy and they need to be honest with you. Science still has a lot to learn about multiple pregnancy, and many medical recommendations and treatments for apparent complications of multiple pregnancy are unproven or controversial. Don't be afraid to ask questions—lots of questions.

You may feel more confident in your health care provider if soon after the diagnosis you schedule time for an in-depth discussion about many of the aspects of multiple pregnancy discussed in the first few chapters of this book. For instance, you need and have a right to know how many sets of twins or supertwins a particular doctor or midwife has delivered. You may want to find out how many sets the health care provider delivered vaginally and how many were surgically delivered, and what criteria may be used to determine the method of delivery. Ask whether the health care provider approaches multiple pregnancy differently than a single-infant pregnancy. If the answer is "yes," ask about the differences. A "no" answer should be followed with a "why not?" since birth outcomes are not the same for multiples from a statistical standpoint. The physician or midwife who has always provided your gynecologic care, or who delivered your previous baby, may or may not be the best care provider for a multiple pregnancy and birth. If your care provider is a midwife, you and she will likely work closely with a physician specialist, such as an obstetrician or perinatologist.

Those who have undergone fertility enhancement treatment may find they must now interview a new obstetrical care provider. Specialists in the field of reproductive medicine often do not provide obstetrical care after their clients have conceived. Having built a relationship with one physician, it is not always easy to start over with someone new or with a care provider you haven't seen in a while. It's okay to

---

** To simplify and be more concise the terms **health care provider, obstetrical health care provider,** and **pediatric care provider** are used in this book to avoid repeating a list of physician, nurse, or certified lay providers who typically provide health care to women and children.

feel excited about the pregnancy yet feel sad that you will no longer be sharing your ups and downs with a provider you've learned to trust. You won't want to wait too long to find an obstetric care provider and your fertility specialist may share recommendations. Still, you may want to interview potential care providers in order to find one who best meets your and your unborn babies' needs for health care.

It is important for you to have confidence in your health care provider(s) and in the health care setting where you will give birth.

KEY POINTS

- ❑ The rates of twin and higher-order multiple births have steadily increased since 1980.
- ❑ There are two kinds of twinning:
  - Monozygotic (MZ) or "one egg" twins are also know as identical twins.
  - Dizygotic (DZ) means "two egg" twins who are also called fraternal twins.
- ❑ Early diagnosis gives an expectant mother more time to prepare and care for her babies by improving her own health habits.
- ❑ Women pregnant with twins, triplets, or more will see their obstetrical health care providers more often. Be sure to go to a care provider you trust for care with a multiple pregnancy and birth.

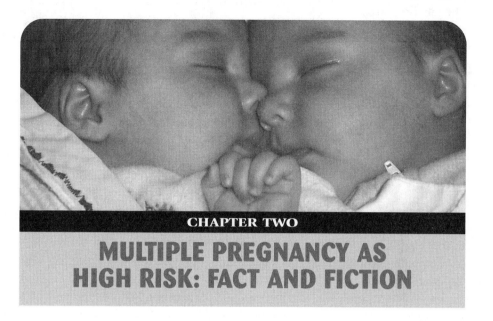

CHAPTER TWO

MULTIPLE PREGNANCY AS HIGH RISK: FACT AND FICTION

Multiple pregnancy shares many similarities with single-infant pregnancy, but multiple pregnancy also is different. Historically, the survival of the human species has depended on carrying and giving birth to only one offspring with each pregnancy. There is additional physical stress for a mother and her babies during a multiple pregnancy.

Because of the additional stressors, most health care providers now label any multiple pregnancy as a "high risk" pregnancy. However, the label of "high risk" only means that certain complications or conditions are more likely to occur with a multiple pregnancy than with a typical single-infant pregnancy. It does not mean a complication or condition will occur. Placing a label on multiple pregnancies merely reminds obstetrical care providers that they must screen more carefully for conditions or complications seen more often with multiple pregnancy.

Maternal Stressors

Even an ideal multiple pregnancy is more physically stressful than a single-infant pregnancy. Typical early pregnancy symptoms, such as nausea, fatigue, and constipation, are often exaggerated during multiple pregnancies. Later in pregnancy, heartburn, backache, and quick tiring or shortness of breath with activity also occur more frequently. These symptoms are more common because of the higher levels of pregnancy hormones and volume of blood circulating within a woman's body

> The label of "high risk" only means that certain complications or conditions are more likely to occur it does not mean they will occur.

and to the increased space two or more growing babies take up. During the last trimester of a multiple pregnancy many women find they've outgrown most maternity clothes and can no longer see their feet when standing upright. Even turning over in bed requires strategic planning!

To screen for the conditions seen more often in multiple pregnancy, your health care provider probably will want to see you more frequently, especially during the last half of pregnancy. Your blood may be drawn and monitored more often since pregnancy-related anemia is more common with multiple pregnancy. Your blood sugar may also be checked periodically because there is a slight increase in the incidence of gestational diabetes with multiple pregnancy. Pregnancy-induced hypertension (PIH), sometimes called preeclampsia or toxemia, occurs more often with multiple pregnancy, so the doctor or midwife will frequently check your weight gain, blood pressure, deep tendon reflexes, and urine. (See Chapter 4, "What To Do If...")

Physical stress isn't the only kind you may experience. Many expectant mothers feel ambivalent about a multiple pregnancy. Whether your multiple pregnancy was a complete surprise or required years of treatment for infertility, it is normal to have mixed feelings about getting more than you bargained for! The thought of multiples may sound exciting one minute, and only a few minutes later the thought of caring for two or more newborns may lead to feelings of mild panic. A concern about giving birth too early may alternate with a sense of awe that your body is nourishing two or more infants so well within it. You sometimes might wonder how multiples will affect your birth plans, how you will manage breastfeeding, how your older children will react, and how much two or more babies will strain the family budget. Don't be surprised if your feelings about the pregnancy and the thought of having multiple babies fluctuate not only from day to day, but also from minute to minute. If you find your emotions about the pregnancy and being the mother of multiples vacillating, you are in good company. Such feelings are very common!

Infants' Stressors

Sharing a uterus is physically more stressful for babies, too. Multiples are more likely to be born early. In the US the average length for a twin pregnancy, or gestation, in 2002 was 35.3 weeks compared with 38.8 weeks for a single-infant pregnancy. Length of gestation averaged 32.2 weeks with triplets, just below 30 weeks for quadruplets, and 28.5 weeks for quintuplets. (This is a decrease of almost a week less in the womb for twins and all supertwin types, and half a week less for singletons among US newborns over the last decade.) Multiples also tend to weigh less than single babies at the same week of pregnancy (same gestational age). More than 55 percent of all twins and 96 percent of higher-order multiples weighed less than

2500 gm (5 lb 8 oz), at birth compared with only six percent of single-born infants. Only one percent of singletons born in the US were "very low birth weight" (VLBW), which is 1500 gm (3 lb 5 oz) or less, while ten percent of twins, 34.5 percent of triplets, 61 percent of quadruplets, and 84 percent of quintuplets were VLBW at birth. It isn't surprising then that a disproportionate number of newborn multiples spend hours to weeks in a newborn intensive care unit (NICU).

Your obstetrical care provider will watch closely and probably test for the physical signs that may come before preterm labor. Many care providers use regular ultrasound exams as a way to check on the health of the placenta(s) and for a slowing down in the growth rate of any of the babies.

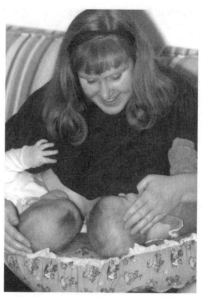

There is every reason to think positive when a multiple pregnancy is discovered.

Think Positive

There is every reason to think positive when multiples are discovered during pregnancy. Many women have healthy multiple pregnancies and deliver two, three, or more healthy babies. Almost 15 percent of twin pregnancies are full-term. It is not unusual for a woman to give birth to twins having average birth weights over 2725 gm, or 6 pounds. Occasionally each of a set of twins weighs 3400 to 4100 gm, or 7 to 9 pounds at birth. And many multiples who are born between 34 and 38 weeks and who are small for gestational age are still healthy at birth.

> **Many women have healthy multiple pregnancies and deliver two, three, or more healthy babies.**

Improving the Odds

There is no point in ignoring risk factors. As the saying goes, "Forewarned is forearmed." However, you can take action to decrease some risks. The earlier a diagnosis of multiple pregnancy is made, the earlier you can begin working to improve the outcome. Ideas for taking care of yourself and your babies before they are born can be found in Chapter 3, so all of you will be ready to get to know one another and begin breastfeeding.

KEY POINTS

❏ Multiple pregnancies are considered "high risk" due to a higher rate of complications.

❏ Multiple pregnancy is more stressful for a woman's body, and many women find it more emotionally stressful as well.

❏ Sharing a single womb, or uterus, is also more stressful for the two or more babies involved.

❏ Expectant mothers of multiples can take action to improve the likelihood that:

- The multiple pregnancy will last until full term or close to it.

- Each of her babies will be among the 45 percent who weigh at least 2500 gm (5 lb 8 oz).

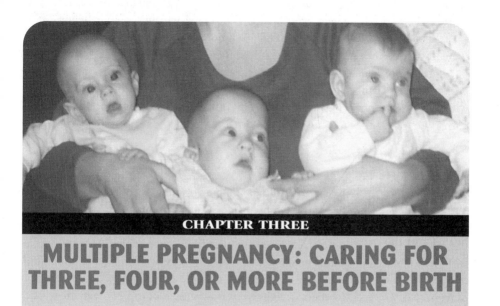

CHAPTER THREE

MULTIPLE PREGNANCY: CARING FOR THREE, FOUR, OR MORE BEFORE BIRTH

Many women have essentially normal, uncomplicated multiple pregnancies, labors, and births. Many multiples are born at term and are of average birth weights or close to term and close to 2500 gm (5 lb 8 oz). And many multiple sets and their mothers are eager and able to breastfeed within an hour or two of birth. There are actions you can take to improve the odds of a good outcome for you and your babies, and to minimize both the risk of complications and their consequences so you can all get off to the best breastfeeding start.

Don't wait and simply hope that all goes well during your multiple pregnancy. There are several contributions only you can make, and they can affect all of you during pregnancy and after the babies are born. To improve the chances of a full-term, or close to full-term, pregnancy and babies with normal weights for gestational age, take an active role in promoting your health and the health of the babies and their placenta(s).

A placenta's job is to keep an in-utero baby supplied with essential oxygen and nutrients, and get rid of waste products. It depends on a mother's healthy cardio-vascular system to do its crucial job. A decrease in placental function, which may affect one or more placentas in a multiple pregnancy, is associated with preterm labor, slower growth rates in affected babies, and maternal complications, such as pregnancy-induced hypertension (pre-eclampsia). There are many aspects of multiple pregnancy outside of your control, but you can take an active role in keeping the placentas as healthy as possible by eating well, avoiding harmful substances, exercising as your pregnancy allows, and relaxing as needed. You already have an advantage if you are: 1) of average weight for your height, 2) at least 62 inches (5 ft 2 in; 1.6 meters) tall, 3) a nonsmoker/non-tobacco user and not regularly exposed to secondhand smoke, 4) free of gum and vaginal or urinary tract inflammation or infection, 5) not anemic when you conceive, and 6) someone who deals positively with stress. Your risks may also be lower if you conceived multiples without fertility enhancing techniques, have carried a previous pregnancy to full term, and your babies are dizygotic (fraternal).

A Good Diet

Take an active role in promoting your health and the health of the babies and their placenta(s).

Eating a nutritious diet and gaining adequate weight during the first twenty weeks and throughout your multiple pregnancy are probably the most important things you can do to take care of yourself and your babies. Although there still is much to learn about the association between diet and a healthy outcome for multiple pregnancy, the link between mothers' weight gains during twin or triplet pregnancies and babies' birth weights is well established. Also, there may be a relationship between an expectant mother's weight gain and the length of multiple pregnancy.

It takes a lot of good food to support the growth and development of two or more unborn babies, and keep one or more placenta(s) healthy! A woman's nutritional requirements are higher during any pregnancy, but nutritional requirements continue to multiply along with the number of babies a woman carries. Pre-pregnancy general health and weight-for-height, which is measurable using the basal metabolic index (BMI),* also influence pregnancy nutritional requirements.

Pre-pregnancy guidelines recommend that a woman with an average BMI take in at least 1800 to 2200 calories from food a day. Current calorie recommendations for singleton pregnancy suggest a daily minimum of 2500 calories with daily minimums of 3500 calories for twin pregnancy and 4500 calories for triplet or quadruplet pregnancies. In addition, some sources advise from 300 to 600 extra calories per day for each additional multiple. If you aren't a calorie counter, eating more of the right kinds of foods and including frequent protein and carbohydrate snacks between meals should help you meet multiple pregnancy weight gain goals. (See "Nutrition Hints" below.)

---

* Ask your obstetric care provider for a chart to calculate BMI or go to the National Institutes of Health Web site for both a metric and standard US BMI calculator at: http://nhlbisupport.com/bmi/bminojs.htm

For twin pregnancy the goal for a woman with an average pre-pregnant BMI (18.5 to 24.9) is to gain about 454 to 705 gm (1 to 1 1/2 pounds) a week for the first 20 weeks and about 570 to 680 gm (1 1/4 to 2 pounds) for each of the next 10 weeks, or up to 30 weeks. The weight gain recommendation for the remainder of twin pregnancy is about the same as for the first 20 weeks. Women having a pre-pregnant BMI of below average (less than 18.5) are considered underweight and are expected to gain an additional 225 to 340 gm (1/2 to 3/4 pound) each week. If

In cultures where "thin is in," it may be difficult to remember that pregnancy weight gain is very different than other weight gains.

a woman is overweight (BMI over 25) when she conceives twins, the weight gain recommendation is about 225 to 340 gm (1/2 to 3/4 pound) less each week than for a woman with an average BMI. Recommendations for total weight gain during twin pregnancy are summarized on the chart included in this chapter. Less is known about weekly weight gain for women pregnant with triplets and other higher-order multiples, but calorie and total weight gain recommendations increase to meet suggested total pregnancy weight gain guidelines.

Although achieving the "average" weight gain may include some week-to-week variation, small weight gains for two consecutive months, a failure to gain any weight during one month, or an actual weight loss in any given month should be looked at carefully by health care providers. Women in Cincinnati's La Leche League Multiples' group who have delivered at full term and whose twins were of average birth weight typically gained 22.5 to 27 kg (50 to 60 pounds) during their pregnancies.

For single-infant pregnancies it is usually enough to recommend expectant mothers "eat to appetite." This suggestion can backfire when made to someone expecting multiples. Feelings of nausea may be exaggerated early in multiple pregnancies. Later in multiple pregnancy some women experience feelings of extreme fullness after eating even small amounts of food.

Although quantity is important when working toward a weight gain associated with better outcomes, the emphasis should be on the quality of the foods you eat. Ideas for eating quality foods and meeting nutritional requirements during multiple pregnancy follow in "Nutrition Hints." Acupuncture also has been used to relieve some pregnancy-related diet difficulties, such as severe pregnancy-related nausea or vomiting.

In Western cultures where "thin is in," it may be difficult to remember that pregnancy weight gain is very different than other weight gains. The babies' weights make up only a percentage of the total pregnancy weight gain. Other necessary physical adaptations to meet the body's demands of multiple pregnancy and the fact that your body is planning ahead for breastfeeding add important pounds. It is not unusual for mothers of multiples to lose two-thirds or more of the weight they gained during pregnancy within a week or two of delivery. The rest may "fall off"

Suggested Total Weight Gain for Multiple Pregnancy

Prepregnant	Twins	Triplets	Quadruplets
Underweight (BMI <18.5)	22.5 to 29.5 kg (50 to 65 lb)		
Average (BMI 18.5 to 24.9)	18.2 to 25 kg (40 to 55 lb)	22.5 to 27 kg (>50 to 60 lb)	29.5 to 41 kg (65 to 90 lb)
Overweight (BMI 25 to 29.9)	16 to 20.5 kg (35 to 45 lb)		
Obese (BMI >30)	13.5 to 18 kg (30 to 40 lb)		

within weeks of giving birth or melt away more slowly during the first year of breastfeeding.

If you or others in your life sometimes lose sight of the importance of a large weight gain during a multiple pregnancy, post signs around your home to help you maintain the proper perspective. Signs might say: "I'm eating for three (or four or more)!" or "I'm not getting fat; I'm growing healthy babies (and keeping their placentas in good working order)."

Nutrition Hints

What to Eat

A well-balanced diet is the goal during multiple pregnancy. Foods high in protein are especially important for building babies' bodies and keeping placenta(s) working well. Protein requirements rise from 110 gm daily for a singleton pregnancy to more than 150 gm daily for twin pregnancy and 200 gm or more for triplet and other higher multiple pregnancies. Meat, fish and other seafood, dairy products, eggs, nuts or nut butters, and legumes are good sources of protein. In addition to extra protein many of the calories you take in should be in the form of complex carbohydrates, such as pastas, rice, and whole grain breads or cereals. Your body uses the energy from carbohydrates to fuel its usual functions, which frees the protein to "build" healthy babies and maintain the placenta(s). Fats are also used for fuel, plus they are a crucial building block in each baby's brain and nervous system development.

Certain nutrients help minimize maternal anemia, which in turn helps maintain the health of your babies and their placentas. Most doctors and midwives recommend a multi-vitamin and mineral supplement during pregnancy. Sometimes higher doses of certain vitamins or minerals are suggested during a multiple pregnancy. However, *do not take additional vitamins or minerals without first discussing it with your health care provider* and possibly a dietitian specializing in perinatal nutrition, as some vitamins and minerals are toxic in higher doses. If

Many large medical centers now employ dietitians who specialize in pregnancy and postpartum nutrition. Consulting with such a dietitian is important for any woman expecting multiples, but it is crucial if you:

- Are carrying higher-order multiples,
- Were significantly under or over weight-for-height (per BMI) prior to pregnancy,
- Are anemic,
- Smoke (or your partner does),
- Are vegetarian,
- Are currently breastfeeding an infant or toddler (see "Breastfeeding while pregnant" in this chapter),
- Have a history of an eating disorder (or think you ever had),
- Have a family history of allergies (or your partner does),
- Have had gastric bypass surgery,
- Have a pre-existing health condition that is affected by diet in any way, such as high blood pressure, type I or II diabetes,
- Develop a health condition that is or may be affected by diet, such as gestational diabetes or pregnancy-induced hypertension (PIH/preeclampsia),
- Are preoccupied with your body size or weight gain,
- Often find it difficult to eat enough for any reason.

Eating a nutritious diet and gaining adequate weight are probably the most important things you can do to take care of yourself and your babies.

additional vitamins and minerals are advised during your multiple pregnancy, such supplements *do not* replace the essential nutrients and calories in food. Continue to eat a well-balanced diet that enables you to gain necessary weight.

The US Departments of Agriculture and Health and Human Services developed a food pyramid as a guide to making healthful food choices for optimal nutrition. Meeting daily pyramid guidelines is simpler than counting calories. The chart on page 17 compares pre-pregnancy and single pregnancy nutrition with that for multiple pregnancies. (The amounts indicated are only an approximation.)

Don't panic if the amount of food seems overwhelming. Most single-serving sizes on the chart are small compared to the servings many persons usually eat. For example, a typical bowl of pasta would meet the requirement for three to four servings from the grain group.

Make the most of meals and snacks by eating foods in as close to their natural state as possible. Focus on lean meats, low-fat dairy products, whole grain breads, cereals and pastas, and fresh fruits, vegetables, and 100 percent juices. Foods rich

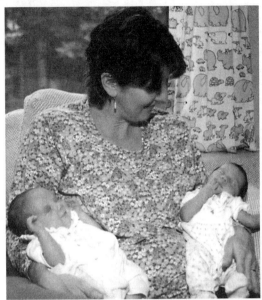

Eating a nutritious diet and gaining adequate weight helps you to grow healthy babies.

in animal protein, including dairy products and eggs, will usually supply most of the daily requirement for fats. However, don't be afraid of "good" fats during a multiple pregnancy. Sauté or fry foods in an unhydrogenated vegetable oil, such as olive oil rather than a saturated fat, such as lard. Eat fewer processed or canned foods, which often are higher in saturated fats and trans fatty acids, salt, and refined sugars, and have lost vitamins and minerals in the manufacturing process.

Try eating smaller amounts frequently—nibble all day long! This is especially helpful if you

> **Foods high in protein are especially important for building babies' bodies and keeping placenta(s) working well.**

regularly experience nausea, quickly feel overfull, or are put on bed rest. Even if you eat several larger meals, also snack between meals. A healthy snack could consist of a half sandwich of lean meat, liverwurst (braunschweiger), peanut butter, or egg salad on whole grain bread or crackers. Follow the high-protein snack immediately, or within an hour, with a fresh fruit or vegetable or 100 percent juice.

A liquid food, such as soup, may be easier on a stomach that has little extra room. Meat, poultry, fish, lentil, split pea, and bean soups are good choices because they are rich in protein. A salad containing a variety of greens and other vegetables or legumes is another nutritious but lightweight meal. Toss slices of lean meat, poultry, fish, tofu, or cheese with salad greens for extra protein. Middle Eastern and Asian cuisines generally are highly nutritious, light on the stomach, and known for many complete-protein vegetarian dishes.

Don't forget the nutritional power packed in every egg. Eggs are an excellent source of protein and several vitamins and minerals. Cook eggs first—whether scrambled, fried, or boiled—because raw egg may carry bacteria that cause food poisoning.

Blending milk or yogurt with fruit makes a nutritious, high-protein shake drink that should not overfill. Some women add powdered milk, wheat germ, or a protein powder to boost the nutrition in shakes or smoothies without adding volume in their stomachs. If you've thought about adding protein powder to food or buying high-protein beverages, be aware that not all brands are created equal. Before trying a

MINIMUM Number of Daily Servings Chart

	Pre-pregnancy	Single Pregnancy	Twin Pregnancy	Triplet Pregnancy**
Grains Group: **Bread, Cereal,** **Rice & Pasta** One serving= 1 slice bread, 1/2 oz. pasta, rice 1 oz./1C cereal 1oz.=30 ml/30gm	6-11	7-11	8-12	9-12
Vegetable & **Fruit Groups** One Serving= 1 whole/1C./8oz. Raw, 1/2C./4oz. cooked, 3/4C./6oz. juice	3V & 2F	4V & 3F	4-5V/3-4F	5V/4F
Dairy Group; **Milk, Yogurt &** **Cheese** One serving= 1C./8oz. milk 1C./8oz. yogurt 1oz. cheese	2-3	3-4	4-5	5-6
Meat, Poultry, **Fish, Eggs, Dry** **Beans & Nuts** **Group** One serving= 2oz., meat, poultry, fish, 2 eggs, 1C./8oz. dry beans, 4 Tbsp. peanut butter	2-3	3-4	4-5	5-6
Fats Group Oils, Processed Snack Foods & sweets	Use sparingly	Get from meat, eggs, dairy products, monounsaturated fats, such as, olive oil and canola oil, and certain fish oils.		
Non-alcoholic, **uncaffeinated** **beverages** One Serving=8oz./ 1 cup	6+	Enough so that urine remains pale yellow.		

commercially prepared drink, discuss the potential advantages and disadvantages of different brands with your health care provider or with a perinatal dietitian. Again, these beverages cannot replace the nutrition in well-balanced meals and snacks.

Fluid is also important during a multiple pregnancy. You are less likely to experience constipation, urinary tract infections, and preterm labor if you drink enough liquid. As long as the color of your urine appears pale yellow, you probably are getting enough. Add fluid to your diet if your urine becomes dark yellow in color. (Be aware that some vitamins or medications pass into urine and change its color.)

To get adequate fluid, pour water into a large sports mug–the kind with a self-contained straw–and keep it nearby during the day and on a bedside table at night. For extra vitamin C, squeeze the juice from lemon or lime wedges into your mug of water. Or alternate lemon water with 100 percent juices. This large mug will become indispensable during the early months of breastfeeding.

Taking Charge in Other Ways

Inflammation or Mild Infection

There may be a link between premature labor or birth with bacteria that an expectant mother can carry in her mouth, urinary tract, or vaginal area. Because inflammation or mild infection may not cause uncomfortable symptoms, a woman may not be aware there is a problem. Since preterm labor is more of a risk with multiple pregnancy, see your dentist during early pregnancy to rule out or begin treatment for any problem in the mouth and gums. Also, your obstetrical care provider can check for bacteria in the urine or vagina.

Normal Activity and Exercise

Ask your doctor or midwife about exercise during multiple pregnancy. Activity can increase appetite and improve general health. However, most women have to modify exercise routines and curtail vigorous activities earlier with a multiple pregnancy. Raising core body temperature through strenuous aerobic exercise can have harmful effects throughout pregnancy, and you also may be cautioned to stay out of hot tubs while pregnant. An earlier employment leave of absence may be recommended if your job is strenuous or if you are unable to take periodic rest breaks after the 24th week of pregnancy.

Multiple pregnancy often has a greater effect on pregnancy-related physical changes that affect motor skills, especially during the last trimester. Your center of gravity shifts earlier and more significantly during multiple pregnancy, which can affect your balance. And you are receiving higher "doses" of those pregnancy hormones that loosen ligaments.

Women expecting multiples often tire more easily or feel short of breath with activity. If you're anemic, this may be exaggerated. Also, two or more babies "take over" space in your upper abdomen, which is usually occupied by the lungs—

among other organs in the vicinity, giving the lungs less room to expand at a time when you're breathing for three or more.

Most women continue to perform normal daily activities throughout twin, and some triplet, pregnancies. However, most also find their bodies tell them to slow down by 24 or 25 weeks. *Listen to your body* when it tells you to sit down and prop your feet up, even if you are used to being active and feel guilty resting in the middle of the day! Intermittent rest breaks take the weight of the babies off of your pelvic area. And rest breaks help your body use food energy more efficiently.

> **Multiple pregnancy often has a greater effect on pregnancy-related physical changes that affect motor skills, especially during the last trimester.**

You may be more comfortable during the last trimester of pregnancy if you wear a maternity support belt. By "cradling" some of the weight of the growing babies in your lower abdomen, these wide, elasticized bands help decrease aches in the lower back and pelvic area. Ask your obstetric care provider about the possible advantages or disadvantages of such belts in your particular case.

Breastfeeding while Pregnant

If you are currently breastfeeding an infant, toddler, or older child, immediate weaning is often advised once multiples are diagnosed. Breastfeeding during pregnancy, in and of itself, is not considered a risk factor for preterm labor. However, it may add risk in the presence of any other factor associated with preterm labor and birth, and multiple pregnancy is highly associated with preterm labor and birth.

It is vitally important to the health of your unborn babies, the current nursling, and yourself that you be completely honest with your obstetric and pediatric care providers about the current nursling's breastfeeding pattern and needs. If you are concerned about an abrupt weaning, discuss with your care providers the risks and benefits of a more gradual weaning process during the first half (up to 20 weeks) of an apparently healthy twin pregnancy. (Gradual weaning is less likely to be considered an option during higher-order multiple pregnancy.) A natural weaning often occurs before the second trimester because milk production often decreases as the placenta(s) assumes production of the hormones that maintain pregnancy.

The healthy growth of two or more developing fetuses and their best chance for full term delivery may make for difficult decision-making. You and your child's pediatric care provider must also consider the nutritional needs of the current nursling, especially if this is an infant who still depends mostly on your milk for growth needs. The increased physical demands of multiple pregnancy on your body may interfere with providing for a breastfeeding infant, but it may be considered compatible if a toddler or preschooler breastfeeds occasionally.

If, after weighing the risks and benefits, immediate weaning is warranted, contact a La Leche League Leader or an International Board Certified Lactation Consultant (IBCLC) for ideas to minimize physical or emotional discomforts for you and your nursling. (See Resources.) Should a more gradual weaning be deemed as safe, you still may want to speak with a Leader or IBCLC for ideas to begin decreasing the daily number of breastfeedings. You also may need to add several hundred daily calories and extra protein to your multiple pregnancy diet until weaning is complete.

What to Avoid

You will want to keep the babies and their placenta(s) free of all harmful substances. Tobacco, alcohol, and street drug use are associated with preterm delivery and low birth weight newborns for single pregnancies, so it isn't difficult to imagine their effect on multiple pregnancies. Never take a medication unless you've checked on its safety with your doctor or midwife. Let your health care provider know if you or your spouse regularly smokes or drinks alcoholic beverages, or if either of you recently used or took any prescription, over-the-counter, herbal, or street drugs.

Tobacco use is the most common among harmful substance abuses. Smoking decreases the amount of oxygen reaching the placenta(s), and therefore, the babies receive less oxygen, too. Smoking can interfere with appetite and it reduces your body's ability to use many vitamins and minerals, so it also affects the kinds and amount of nutrients the babies and the placenta(s) receive and contributes to maternal anemia. Over time, areas of the placenta(s) deteriorate due to the decreases in oxygen and necessary nutrients.

You won't want to expose yourself and your unborn babies to secondhand smoke either, since it also interferes with placental blood flow. Ask smokers to go outdoors. Babies and young children exposed to secondhand smoke are more likely to suffer from colds, croup, bronchitis, other respiratory illnesses, and Sudden Infant Death Syndrome (SIDS). If you insist on a smoke-free home to improve the health of you and your babies during pregnancy, it will have become a habit by the time you bring your babies home. And feel free to gently remind those who must step outside to smoke that they will soon be role models for two or more curious children. Of course, they wouldn't have to go outside at all if they quit.

Mind-Body Connection

Is it possible that women expecting multiples deliver prematurely more often than need be partly because their health care providers, family, and friends keep telling them it will happen? No one has studied whether these dire predictions might contribute to the creation of a self-fulfilling prophecy. But it certainly can't help, and there is evidence that stress can contribute to preterm labor or birth. Many mothers mention the anxiety they felt due to a constant repetition of the "you'll give birth early" message. Instead of imagining a joyful birth followed by immediate breastfeeding, there often is an expectation of pregnancy and birth problems with newborn intensive care unit (NICU) stays for the babies.

> You can be prepared for potential problems without becoming preoccupied by them.

You can be prepared for potential problems without becoming preoccupied by them. If you are eating well, avoiding potentially harmful substances, and being sensible about exercise and rest, you are doing all that is within your power to give birth to healthy babies. Worrying about what might happen wastes mental energy on factors beyond your control, and worry improves nothing even if you eventually do experience a sign of some complication.

Instead of worrying, invest a few minutes several times a day on relaxation and visualization exercises that decrease anxiety and improve the function of your cardiac and respiratory systems. This increases the amount of oxygen and nutrients available to the babies via their placenta(s). Take advantage of frequent rest breaks to practice these exercises.

Guided Imagery Exercise

There are many relaxation and visualization—guided imagery—scenarios; this one is fairly simple. It will take longer to read the following script than to actually practice it.

- Close your eyes and take two or three deep breaths, breathing in through your nose and out through your mouth.
- Beginning with the crown of your head, work down your body; relax your muscles. Go from face to neck and back to upper extremities to abdomen to pelvis and finally to lower extremities. Let tension melt away as you move downward, until all built-up tension exits through the bottoms of your feet.
- With your mind's eye watch the air you breathe in as it enters your nose, travels to your lungs, passes into your circulation, and moves throughout your body—picking up different-colored nutrients from your food as it flows through your intestinal tract.
- Follow the flow of oxygen and nutrients as they leave your circulation, enter placental circulation, and spread through the placenta(s), keeping the tissues healthy.
- Visualize oxygen and nutrients entering each baby's cord. Watch each multiple literally grow within your uterus as the oxygen and nutrients circulate and are used by their bodies.
- Talk to your babies—mental conversations work. Tell them how much you love them and that you are doing everything you can to help them grow and develop.

- When you are ready to leave them, travel with returning blood flow back to your lungs. Become aware of your breathing again. And as you breathe out through your mouth, release any worry or anxiety with each breath.
- Once you feel calm and relaxed, open your eyes if they've been closed, stretch and move around again.

In addition to guided imagery exercises, massage, aromatherapy, acupressure, biofeedback, and similar complementary health care interventions promote relaxation and reduce stress. Some expectant mothers of multiples report they found meditation or writing in a journal to be relaxing. Some research has found such therapies, particularly massage, may lower the risk of preterm birth.

If you believe in a higher spiritual power, place yourself and your babies in the "hands" of that being. As you pray or meditate, ask that higher power to take on any tension and worry for you. You literally may feel your tension and worries lift away. Many expectant mothers say this method has helped reduce anxiety about any risks of multiple pregnancy.

KEY POINTS

- ❏ Your health habits influence your babies' growth and development as well as your body's ability to care for them in your womb/uterus.
- ❏ Eating well is the most important thing you can do for yourself and your growing babies during multiple pregnancy
  - Eating well means eating often.
  - Eating well means eating a lot of good, healthy foods with a special focus on protein.
  - See a dietitian/nutritionist who specializes in pregnancy nutrition.
- ❏ See your dentist during early pregnancy and ask your obstetric care provider to check for possible signs of infection in urine and vaginal fluids.
- ❏ Stay active but listen to your body when it tells you to rest or slow down.
- ❏ If breastfeeding another infant or child, be sure your obstetric care provider knows it.
  - Discuss pros and cons if weaning is advised.
  - Speak with an LLL Leader or IBCLC for helpful hints if needed.
- ❏ Lowering the amount of stress in your life may have a positive effect on multiple pregnancy.
  - Relaxation exercises, such as guided imagery, massage, acupressure, and similar activities have been shown to be helpful for reducing stress in higher risk pregnancies.

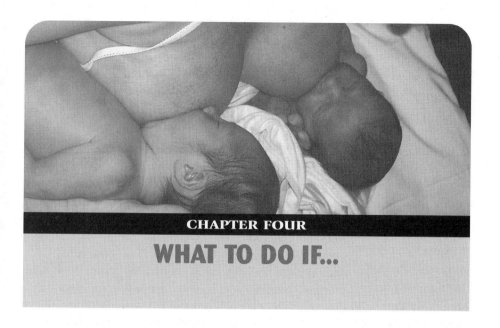

CHAPTER FOUR

WHAT TO DO IF...

It would be wonderful if you could be assured of giving birth to full-term multiples, each weighing more than 2500 gm (5 lb 8 oz), rooting eagerly at your breast soon after birth, simply by eating well and gaining sufficient weight, exercising sensibly and avoiding harmful substances. However, there are no guarantees. A woman can do everything "right" during multiple pregnancy and still experience a complication, because many aspects of multiple pregnancy are beyond the expectant mother's control.

If you're now asking, "What's the point of doing everything right?" know that the consequences of complications may be less severe when you maintain your health during pregnancy, build strong baby bodies, and provide for optimal function of the placenta(s). Following the diet and exercise recommendations presented in Chapter 3 should lead to the healthiest outcome possible for you and your babies even if a complication occurs. You will also have the satisfaction of knowing you did everything possible for yourself and all your babies.

Recognizing the early signs of common complications can also make a difference, since getting immediate treatment will often stop or slow the progress of several of the most common complications, such as preterm labor and delivery, and allow the pregnancy to continue longer. Sometimes an extra week or two of pregnancy makes a big, positive difference for the babies' health. For other complications, the obstetrical care provider may recommend delivering multiples early as immediate treatment. For instance, little or no growth of one or more of the babies for days to weeks may mean that it is safer for the babies to be outside the uterus than in it.

Signs to Watch and Report

Preterm Labor

Preterm labor, or labor occurring before the 37th week of pregnancy, is one of the most common complications of multiple pregnancy. When labor progresses and is followed by preterm birth, babies' immature physical systems are not ready to function optimally outside the uterus. The earlier the preterm birth, the more likely infant complications are to occur. Fortunately, early intervention can often halt preterm labor or at least postpone delivery.

> A woman can do everything "right" during multiple pregnancy and still experience a complication.

Cervical changes. The cervix of the uterus, the end that opens to the vagina and is also called the birth canal, thins and opens so the baby can be born at the end of labor. With full-term pregnancy the cervix remains long, thick, and closed until at least two to three weeks before labor. When the cervix begins to shorten, soften, or open too early, preterm labor and birth are more likely. An obstetric care provider may suggest periodic transvaginal ultrasound exams to watch for early signs of cervical shortening or "funneling," which are associated with preterm labor and birth.

Fetal fibronectin. Your obstetric care provider may recommend periodic testing of vaginal secretions for a protein called "fetal fibronectin" (fFN) from about the 24th to 34th week of pregnancy. This protein is common in vaginal secretions until about the 20th week of pregnancy, but fFN should not be found in secretions after this time until at least the 34th week of pregnancy. Research has shown that an increase in fFN after the 20th week of pregnancy is associated with a high incidence of preterm labor. Obtaining a sample of the vaginal secretions is similar to the procedure for any pelvic exam. The care provider inserts a speculum into the vagina and wipes the secretions with special swabs, which are then tested for fFN. A negative sample is considered reassuring, and in the absence of cervical shortening, a woman is usually able to go about her usual activities for another two weeks.

Contractions. Uterine contractions can be a sign of preterm labor. If you have, or think you are having, more than two or three contractions an hour: 1) begin timing how often one occurs and how long each lasts, 2) empty your bladder, 3) drink several glasses of water, and 4) lie on your left side. Once you've had four contractions within an hour, whether you feel any pain with them or not, call your care provider—*now.* Do not wait to see if they stop, increase in number, or get stronger.

Bleeding. Should you experience any vaginal bleeding, with or without contractions, call your care provider immediately. Bleeding may be associated with certain complications of the placenta(s). Such complications are more common in multiple pregnancy because the placenta(s) cover more space.

Treatment for Preterm Labor

Preterm labor, or labor occurring before the 37th week of pregnancy, is one of the most common complications of multiple pregnancy.

Obstetric care providers often recommend immediate hospitalization for suspected preterm labor. They will want to determine whether the contractions are true labor contractions—contractions that cause cervical change, particularly cervical dilatation. Bed rest, fluids often given intravenously (IV), and special tocolytic medications to decrease the "irritability" of the uterus are usually used to stop true preterm labor. You are likely to be given an injection of a corticosteroid that has been shown to enhance the maturity of babies' lungs. Due to the potential harm for mother and babies, repeat dosing is not recommended as a matter of routine or "just in case" preterm labor recurs.

Women often are given extra fluids when admitted to the hospital in preterm labor. This is because dehydration is associated with contractions. Quickly hydrating a woman often helps decrease contractions short term. Some women think it then follows that preterm labor and delivery can be avoided and pregnancy weight gains safely limited simply by drinking large amounts of fluid. Wrong! Poor diet and inadequate food intake are also associated with preterm labor contractions. You, your babies, and their placenta(s) depend on your well-balanced diet—one that includes varied nutrients, plenty of calories, and sufficient fluid.

Most women are discharged once contractions stop, but many continue on partial or full bed rest and tocolytic medication at home. These treatments have been found to prolong a pregnancy after a confirmed episode of preterm labor. Home treatment may include a system to monitor further contractions or uterine activity, such as bringing in a home health nurse to make regular calls or home visits. The nurse often becomes a resource for answering questions and a sounding board for sharing your concerns.

Prescribing bed rest or tocolytic medication to prevent preterm labor during the last trimester of a multiple pregnancy is common in some areas; however, the use of either treatment as a preventive measure is controversial. The thinking is that bed rest shifts the weight of the babies off of the cervix and increases blood flow to the uterus and the placenta(s). Routine tocolytic use is thought to lessen uterine activity, and therefore contractions, during the remainder of the pregnancy. Yet, there is no solid evidence to support the use of either bed rest or tocolytic medication for the prevention of preterm labor and birth during twin pregnancy. The preventive effect of bed rest for higher-order multiple pregnancies is less controversial,

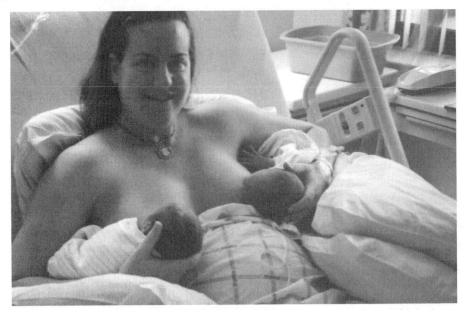

The goal is to give birth to healthy babies who will be ready to breastfeed soon after birth.

although questions about its effectiveness remain. If carrying triplets or more, don't be surprised if strict bed rest is recommended before the 28th week of pregnancy.

Strict bed rest regimens and tocolysis are associated with profound side-effects for pregnant women. Strict bed rest is associated with maternal muscle weakening, diminished appetite with decreased food intake, and depressed mood. Any of these consequences may affect a woman's physical and mental health for the remainder of the pregnancy, her babies' birth outcomes, and her physical and emotional ability to care for her babies after delivery. Tocolytic medications are associated with mild to severe side effects, which differ depending on the action of the particular drug or combination of drugs.

It is crucial to discuss all aspects of preterm labor treatment with your health care provider. Ask why tocolysis or strict bed rest is recommended, and request research reports that support either treatment. Discuss the potential benefits, risks, and possible side effects of any treatment plan. Be sure you understand the signs and symptoms of all possible side effects.

When bed rest is prescribed, find out exactly what your care provider means by this term. Different health care providers define "bed rest" differently. (Several bed rest Web sites listed in the Resources offer checklists to review with your care provider.) Bed rest may mean anything from restricting physical activities and propping your feet up during extended rest periods to lying on your left side and staying off your feet completely. Most definitions of bed rest include a recommendation for an immediate leave of absence from a woman's place of employment. If your obstetric care provider does not mention it, ask if you may consult with a physical therapist to learn exercises that will help avoid a loss of muscle and physical strength.

If "in bed" bed rest is prescribed, ask the OB care provider if exercises focusing on the upper and lower extremities, while avoiding pressure in the pelvic area, may be performed. Exercising extremities may help prevent some loss of muscle mass, which may help with recovery after delivery. Exercising may also enhance a mother's appetite so that she can continue to gain weight. Resistance exercises, using bands or small weights, may be possible, although there may be restrictions on positions that can be used. Again, exercises recommended by a physical therapist may help minimize these issues. (See Resources, "Books: Pregnancy and Birth" for exercise suggestions.)

If bed rest is prescribed after preterm labor is diagnosed, ask your care provider for the names of other mothers who have been on bed rest during pregnancy. They may be able to share tips for maintaining perspective, accomplishing work, and making time seem to go faster. Local and Internet support groups for parents of multiples often have such information or contacts. There are specific "bed rest during pregnancy" Web sites for mothers. (See Resources.)

Fetal Well-Being

Fetal Growth Restriction

Multiple babies essentially "compete" for space and nutrients during pregnancy. Sometimes one receives more nutrients and grows better than another because of where or the way the placenta(s) or umbilical cord(s) attach or develop. When any baby is not growing well, it is said to be affected by fetal growth restriction (FGR), which may also be called intrauterine growth restriction (IUGR). If one or more is smaller than he or she should be for the week of pregnancy, it is also referred to as small for gestational age (SGA). Differences, or discordancy, in babies' growth rates typically begin to show up at 28 weeks of pregnancy or later—about the time growth rates slow down for twins or

> When any baby is not growing well, it is said to be affected by fetal growth restriction (FGR), which may also be called intrauterine growth restriction (IUGR).

triplets when compared to a single baby during later pregnancy. (This may occur earlier for a few sets of twins and for higher-order multiples.) Because of this, health care providers want to keep a close eye on each baby, which gets rather tricky since one may be hiding behind, below, or above another.

Twin-to-Twin Transfusion Syndrome (TTTS)

TTTS occurs mainly in MZ (identical) twins who share a placenta. Of the 75 percent of MZ twins who share a placenta, about 75 percent will develop blood vessel connections within the shared placenta and, for approximately 15 percent of that group, the vessel connections influence the amount and direction of blood flow. Depending on the type of vascular connections, the effects may range in severity from minor to life threatening, or even death, for one or both MZ twins. The twin receiving increased blood flow is always called the recipient twin and the one receiving less is termed the donor twin.

The recipient twin receives too much fluid, which may overload his cardiovascular system and, in severe cases, lead to congestive heart failure or stroke. Since the donor twin receives less fluid, he is anemic, which may vary from mild to severe. The recipient twin is significantly larger and has too much fluid in his amniotic sac. The donor twin is growth-restricted and his amniotic sac contains too little fluid. MZ twins suspected or known to have TTTS will be followed closely during pregnancy. Some TTTS symptoms may be treated during the pregnancy, but if staying in the uterus becomes more of a danger for the babies, it may be necessary to deliver them prematurely.

Diagnostic Testing during Multiple Pregnancy

Ultrasonography

Ultrasound is considered a valid and important diagnostic tool during multiple pregnancy.

When an early prenatal physical examination or an evaluation of a woman's blood sample points to multiples, an ultrasound exam is usually recommended to confirm whether a woman is carrying two or more babies. Ultrasound allows obstetrical care providers to "see" the babies by "bouncing" sound waves off of each baby's body tissues. This creates "pictures," or a sonogram, of the developing babies which can help care providers determine the number of babies as well as measure the growth and development of the babies while in the uterus.

Ultrasound has confirmed multiple pregnancies as early as three weeks after conception when multiple sacs may be seen with vaginal ultrasound. Abdominal ultrasound can often pick up babies' individual heart activity at five to six weeks. In addition, first trimester ultrasound can be used to determine whether twins share a single placenta and outer sac (chorion) and are, therefore, definitely MZ. Knowing twins share a placenta alerts OB care providers to watch closely as pregnancy progresses for TTTS and certain other complications that sometimes occur only with this group of MZ twins.

First trimester diagnosis has resulted in an interesting side-effect of ultrasound's role in the early confirmation of multiple pregnancy—the discovery of a vanishing twin syndrome in which at least one multiple confirmed early in a pregnancy has "disappeared" on a later ultrasound. Some instances of early pregnancy bleeding now are thought to be related to the miscarrying of a multiple, but not all cases of "vanishing" multiples are associated with bleeding. When a multiple does "vanish," the development of the remaining multiple(s) usually progresses normally, but many women still experience feelings of disappointment or deep sadness and loss.

Once multiples are definitely diagnosed, the babies' initial measurements are taken to help establish gestational (pregnancy) age and a "due date." Additional ultrasounds may be recommended by 20 weeks for higher-order multiple pregnancy and MZ sets with a single placenta and after 24 weeks for other twins. At this point care providers may recommend serial ultrasounds—ultrasound examination at regular two to three week intervals. Frequent ultrasound will also be suggested if an extreme change is seen in the growth rate of one or more babies. If you hear the obstetric care provider refer to a level II ultrasound, it simply means the care provider wants a more comprehensive and detailed "picture" of what is happening in your uterus.

During the last 10 to 12 weeks of pregnancy your care provider may suggest an in-depth ultrasound exam that is combined with a nonstress test, referred to as a biophysical profile (BPP), to evaluate the babies' breathing and body movements, the amount of fluid in their amniotic sacs, and the function of the placenta(s) and umbilical cord(s). Ultrasound also may be used for Doppler flow studies, which allow health practitioners to visualize blood flow in a baby's umbilical cord. These studies can help them determine how well the placenta(s) are functioning.

There has been some controversy regarding the routine use of ultrasound during pregnancy since its introduction in the US in the mid-1970s. However, ultrasound is considered a valid and important diagnostic tool during multiple pregnancy. Early confirmation and monitoring of the individual babies' growth later in pregnancy can have a significant effect on the health of the babies and mother. In addition, the low-frequency sound waves used for pregnancy ultrasound are not associated with any ill effects for babies/children or their mothers.

Nonstress Test

Another test care providers may recommend during the last weeks of pregnancy is a nonstress test (NST), which is a way of keeping an eye on the babies' well-being. During the NST you recline in a semi-sitting position and belts equipped with special monitors are fastened around your abdomen. One belt picks up uterine contractions and babies' movements. The other belts, and the number depends on the number of babies you're carrying, record babies' heart rates. The belts are attached to a machine that translates the information into a written recording.

A nonstress test may be recommended to keep an eye on the babies' well-being.

Care providers look at the tracing of each baby's heart rate and compare it with uterine and baby activity. This gives them an idea of how the individual babies are responding to change. Certain heart rate patterns are associated with a baby's healthy response to environmental changes; other patterns may indicate that one or more babies is having some difficulty. Depending on the perceived problem, a repeat NST or an immediate high-level ultrasound may be added to get more complete information.

A similar test induces uterine contractions by using a synthetic oxytocin (Pitocin) or nipple stimulation. It is called a contraction stress test (CST). When oxytocin (Pitocin) is used, CST may be referred to as an oxytocin challenge test (OCT). CST using breast stimulation to induce contractions is called a breast self-stimulation test (BSST). Because of the risk of inducing preterm labor, CST is *not* recommended during multiple pregnancy.

Counting Fetal Movements

There is a simple exercise that you can do to help care providers keep an eye on your babies' development—become aware of each baby's movements. You may have noticed that each seems to move in a certain spot and has a particular pattern of movement during the course of a day. If you haven't paid attention to this yet, you may be surprised how easy it may be to identify each baby.

To do a "kick count," begin at about 28 weeks of pregnancy, or possibly a little earlier with higher-order multiple pregnancies, and:

- Count each baby's movements at about the same time each day until each has moved 10 times;
- Track, on a separate sheet for each baby, how long it takes each to move 10 times—most babies will move 10 times within a two-hour period;
- Chart the types of movements noticed for each, such as vigorous "kicking" versus a more rhythmic turning. If any of the babies does not move 10 times in two hours or it takes longer each day for any to reach the 10 movements, contact your obstetrical care provider. Should one suddenly make very strong movements that are followed by a sudden halt in movement, call your care provider.

Difficulty counting a baby's movements may mean that one or more babies is napping at the time you've chosen or one simply may be harder to identify because of the babies' positions in the uterus. If you cannot distinguish which baby is which, you may be able to develop a sensitivity to their general patterns of movement at certain times of the day. Report any real change in the babies' patterns. It never hurts to report questionable findings.

Maternal Issues

Pregnancy-Induced Hypertension (PIH)

PIH, or the development of high maternal blood pressure during pregnancy, may also be referred to as preeclampsia or toxemia. It is the most common maternal complication of multiple pregnancy, occurring two to three times more often in multiple pregnancies. The cause(s) of PIH and why it is more common in multiple pregnancy still are not well understood, although researchers are looking more closely at a relationship to placental function. Awareness of PIH's early signs can lead to earlier diagnosis and intervention. Obstetrical care providers check for PIH during each prenatal visit by weighing you, testing your urine for protein, taking your blood pressure, and checking your reflexes. The warning signs of mild or early PIH include:

The typical early warning signs of PIH/preeclampsia may not occur in multiple pregnancy, and PIH tends to progress more quickly.

- Sudden, sustained increase in an expectant mother's blood pressure,
- Sudden swelling or puffiness in the face and hands related to extreme fluid retention,
- Swelling of the ankles or lower legs that is unrelieved after propping the feet and legs up,
- Sudden and excessive weight gain that is related to the fluid retention.

The development of any of these symptoms should be reported to the care provider immediately. Unfortunately, the typical early warning signs of PIH may not occur in multiple pregnancy, and PIH tends to progress more quickly. Often the first signs of PIH are those associated with severe PIH, such as:

- Headache, blurred vision, or seeing spots in front of the eyes,
- Pain in the area of the stomach or left, upper abdomen (epigastric pain),
- Nausea and vomiting,
- Shortness of breath or "wet" breath sounds,
- Exaggerated feelings of tension or irritability.

Contact your care provider immediately if you experience any symptom of severe PIH whether or not you have experienced or been treated for milder PIH. Severe PIH increases the risk of maternal seizures (eclampsia), which can affect the babies' oxygen supply.

Treatment for PIH depends on its severity. Mild PIH often is treated at home. Bed rest may be recommended and your diet may be reviewed for adequate protein. Your care provider probably will want to see you more frequently and ultrasound testing to check on the babies' wellbeing might be recommended more often.

If some change occurs, whether it is obvious, "just a feeling," or a sense that something isn't quite right, contact your obstetrical care provider right away.

Severe PIH is treated in the hospital with strict bed rest and IV medications to decrease the risk of a seizure. A medication to lower blood pressure may be prescribed. Sometimes a sedative is suggested if feelings of tension or irritability continue. The babies' conditions will be monitored closely.

Preterm Delivery
Unavoidable Preterm Birth

Sometimes preterm labor cannot be halted or prenatal testing indicates the babies can no longer remain safely in the uterus.

Sometimes preterm labor cannot be halted or prenatal testing indicates the babies can no longer remain safely in the uterus. Unless labor is progressing rapidly or any multiple is in such distress that birth must occur immediately, your care provider will likely recommend additional tests or treatments. Usually an injection of a steroid is given to quickly advance lung maturation in the unborn babies.

Doctors may want to do an amniocentesis to test amniotic fluid from each baby's sac for substances that indicate whether the babies' lungs are mature enough for them to breathe without assistance outside the uterus. By using ultrasound and then injecting a small amount of a harmless dye into a sac from which amniotic fluid already has been drawn, doctors can be sure they test the fluid of each baby and do not retest the same baby. Some research indicates that unborn multiples' lungs may mature a little earlier in pregnancy than those of single-born infants.

If the tests show that the lungs of one or more babies are not yet mature, obstetric and neonatal care providers should include you in a discussion to weigh the risks of preterm delivery with those of remaining in a less safe uterine environment.

It is scary to think about the possibility of complications. However, it is even scarier to be faced with a complication after missing the early warning signs that might have minimized the consequences. When it comes to your health and that of your unborn babies, you are likely to be the first one who becomes aware when something is not "right."

Trust your knowledge of yourself and your babies. You know your body, its response to the pregnancy so far, and the behaviors or responses of your unborn babies better than anyone. If some change occurs, whether it is obvious, "just a feeling," or a sense that something isn't quite right, contact your obstetrical care provider right away. And if your care provider recommends a treatment that you don't yet feel comfortable with, advocate for yourself and your babies. Ask questions, discuss benefits and risks, and explore possible alternatives until you clearly understand that a test or treatment is in your and your babies' best interests.

KEY POINTS

❑ Complications are more common in twin and higher-multiple pregnancy, even when an expectant mother eats well, rests, and does everything "right."

❑ Preterm labor and birth are the most common complication of multiple pregnancy.

❑ It is important to know the warning signs of preterm labor; Call your OB care provider immediately if any occur.

❑ Fetal growth restriction (FGR) is also common for one or more of a set of multiples.

❑ When one or more multiples is smaller than he or she should be for week of pregnancy, it is also called "small for gestational age" (SGA).

❑ A condition called twin-to-twin transfusion syndrome (TTTS) sometimes affects monozygotic (MZ/identical) twins sharing a single placenta; it causes growth restriction in the twin receiving less blood flow.

❑ Strict bed rest is often recommended during multiple pregnancy, but it is still not known whether it is helpful.

   • Women experience many side effects when on strict bed rest.

   • When suggesting bed rest, the OB care provider should tell you how it will help your pregnancy and exactly what he/she means by "bed rest."

❑ Because of the greater chance of complications, your care provider may want to do more testing in order to watch the babies more closely and pick up on early warning signs for preterm labor.

❑ Pregnancy-induced hypertension (PIH/preeclampsia/toxemia) occurs 2 to 3 times more often in women expecting twins or higher multiples.

   • With multiple pregnancy, PIH may not show any early warning signs and go straight to a more severe form.

   • Call your doctor if you get a severe headache or stomach ache, see spots in front of your eyes, or feel extremely irritable or tense.

❑ Occasionally doctors must deliver multiples early because of some pregnancy complication. However, the doctor should tell you why it would be better to deliver the babies early and discuss the risks as well as benefits.

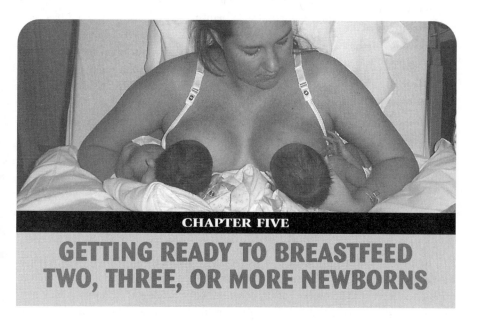

CHAPTER FIVE

GETTING READY TO BREASTFEED TWO, THREE, OR MORE NEWBORNS

Breastfeeding is the ideal way to feed and nurture a human baby whether that baby comes alone or as part of a set. There is no reason to change your decision to breastfeed simply because multiples are expected. Many mothers have breastfed multiples in sets of two, three, or more babies.

No matter what the circumstances of your babies' births, it is possible to breastfeed. Women have breastfed twins and higher-order multiples after surgical deliveries, "surprise" twins, preterm births, multiples requiring long-term special care, personal complications, other small children at home, little or no household help, employment outside the home, or combinations of the above. Have confidence in your body's ability to adapt no matter what your particular situation.

Advantages of Breastfeeding Multiples

Nature worked hard over tens of thousands of years to make a mother's own milk the perfect food for her babies. Breastfeeding provides numerous benefits for both babies and mother. Those benefits are even more important and intense for multiples. Babies tend to be happier and easier to care for when they are healthy, and human milk is associated with better infant health.

Human milk is the most nutritious and balanced food available for human infants. It contains everything full-term babies need for growth and development during the first six months, and it continues to provide important nutrients as other

No matter what the circumstances of your babies' births, it is possible to breastfeed.

foods are added to the diet after six months. Because human milk is made for human babies, sensitivity to mother's milk is highly unlikely. Breastfed babies also tend to develop fewer allergies. Companies producing infant formulas strive to make their products more like human milk, but they will never achieve a perfect match, because a mother's milk adapts to her own particular babies.

Babies digest human milk more easily and quickly, and they use its nutrients more completely. For instance, the fats in human milk are tailor-made for human brain and nervous system development, and these fats are in a form that a baby's body can easily use—even if born preterm. Human milk is easier for babies' body systems to use, or metabolize—from heart and lungs to intestinal tract and kidneys. This is especially important for preterm or sick newborn multiples, but is beneficial for all young babies. It is rare for fully breastfed babies to become constipated or suffer from diarrhea.

Immunity (antibody) factors in human milk help protect babies against many illnesses, which is especially important when multiples are preterm or when uterine conditions were less favorable for one or more babies. Substances in your milk also help in the development of each baby's own immune system. Since one sick multiple usually means the other(s) will soon catch it, you will appreciate the antibody protection of breastfeeding more than most. It can also save quite a few dollars on visits to the babies' pediatric care provider or prescription medications.

Breastfeeding ensures maximum skin contact with each baby. This is particularly important with multiples whether they are fully or partially breastfed. It even applies when two babies always breastfeed simultaneously. No matter how hard you try, it is difficult, if not impossible, to give each multiple the time and attention you could give a single baby. Yet each multiple has the same needs as any single baby. Breastfeeding is the perfect way to meet the babies' need for food and their mother's arms.

Breastfeeding lets you invest time in the babies instead of in preparation and cleanup. It is more than twice as nice to curl up at night for feedings in your warm bed, rather than wake to crying babies who must wait while you heat their meals. Breastfeeding is a one-handed task, which means you still have a free hand to tend to another multiple or you can feed two at once.

Cost is an important consideration. You will save twice (or more) on the cost of infant formula and feeding equipment. Even if you must rent or buy a breast pump and related equipment, the cost of formula-feeding is much higher. The average estimated cost of formula for the first year is at least $200 per baby per month with ready-to-feed varieties costing more than powdered* ones. You will spend even more if preterm multiples or one with another health condition requires a special formula.

*If using powdered formula to complement/supplement breastfeeding, discuss proper preparation with the pediatric care provider due to possible bacterial contamination during the canning process. This is more of a risk for preterm babies and during the first month for term babies.

Breastfeeding Goals

Breastfeeding is the perfect way to meet the babies' need for food and their mother's arms.

Have you thought about your goals for breastfeeding multiples? A breastfeeding goal is more likely to be achieved if you are aware of it. A goal is like a destination for a trip. If you don't know where you want to go, it's going to be difficult to get there.

Committing a goal to paper is like marking the destination on a map. You are more likely to reach your breastfeeding destination if your plan includes both direct and alternate routes. Mapping optional routes helps you plan for potential breastfeeding detours or dead-ends, and you will have some idea about what to do if you find yourself on the long and scenic route when your original plan was to take the super highway. A map for breastfeeding multiples may cover "how much," such as full or partial breastfeeding, and for "how long"—baby-led weaning versus a specific time period—as well as plans to accommodate babies that arrive early and need extra time to learn to breastfeed.

Early postpartum is a time of confusion after the birth of even a single baby. It can be even more chaotic when bringing home two or more newborns. If one or more babies requires special care in a NICU, you may feel pulled in several directions at once.

Many mothers question the decision to breastfeed during the early weeks when they and their babies are still learning to coordinate at least twice as many breastfeedings each day. Sleep deprivation may fog thinking and make it difficult to remember that caring for two, three, four, or more newborns takes more time no matter how they are fed.

Importance of Commitment

A commitment to breastfeeding may be the single most important element in reaching your final breastfeeding destination. No one would say, "I'm going to try to make it to the city for my family reunion, but if something comes up, I'll stop or turn around." Travel often includes unexpected glitches, so once committed to making the trip, the traveler anticipates and prepares to handle a detour, flat tire, or some other difficulty that may occur.

A commitment to breastfeeding may be the single most important element in reaching your final breastfeeding destination.

To reach a breastfeeding destination, be positive about making the trip. Say to yourself and others, "I am going to breastfeed my babies," instead of, "I want to try to breastfeed." Plan the trip and prepare for obstacles along

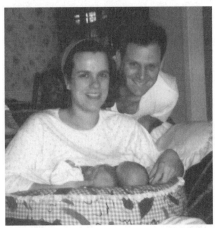

A father's support can be essential to a mother who is breastfeeding multiples.

the way. You may be surprised at how much more confident you feel when you have a positive attitude and a detailed "map."

Planning a "trip" with multiples involves developing short-term breastfeeding goals. These are like the stages of the route and mark specific distances toward the final destination. When reaching the final destination seems overwhelming, traveling one stage, or leg of the journey, usually appears manageable. Short-term breastfeeding goals keep a mother moving—another day, another week, another month. Achieving one goal motivates one to stay on the route until the next stage is reached.

An initial short-term goal may be to establish and maintain milk production for multiples, whether babies go directly to breast or milk must be expressed for preterm or sick babies. Your next goal may be to continue for a certain number of weeks before re-evaluating the route. The second goal should allow enough time for you and the babies to learn to breastfeed well.

Most mothers of multiples suggest setting an initial breastfeeding goal of at least six weeks, because it takes at least that long to recover from the birth and give everyone involved time to learn to breastfeed. Other mothers set a shorter initial short-term goal. They commit to breastfeeding (or expressing/pumping their milk) for one week. When they meet the one-week goal, they re-establish that same goal for one more week, and so on.

Put your short-term goals in writing and sign it like a contract and specify how you plan to reward yourself each time you meet a short-term goal. You should invest at least some of the money saved by breastfeeding multiples to reward yourself for providing your babies with nature's perfect food.

It is best to anticipate that you may face an occasional detour or wrong turn when multiple babies are along for the trip. Check out alternate breastfeeding routes in advance by reading this book and other materials about breastfeeding and multiples. You will want to be free to concentrate, especially for the first leg or two on the journey. Arrange now for someone else to take over household tasks, such as cooking, doing laundry, or caring for an older child. It also helps to have extra arms to hold a baby or two at times. (For more ideas, see Chapter 7, "Getting Ready: Preparing for Multiples.")

Family and friends can make travel easier or more difficult. To gain their support, share information about breastfeeding with them and let them know how important breastfeeding is to you and the babies. When passengers understand the route and why you wish to take it, they are more likely to help you navigate and to cheer you on if an obstacle arises.

There are "mechanics" available if you want help with a mechanical problem or if you ever feel lost along the road. La Leche League (LLL) Leaders and board-certified lactation consultants help mothers with breastfeeding questions or problems. (You will read more about them in the next section.) Post their numbers near a convenient telephone. In addition, it's always helpful to talk to a mother who has traveled the same road. Talking to someone else can help you regain "big picture" perspective on days when you worry that one or more baby will never learn to breastfeed well or when babies stage a breastfeeding marathon.

Most mothers of multiples suggest setting an initial breastfeeding goal of at least six weeks.

Once you develop your basic plan, refuse to listen if anyone tells you the trip can't be made. It can and it has. Many, many times. You know the route is flexible. If a detour pops up along the route, you can revise the plan to fit the circumstances. Who knows? You may have two, three, or even four storybook babies who are happy to adapt to any realistic breastfeeding routine. Then again, you may have to adapt the plan, perhaps only temporarily, if two, three, or four babies need extra time to learn to breastfeed or they consistently stagger feedings around the clock. Wait and see.

Additional Tools for Mapping Your Route
Written Information

There are numerous books and pamphlets containing good, general information about breastfeeding and lactation, the body's process of producing milk. THE WOMANLY ART OF BREASTFEEDING published by La Leche League International, has been a popular breastfeeding guide for almost 50 years. The seventh revised edition was published in 2003. The basic process of breastfeeding is the same no matter how many babies you will be feeding, so read, read, and read some more. Be sure to share written information with your husband, family, and friends.

Many childbirth classes incorporate breastfeeding information as part of the curriculum. Others offer separate breastfeeding classes. As much as your multiple pregnancy allows, take advantage of any such opportunities.

La Leche League (LLL) Group Support Meetings

The most valuable breastfeeding help is available at La Leche League (LLL) monthly meetings. In many areas an LLL meeting is the only place where a woman can actually see babies breastfeed and hear real mothers discuss the joys of nurturing babies this way. You can watch mothers handle babies and see how they position them for breastfeeding. It can be reassuring to observe how babies of the same age are as different as they are similar, which may be of particular interest if your multiples are dizygotic/fraternal.

Many mothers have breastfed multiples and you can do it, too.

Begin attending LLL meetings before 20 to 24 weeks if possible, because your activities may be restricted later in pregnancy. If you are unable to attend meetings, contact a local LLL Leader and talk. The Leader will have information that will help you begin breastfeeding multiples. She may also know of a Leader or mother who has already breastfed multiple infants. It is really helpful to talk to someone who has "been there."

La Leche League now offers a variety of online resources which can be helpful to you if you are unable to attend meetings or if you are put on bed rest. There are online discussions as well as answers to Frequently Asked Questions (FAQs), an online Catalogue, and Help Forms that are answered personally by online LLL Leaders. See www.llli.org.

Being Prepared for Anything

Multiples are more likely than single infants to initially be cared for in a newborn intensive care unit (NICU), so there is a greater chance that you will have to express or pump your milk for one or more of your babies during the early postpartum period. To prepare for this possibility, ask your obstetrical care provider if the hospital where you are to deliver has full size, hospital-grade, automatic-cycling electric breast pumps and double milk collection kits available. The double kit will allow you to pump milk from both breasts at once, which can save time and increase milk production. LLL Leaders usually know about equipment available in local hospitals or you can contact the hospital and ask to speak with a lactation consultant or nurse on the postpartum unit. They should have this information.

Ideally, the hospital will have an International Board Certified Lactation Consultant (IBCLC) on staff. She can give you an idea of what to expect at the hospital and how to get the help you need when you are on the postpartum unit. You may want to ask if nurses routinely apply a breast pump when a mother's condition initially makes it difficult for her to do so or whether you need to include that request on a birth plan. The LLL Leader or IBCLC will also know where you can rent a breast pump or buy a collection kit if you must continue to pump after hospital discharge. If the hospital does not have an IBCLC on staff, you might want to locate a lactation consultant who practices in your community. An LLL Leader usually is aware of IBCLCs working in an area or you can contact the professional organization for lactation consultants listed in Resources.

Physical Preparation

A breast assessment specific for breastfeeding and lactation can identify potential physical factors, such as flat or inverted nipples, that may affect breastfeeding initiation. Many such factors resolve without treatment by the end of pregnancy. Also, treatments currently recommended for flat or inverted nipples or as prenatal preparation for breastfeeding have not been proven to be effective and may carry risks if

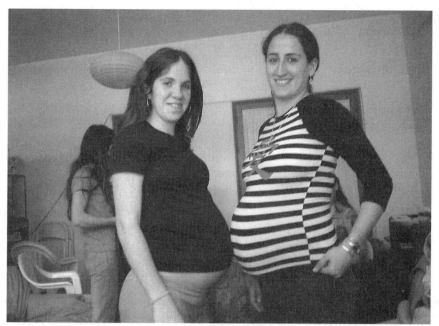

Being in touch with other mothers provides support and reassurance as
you plan your breastfeeding goals.

used during a multiple pregnancy.

Due to the increased risk of preterm labor and delivery during multiple pregnancy, prenatal nipple care and all nipple "exercises" or techniques that involve any type of nipple stimulation or nipple stretching should be avoided. Nipple stimulation may stimulate uterine contractions. The use of breast shells, which exert a gentle but steady suction pressure to draw out flat or inverted nipples, could also cause problems. In addition, prenatal nipple care has been found to be of no value in the prevention of sore nipples and may actually damage a protective layer of cells on the nipples and areola.

> **Determine your goal, or "final destination," for breastfeeding and then develop a flexible plan to reach it.**

A physical factor, such as a flat or inverted nipple, that persists after the babies are born usually can be overcome with appropriate support from an experienced LLL Leader or a lactation consultant. For some of these situations, multiple babies can be part of the solution. A factor that causes a problem for one multiple may create no impediment for another. Actually, the "work" of one multiple often helps another breastfeed better.

Many mothers have breastfed multiples and you can do it, too. Determine your goal, or "final destination," for breastfeeding and then develop a flexible plan to reach it. You can learn about possible routes by reading information about breastfeeding, going to special classes, and attending La Leche League meetings.

Achieving short-term goals, or stages, may be motivating on days when the final destination seems out of reach. It also helps to know where to get help if you meet an obstacle in the road.

One final note about reaching your destination—your multiple passengers will greatly influence the ultimate breastfeeding route you follow, but you don't really get to meet them until you begin the trip. Therefore, accept that it is impossible to anticipate every situation that may arise. There is no point in wasting time now worrying about potential problems that may, but then again may not, be down the road. You've done what you can to get ready for the trip. La Leche League Leaders and lactation consultants are prepared to assist you if a contingency plan becomes necessary. So relax and enjoy the rest of your pregnancy.

For an extensive discussion of the physical benefits of breastfeeding, read La Leche League International's THE WOMANLY ART OF BREASTFEEDING. Also, check the Resources section at the end of this book for information about obtaining additional reading material, contacting LLL Leaders and lactation consultants, renting or purchasing breast pumps or other breastfeeding aids or devices, and other helpful tips.

KEY POINTS

❏ Mothers can and do breastfeed twins, triplets, or more—fully or partially.

❏ Nature made your milk to be the best first food for your babies. In addition to the nutrition your milk provides, it also:

- Contains antibodies that prevent or fight disease in babies and children.

- Allows you to spend your time with your babies instead of preparing their food and cleaning feeding equipment.

- Is the deal of a lifetime when you realize it costs little, or nothing, compared to other food choices—the only time a person gets the best product for the least money!

❏ Commit to breastfeeding your multiples and say, "I *will* breastfeed my twins (triplets, quadruplets, etc.)" instead of "I'll *try* to breastfeed."

- Plan ahead for breastfeeding multiples.

- Develop goals. For instance, do you want your babies to receive only your milk for their first several months? How long do you want them to get your milk? Your answers are breastfeeding goals.

- Learn about breastfeeding multiples by reading, talking to persons supportive of breastfeeding, and getting in touch with other mothers who have breastfed multiples.

- Be prepared for difficulties at times. You will have two or more times the usual number of babies, and they are more likely to be born early and less mature than term babies.

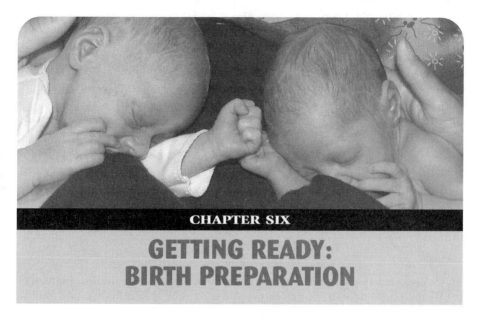

CHAPTER SIX

GETTING READY: BIRTH PREPARATION

A diagnosis of multiples has been made, your initial questions about multiple pregnancy have been answered, and you know you are doing all you can to help your babies grow while they reside inside you. To learn more about the "how-to" of breastfeeding multiples, you have been attending La Leche League meetings in person or online or you are talking to an LLL Leader or a lactation consultant by telephone. Now your thoughts may turn toward giving birth and other baby care issues for two or more newborns. What can you expect? How do you get ready?

Preparation for Birth

Obstetric care providers often view the labor and delivery of multiples differently than a single-infant birth. You, your partner, and your care provider may have to spend more time discussing possible labor and birth scenarios if you are to work together to achieve an optimal birth experience as well as optimal physical outcomes for you and each of your babies. A good first step is to learn about the process of childbirth and explore your thoughts and feelings about labor and birth. Share information and feelings with your partner. Determine the kind of birth experience you consider to be ideal or meaningful. Discuss your views about birth with your doctor or midwife and ask for her/his view, especially for multiple births. If the care provider's view is not compatible with yours, ask for explanations. You and your partner will want to understand the rationale when the care provider's approach to multiple birth differs from yours. It is your task to clear up any questions related to differences between those points of view so you can experience childbirth in a way that is both safe and meaningful to you.

Vaginal vs. Surgical Birth

Learn about the process of childbirth and explore your thoughts and feelings about labor and birth.

Surgical, or cesarean,* delivery is more common with multiple births. Almost 50 percent of US twin births are surgical deliveries and, in another 10 percent, the first twin is delivered vaginally and the second is a surgical birth. Some increase in surgical births for twins would be expected because there are more instances of complications for babies and mothers, but such a high rate of surgical delivery for twins has been questioned. It seems to be due mostly to an increase in the "routine" surgical delivery of twins by some care providers.

The routine surgical delivery of twins appears to be unnecessary. Vaginal delivery is a reasonable consideration and outcomes are as good for the second twin in otherwise uncomplicated twin pregnancies when:

- Pregnancy is at least at 32 weeks,
- Each baby is estimated to weigh at least 2000 gm (4 lb 7 oz),
- The first baby presents in the vertex, or head down, position. (The first twin is vertex in more than 80 percent of sets.)

However, research indicates that surgical delivery leads to better outcomes when the first twin is nonvertex (breech or transverse) and for the small percentage of identical twins who are in the same inner sac, or amnion, and are called monoamniotic twins. (Most identical twins share the outer sac, or chorion, but this does not create a problem at birth.) Surgical delivery is also associated with better outcomes for higher-order multiple sets.

Birth Setting

A hospital birth is generally recommended for multiple births. Even when a twin or triplet pregnancy is full-term, all babies are estimated to be over 2500 gm (5 lb 8 oz) and the first baby is well "engaged" in a vertex presentation, there are increased risks for babies and mother during a multiple labor and birth. Because of the unpredictability of any subsequent (second or third) baby's position, the potential for pressure on its umbilical cord, and a concern about excessive maternal bleeding, obstetric care providers prefer to deliver multiples where they are prepared for any emergency.

---

* This book uses the term "surgical" birth or delivery instead of cesarean birth. It is more accurate and it reminds all involved that the mother is recovering from major surgery while assuming the care of two or more infants.

The precise presentation of the second (and third) baby cannot be determined until after the previous multiple's birth. Although few second (or third) babies do a complete flip of position during labor, it is fairly common for the second (or third) baby to find itself somewhat crooked as it enters the birth canal, even if vertex/head down. Such malpositioning, or "malpresentation," can increase the physical stress for an unborn baby and its mother. An umbilical cord prolapse is always a serious concern with each multiple after the first. A prolapsed cord results in compression of the baby's umbilical cord, which drastically decreases that baby's oxygen supply. It is more common if a multiple is in a breech or transverse position but it can occur as a second (or third) baby is becoming engaged in a vertex position. Also, the delivery of one very large or two (or more) placenta(s) from a more "stretched out" uterus is associated with more postpartum hemorrhage for women after giving birth to twins and higher-order multiples.

> **Most care providers prefer to deliver higher-order multiples in high level, or regional, health care centers.**

Many care providers will monitor labor and "catch" twins in a hospital birthing room. Unmedicated birth can be ideal for the vaginal birth with twins or triplet sets. You, your contracting uterus, and gravity can work together to push out each baby, thereby minimizing the need for artificial manipulation, especially for the second (and third) baby.

Ask what level of nursery care is available in the hospital where you are considering giving birth. Multiples are much more likely than single-born infants to spend hours to weeks in a newborn intensive care unit (NICU) because of complications associated with multiple pregnancy, labor, and birth. Not all NICUs provide the same level of care, because it is not cost-effective for every hospital to equip and staff a high level NICU. Smaller hospitals and those with limited number of births usually have lower to medium level NICUs. When extremely sick or very low birth weight (VLBW) preterm babies are born at a hospital that provides a lower level of newborn special care, they are often transported to a hospital with more extensive services.

It is more stressful for mothers when one or more babies must be moved to a different hospital. Since the mother is recovering from a more demanding pregnancy and birth—quite often a surgical delivery—it may be more difficult for her to travel to be with her babies. Frequently babies are "divided" between two different hospitals—one (or more) remains in the birth hospital while the other(s) are transported to a high level NICU. Their mothers feel as divided emotionally as their babies are physically.

You may want to discuss with your care provider the option of delivering in a hospital with a higher level NICU. A lower level medical center may be reasonable for a healthy twin pregnancy, but you may want to reconsider birth sites if you experience symptoms of any infant or maternal complication. Most care providers prefer to deliver higher-order multiples in high level, or regional, health care centers.

Childbirth Classes

Attend childbirth education classes during the second trimester of pregnancy, so you are more likely to complete the course.

More locales now offer childbirth classes designed for parents expecting multiples. Ask your obstetrical care provider, look for "childbirth education" in the yellow pages of your telephone book, or check online for information. Most childbirth education groups will know if special multiple-birth classes are offered in an area, and they will usually provide contact information if available. If there is no multiple-birth class in your area, attend a "standard" childbirth education class. The basic process of birth and how to cope with labor does not change. Let the instructor know that you are expecting multiples. Many will adapt class instruction to accommodate your needs.

Be sure that surgical delivery is included in class discussion. In most childbirth classes, the surgical procedure(s), the types of anesthesia and post-delivery pain medication, and what to expect in the first weeks after the surgery are described. Ideas for getting a good breastfeeding start after surgical delivery often are included.

Attend childbirth education classes during the second trimester of pregnancy (four to six months/13 to 26 weeks), so you are more likely to complete the course. You will also feel more physically comfortable during that time than later in pregnancy. You will want to complete childbirth or surgical delivery classes by 24 weeks if higher-order multiples are expected. Some childbirth educators provide weekend "intensive" courses and others are willing to provide in-home, private instructions. (See Resources for information about childbirth classes for expectant parents of multiples.)

Birth Plans

Include options in any birth plan that take into account common variations for labor and delivery with multiples, which means expecting the unexpected.

A written birth plan can be helpful in ensuring that as many as possible of the aspects you find meaningful are included in your multiples' births. Birth plans should include your preferences for:

- Labor and birth interventions, such as induction, monitoring, IV fluids, etc. (See Chapter 8, "Happy Birthday"),
- Medication and anesthesia,
- Immediate mother-babies interaction,
- Breastfeeding after birth.

Include options in any birth plan that take into account common variations for labor and delivery with multiples, which means expecting the unexpected. You may want to plan for the uncomplicated, full-term (or close to term) vaginal births of all babies, surgical birth of all babies, and a vaginal-surgical birth combination.

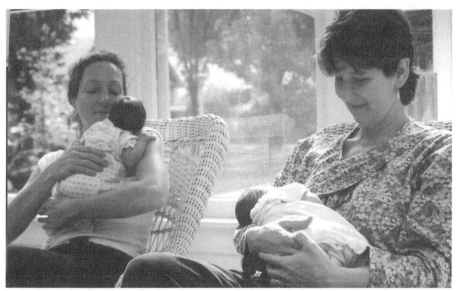

Mothers need lots of support before and after the birth of multiples.

Discuss your birth plan with your partner, your obstetrical care provider, and any other labor/birth support person who will be with you. When care providers know you understand the need for flexibility during labor and birth with multiples, most will do what they can to fulfill the birth plan and help make your birth experience as satisfying as possible. Once you, your partner, and obstetric care provider reach agreement on your birth options, write a final birth plan. Take several copies to the hospital with you. Your partner, care provider, and any additional support person should each keep a copy. Another copy should be attached to your chart. (See Chapter 8, "Happy Birthday," for other aspects of labor and delivery to be considered while developing birth plans.)

Doula Support

A doula is a woman with knowledge and experience about the childbirth process who provides physical and emotional support to a laboring/birthing mother and her partner. Doula support for birth is a "new" old idea! Throughout human history most women have had other experienced women to support them during labor and birth. New research among women having single births reinforces the old idea that the support of an experienced woman is of benefit to mothers and babies—labors tend to be shorter, less medication is required, and surgical births are fewer.

> You would want to find someone knowledgeable about multiple births or a doula willing to learn and adapt to the situation.

The support of a doula during multiple birth is an idea

worth considering, although her role may be slightly different than for a single birth. You would want to find someone knowledgeable about multiple births or a doula willing to learn and adapt to the situation. Contracting with someone who is a certified birth doula means that she has passed a standardized testing process for knowledge in this field. A doula can help you and your partner develop a birth plan and will work with hospital care providers to see that it is fulfilled insofar as possible after admission. Most doulas remain with mothers during the initial recovery period, so your doula can help you begin to breastfeed your healthy babies. (See Resources for information about locating qualified doulas in your area.) If you cannot find a doula in your area, the support of a female relative or friend who understands what you want of the birth could still prove invaluable.

Baby Care Classes

Today many first-time parents give birth with no prior experience handling a newborn or young infant, so expectant parents may be really unsure about where to begin with multiple newborns. You will feel more comfortable cuddling your own babies if you spend time during pregnancy observing other parents, and holding and changing others' babies. La Leche League meetings are a great place to gain some experience.

Baby care classes for expectant parents are offered in many areas and, as with childbirth classes, you should plan to attend during the second trimester of a multiple pregnancy. The dolls often used in these classes don't squirm like the real thing, but they do allow fledgling diaper-changers or baby-bathers to get some idea of how to handle basic baby care tasks. Many expectant parents of multiples also feel more confident after taking an infant cardiopulmonary resuscitation (CPR) class. (See Resources for US agencies offering baby care or CPR classes. Children's hospitals and hospitals with large NICUs often hold classes where you can learn infant CPR.)

Pregnant Memories

Take a photo series of your expanding profile during the last 10 to 12 weeks of pregnancy.

You may think that once the babies arrive you would just as soon forget the details of your multiple pregnancy. Many mothers of multiples say they do not want photographic reminders of their extremely pregnant waistlines, but many of them later express regret that they don't have photos of themselves late in pregnancy. Be sure to take a photographic series of your expanding profile during the last 10 to 12 weeks of pregnancy. As the memory of how it looked and felt to carry multiples fades, these photographs may become a cherished treasure of a special time in your life. Older multiples, curious about where they came from, will enjoy seeing what Mommy looked like when they were inside you.

KEY POINTS

❏ Although a cesarean/surgical birth is more common for multiple births, it should not be "automatic" for the majority of twins.

❏ Because of the extra risk factors for multiple babies and mother during labor and birth, a hospital birth is preferred by most obstetric care providers.

❏ Ask your obstetric care provider about the level of care available at the newborn intensive care unit (NICU) or special care nursery (SCN) at the hospital where you are planning to give birth.

❏ Prepare for your multiple birth by
  • Taking a childbirth education/preparation class.

  • Writing a birth plan that covers the kind of care that is important to you during the labor and birth of your babies.

❏ For a multiple birth, your birth plan should mention options in case a complication occurs.

❏ Consider hiring a certified birth doula who has been trained to support women during labor. Having a doula can be especially helpful during labor and multiple birth.

❏ If you or your partner has had little experience with young babies, you may want to take a baby care class and an infant cardiopulmonary resuscitation (CPR) class during the second trimester of pregnancy.

❏ Take a photo "diary" of your pregnancy. You and your multiples will be glad to have these visual memories in years to come.

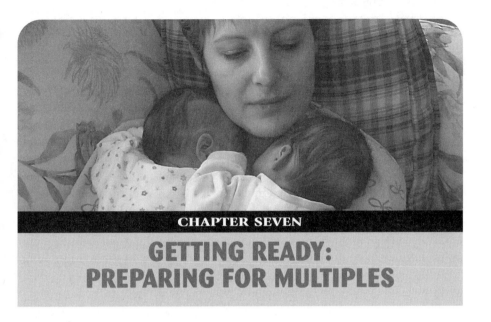

CHAPTER SEVEN

GETTING READY:
PREPARING FOR MULTIPLES

You're reading birth and breastfeeding books, attending classes, watching "caring for multiples" videos, and speaking to an experienced mother about breastfeeding multiples. What else needs to be accomplished before your multiples are born?

Pediatric Care

Pregnancy is the time to "shop" for pediatric care for your babies. Many pediatricians, family physicians, or pediatric nurse practitioners offer a free office interview visit. Others will schedule telephone interview time. Take advantage of these opportunities, but be sure to speak directly to the pediatric care provider you are interested in having for your babies' health care. Office personnel are not acceptable substitutes. Your obstetrical care provider, LLL Leaders, and IBCLCs may be able to recommend local pediatric care providers who are supportive of breastfeeding. If you already have a child, you probably have a pediatric care provider. However, you will want to discuss the impact multiples might have on the type of care provided, especially if this will be your first breastfeeding experience.

Interview Questions

Doing your interview "homework" is especially important since you plan to breastfeed multiples, because the care provider's support and encouragement can affect your confidence. You will want to ask each pediatric care provider you interview what she or he knows about breastfeeding in general and breastfeeding multiples specifically. If your goal is to breastfeed two or more babies completely for several weeks or months, what kind of support can the care provider offer? Does the provider work with LLL Leaders and IBCLCs in the community? How many sets of completely and partially breastfed twins and higher-order multiples has the provider seen? How long did the multiple sets breastfeed? Does the provider believe multiples, especially twins, can be fully breastfed for several months? What are the provider's thoughts about complementing, or "topping off," and supplementing breastfeeding? Will the provider support a decision to express/pump milk and feed it to preterm or sick newborn multiples if any of the babies require NICU care? What does the provider think about "kangaroo care," skin-to-skin parental care for babies in the NICU? What plan does the care provider recommend to transition preterm or sick newborns to direct breastfeeding?

Other Questions

Check the pediatric care provider's business hours and ask about the "call" schedule and how long it usually takes for a phone call to be returned. You will want to know how long you can expect to spend in the waiting room with multiple, and possibly fussy, babies. Ask if you can avoid a long wait if you schedule your babies to be seen at certain appointment times. You may want to know whether an office has an "isolation" waiting area, so your babies are not exposed to children with contagious illnesses. Look into the fee structure. Some care providers charge less for each additional multiple's office visit after the first baby, although each immunization or treatment usually is a set fee.

Location, Location, Location

Visit each care provider's office or clinic to check the location. Unlike a mother of one baby who has a free hand to open doors or hold a stairway handrail, mothers of multiples cannot maneuver two or more babies in or out of a car and building as freely. Depending on accessibility, you may be able to get by with only a multiple stroller or a baby sling/carrier, or you may need to take another adult with you for every trip. Look for a safe play area in the waiting room; it won't be long before your babies are curious and fast-moving toddlers.

Baby Names x 2, 3, 4, +

Pregnancy is the ideal time to begin thinking of your multiples as separate, unique persons. And what is more reflective of an individual than the name that person carries? Consider carefully the names you give each multiple. Your babies' names provide a clue to others, and eventually to the multiples themselves, about how you view these children. Is each considered special in his or her own right, or are they seen as more special because they arrived as a set?

> **Your babies' names provide a clue to others, and eventually to the multiples themselves, about how you view these children.**

Some adult multiples think "twin" names–close-sounding, rhyming, alliterated, or "famous couple/trio" names–are fun. Others resent such names. Naming each from the same category, such as ethnic, Biblical, traditional, unisex names, or family names can give the impression that the babies "go together" yet may avoid the appearance of a "set."

There is no "right" or "wrong" way to name multiples. Some parents have regretted bestowing "twin" names on their babies, but others have never felt it caused a problem. Imagine yourself as a twin or higher-order multiple and explore your feelings about having a name that matches one or more others. Then bestow on your babies the names that you and your partner like best.

Household Help

Having household help before and after a multiple birth is not a luxury; it is a necessity. Mothers of multiples often say in hindsight, "I should have gotten more help," or "I wish I'd had help longer." In cultures stressing feminism and self-reliance, it can be difficult for women and their partners to accept the need for help in the household during a multiple pregnancy and after babies are born. Incorporating a single newborn into a family requires a major investment of time and energy. Multiply the amount of adaptation required when bringing multiple babies into the family. Few mothers of multiples can manage the household routine alone and still feel rested and ready to manage baby care times two, three, or more. Planning for household help will decrease postpartum pandemonium.

> **Having household help before and after a multiple birth is not a luxury; it is a necessity.**

You should be free to get to know your babies and recuperate from multiple pregnancy and birth when you first bring multiples home, so arrange to have at least one full-time, supportive household helper in your home during the first few weeks after discharge. Part-time helpers can also take over some household chores. The more babies you have, the more helpers you will need and the longer you will need them.

The kind of help needed depends on the circumstances; however, most new mothers need someone to cook, clean, and run a washing machine while they care

Planning for household help will decrease postpartum pandemonium.

for babies. If your multiples are first children, you may also want someone who helps you learn to handle, bathe, and change the babies. An experienced mother probably will want someone to help care for older children and keep them occupied. All mothers of multiples can use an extra pair of hands at times to help cuddle fussing babies.

Examine household help options realistically. If dad can take a couple of weeks off work and knows his way around the kitchen and laundry room, he may be the ideal full-time helper. If housework is not his specialty, recruit him to hold babies and run errands, but look elsewhere for someone to cook, clean, and do laundry. The babies' grandparents or new aunts and uncles are often willing and eager to lend a hand. If husband or relatives are likely to be more hindrance than help, look elsewhere!

Hire someone to take over household tasks when family members or friends are unable to stay full time. Hiring help is cost-effective when you consider that it frees you to breastfeed, which in turn is a substantial cost savings. You'll be healthier long term and ready to resume more of the household tasks sooner if you've been given time to recover from multiple pregnancy and birth and to develop a breastfeeding and baby care routine.

An excellent source of help might be through a postpartum doula service. (See Resources for information about finding certified postpartum doula services.) Women have also found help through housecleaning, nanny, or au pair agencies. Others have posted notices or received names for full- or part-time help at churches, senior citizen centers, and junior or senior high schools.

When full-time help is no longer needed, don't be surprised if you still require part-time help–for years. Housecleaning service once or twice a week may be a sanity saver when two or more toddlers or preschoolers are finding creative uses for household items. You may also want to have a mother's helper come in to help with older children or babies for a few hours several times a week.

Families with freezer space may want to get a head start on postpartum meals by doubling recipes or going on a day-long cooking binge now to freeze dinners for later use. Extended family members and friends may also want to contribute to the stockpile. Many mothers of multiples say they appreciate a "supper shower" more than a regular baby shower. Guests at this shower bring meals that can be frozen or it can take the form of coupons to be redeemed at a later date if freezer space is minimal.

Employment Issues

Many women combine parenting, breastfeeding, and outside employment, and many do it well. However, anticipating a return to work after giving birth to multiples adds to the challenge of combining the roles of mother and employee. Multiple pregnancy often results in a woman taking an earlier than anticipated leave of

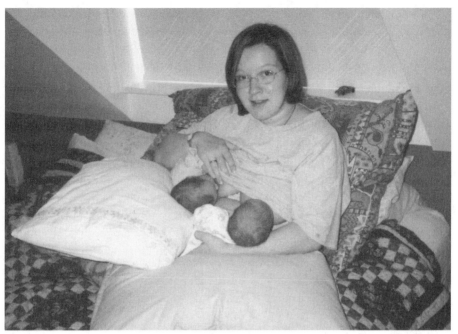

Having household help allows a mother to recuperate from the birth and devote all of her energy to feeding and caring for her babies.

absence. This may add pressure to return to work at an earlier date after a more physically demanding pregnancy and delivery.

You are more likely to need more time rather than less to recuperate after a multiple pregnancy and birth. Of course, you are likely to get less rest instead of more, since multiple babies require more daytime and nighttime care. Because of the increased complexity of returning to work after giving birth to multiples, you may want to spend time during pregnancy considering options for several work-related issues.

Many women combine parenting, breastfeeding, and outside employment.

Leave of Absence

Ideally, mothers of multiples can extend a leave of absence due to the lengthier recovery period. If multiples were born preterm and discharge was delayed, the family will need more time to adapt. In addition, each multiple has the same need as any single infant to develop a strong bond with his or her mother, but it takes more time to get to know and learn to love the individuals within a multiples set. The pressure of returning to work within weeks of delivery can interfere with establishing breastfeeding. Many mothers think they have to "hurry and get it right" when, in reality, most multiples and their mothers need more time to learn to breastfeed as a team.

If a lengthier leave is possible but only if it is an unpaid leave, don't dismiss the idea until you have done some calculations. To consider the effect on the family budget, deduct the costs of child care, transportation to and from work, work clothing costs, and meals during the workday from your salary. This may give you an entirely new perspective.

Alternative Work Plans

The pressure of returning to work within weeks of delivery can interfere with establishing breastfeeding.

Returning to part-time employment is another option to working full-time on top of mothering multiple babies during their first year or two. If dad takes over baby care during mother's work hours, this actually may provide comparable income to a full-time salary after deducting child care costs. Some mothers find they can combine part-time hours at the work site with "at home" hours for paperwork. New computer and Internet technology has made it more realistic to combine work on site and at home or entirely from home. Another idea is to join the increasing number of women who "job share" one full-time position or who arrange to work flexible hours, or flex-time, in order to meet both personal and professional responsibilities.

Examine aspects of your present job during pregnancy. If you find there is potential for a more flexible return-to-work schedule, now is the time to develop and present a plan that outlines how it would work. An idea is more likely to be favorably received if you have considered all the details in advance of the proposal presentation.

Child Care for Multiples

Finding quality day care for multiples is not always easy. Most parents must balance the increased cost of care with a child care provider's ability to meet the physical and emotional needs of two or more babies. Many providers charge less for each multiple after the first, but quality care is costly–sometimes about the same or even more than one parent's salary after deducting other job-related expenses, such as transportation, clothing, and meals. Child care is not, however, the place to trim your budget. Also, some providers may have to be eliminated because they or their facilities are unable to handle multiple infants.

If you will be, or are considering, returning to work during the multiples' first several weeks or months, begin interviewing day care providers during pregnancy. To learn whether an individual care provider's or agency's philosophy of child care is compatible with yours, ask each to share beliefs about meeting infants' and children's physical and emotional needs. Agencies should have written mission and philosophy statements available. When considering day care outside of your home, ask how many other babies are in the care of each care provider. Providing agencies should also explain how they "divide" care for multiples.

Ask potential providers if they often have other breastfed children in their care and whether they are comfortable with having expressed milk brought in for your children. Let potential care providers know if you will be taking breastfeeding breaks with your babies and that you intend to drop in unannounced at times to check on your children. Quality child care providers welcome parents at any time. You will also need to ask what arrangements must be made if any of your multiples is sick. Since multiples often share childhood illnesses, parents can lose a lot of sick days when each becomes ill one at a time.

Ask potential caregivers if they often have other breastfed children in their care and whether they are comfortable with having expressed milk brought in for your children.

Consider what type of child care will work best in your situation–care in your home, day care in an individual provider's home, or a day care center. If you make arrange- ments for day care near your work site, you might be able to take a breastfeeding break with your babies once or twice a day. You will also be separated from the babies for less time each day. Having a child care provider come to your home means the babies are in a familiar environment and there is no exposure to other children and their illnesses.

During pregnancy it may seem difficult to imagine that your babies will ever arrive. Yet they will be here before you know it! Any postpartum preparation that you can accomplish now will help you meet your own and your family's needs later. And it probably will decrease the postpartum pandemonium that is so common after multiple births.

KEY POINTS

❑ Select a pediatric care provider for your babies before they are born by talking to several in person or over the phone.

- Before choosing a pediatric provider, ask about how many breastfed multiples he/she has cared for and what kind of breastfeeding support you can expect from him/her.

- Be sure the pediatric office is convenient and easy to get two or more babies in and out of!

❑ Think about the names you choose for multiples. If you were a twin or triplet, would you want a name that sounded as if it was "matched" with others or would you want a special name of your own?

❑ Plan to have household helpers after you give birth to multiples, so you are freer to breastfeed and get to know each of your babies.

❑ If you will be returning to outside work after your babies' birth, think about:

- A longer leave of absence so your body has time to recuperate, and you and your babies have time to get breastfeeding going well.

- Possible part-time options, since "take home" salary will be affected after subtracting the cost of child care for multiples and other job-related costs.

- Finding a child care provider who shares your beliefs about breastfeeding and meeting babies' physical and emotional needs.

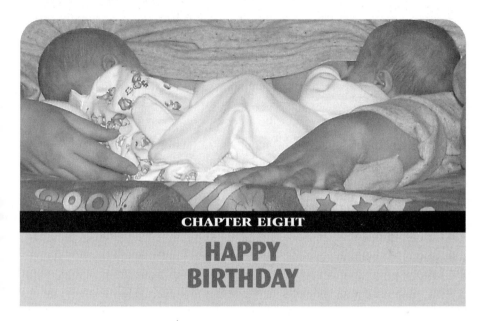

CHAPTER EIGHT

HAPPY BIRTHDAY

Today's the day! Ready or not this is your babies' birthday. You've taken childbirth and breastfeeding preparation classes. You've toured the maternity unit. Your obstetrical care provider has reviewed your birth plan(s) and given the go-ahead. What can you expect when rehearsals end and the actual performance begins?

Labor

The *stages of labor* are essentially the same whether one baby or multiples are born. The uterus, or womb, is a muscle and the establishment of regular contractions of that muscle identifies the *first stage* of labor. Contractions dilate, or open, the lowest portion of the uterus, which is called the cervix. The contractions increase in strength and number as labor progresses until the cervix is completely dilated at 10 cm so that the first baby's presenting part can enter the vagina, or birth canal. With rare exception, the cervix dilates only once for a multiple birth.

During the *second stage* of labor you work with your contractions to push the first baby down and out of the birth canal. Although the cervix remains dilated, the process of pushing begins again once the second baby is in position. After the second baby is born, the process is repeated when a third baby is born vaginally. However, pushing to give birth to the first baby generally takes longer than pushing for a subsequent multiple. The average time interval between the birth of a first twin and that of the second is about 5 to 20 minutes. A longer time is not a prob-

Studies find the overall length of labor when giving birth to multiples tends to be similar to that for single-infant pregnancy.

lem if the fetal monitor shows that the second baby is doing well. No matter how many babies you push into the world at the end of a multiple pregnancy, it is considered a single second stage of labor.

The *third stage* of labor begins when the last multiple baby is born and ends when the last placenta is delivered. Rarely does expulsion of the first baby's placenta precede the birth of the second baby. About 75 percent of identical twins share one large placenta. The remaining 25 percent of identical twins and all fraternal multiples have individual placentas; however, two (or more) placentas often grow until they join/fuse along their borders, which can give the appearance of a single placenta.

The first one to four hours after birth form the *fourth stage* of labor. During this time the uterus begins to adapt to the "loss" of its recent occupants, and the mother's body must adjust rapidly to the sudden change in hormones initiated by the expulsion of the placenta(s).

Women are often told to expect a longer labor with multiples. It is thought that a uterus distended with multiples may contract less effectively. However, studies have found that the overall length of labor tends to be similar to that for single-infant pregnancy, although typical time periods for certain phases within the first stage of labor were different.

Vaginal Birth

The birth of a first multiple in the vertex, or head down, position is essentially like the birth of a single vertex baby. On some labor and delivery units, women may give birth to full-term, vertex multiples in a birthing room. This may be acceptable when the room can be adapted for an emergency surgical delivery or if a surgical suite is within several steps if a problem arises during the birth of the second (or third) baby. When this flexibility is not available, obstetric care providers may prefer that multiple births take place in a delivery room with the mother on a delivery table. Depending on how you feel and the condition of the first baby, you may be able to hold your first baby before labor resumes in earnest with the second baby.

Once the first (or second) baby is born, care providers will continue to monitor any multiple remaining in the uterus. As the second (or third) baby moves into position for birth, it may be necessary to readjust external monitoring belts. (See "Labor Monitoring" in this chapter.) Because of the increased risk of the second (and third) multiple during delivery, care providers may want to apply an internal monitoring electrode once that baby is engaged in the pelvis. The need for medical intervention with the birth of any subsequent multiple depends on that baby's position in the birth canal and whether there is any sign of fetal distress.

Surgical (Cesarean) Birth

Surgical delivery is common with multiple births. (See Chapter 6, "Getting Ready: Birth Preparation.") Surgical delivery may be planned when a first multiple is in the breech or transverse lie position, a placenta covers part of the cervical opening, or there are higher-order multiples. A "repeat" surgical birth is not always necessary when a twin pregnancy follows the surgical delivery of a previous pregnancy. Women have had twins by vaginal birth after cesarean (VBAC), although in many areas it is difficult to find a care provider willing to consider VBAC for twins.

A "trial of labor" may be considered for some of the complications that may occur in multiple pregnancies. These may include maternal conditions, such as pregnancy-induced hypertension (PIH) or gestational diabetes, or when there is greater risk of fetal distress for one or more babies, as with a poorly reactive non-stress test (NST) or a second twin in a breech or transverse position. (See Chapter 4, "What to Do If...") Should fetal distress develop during labor for any multiple or if a mother's condition suddenly worsens, an emergency surgical delivery can be performed.

During a surgical birth each baby is delivered through an incision, or cut, made in a woman's abdominal area. The outside, or skin, incision may run vertically from the umbilicus to the pubic hair line, or it may be a horizontal cut (Pfannenstiel) along the pubic hair, or bikini, line. The skin incision does not necessarily reflect the direction of the uterine incision. Generally a horizontal incision is made in the lower segment of the uterus; however, some care providers prefer a lower segment vertical incision for multiple births, especially if one or both are in unusual positions or when a placenta covers part of the cervical opening.

Multiples delivered surgically are lifted out one at a time, and the time between births usually is closer than during a vaginal birth. There may be a slightly longer time between births when the first multiple is born vaginally and a subsequent one is surgically delivered. Depending on the babies' conditions, some mothers ask that a nurse or a doula massage the babies after delivery to provide skin stimulation in place of that received during passage through the birth canal.

Hospital Routines and First Stage Interventions

Interventions are recommended more often during labor and delivery with multiples, and it was for the special situations more likely to occur with multiples that many interventions were developed. However, all interventions also have consequences or side effects. Sometimes parents and care providers must weigh the potential consequences of a complication or condition with those of an intervention. This makes it more important for you to understand the reasons for, and the potential consequences of, any recommended labor and delivery intervention.

> It was for the special situations more likely to occur with multiple births that many labor and delivery interventions were developed.

An unmedicated birth is feasible when full- or close-to-full-term twins (or triplets) meet the criteria for vaginal birth.

Admission. A prenatal/antenatal form usually is sent to the labor and delivery (L&D) unit so that hospital staff have pertinent information about your pregnancy. Often it is sent during the second trimester. It probably won't include the birth plan(s) you and your partner developed, so tuck an extra copy or two in the bag you've packed to take to the hospital.

In most areas a prep, or shave, of the perineum prior to a vaginal birth is no longer a routine. Likewise, studies have shown that there is no need to administer an enema to a laboring woman. If either is suggested, you may want to ask why.

When admitted for a planned surgical birth, your abdomen will be "prepped"; it will be cleansed with antibacterial soap and then shaved. Also, expect a catheter to be inserted into the bladder to continuously drain urine for the first day or two after birth. Sometimes catheterization is postponed until a woman is anesthetized. These procedures can be performed later in labor if a surgical delivery becomes necessary.

The admission procedure with any labor includes answering a lot of questions and having your temperature, blood pressure, and pulse checked. Usually the nurse or midwife will also do an initial vaginal examination to check the dilatation of the cervix. Blood will be drawn to make sure blood counts are within normal range. It is common with multiple pregnancies to check the positions of the babies and the placenta(s) in the uterus via a portable ultrasound machine.

Early in labor you may be encouraged to walk, because activity has been shown to accelerate labor naturally. Walking may be discouraged if the first baby's presenting part is not firmly engaged in the pelvis, especially if that baby's membranes (amniotic sac or bag of waters) already ruptured, or broke, spontaneously–referred to as spontaneous rupture of membranes (SROM). A spontaneous rupture of the membranes in a full term pregnancy before labor begins may be referred to as premature rupture of membranes (PROM). When labor is preterm, before 37 weeks gestation, this is called preterm premature rupture of membranes (PPROM).

Intravenous line (IV). Because of the extra risks associated with multiple birth, obstetrical care providers may want to insert an IV or a heparin lock during active labor even when an unmedicated birth is planned. The idea is to have a vein immediately available for infusing medication if a complication or emergency develops. The IV may also provide extra fluid during an unmedicated labor and birth.

If you plan to have analgesic (pain) medication or an anesthetic is to be given, obstetric care providers may insist on an IV before administering medication, because these medications include some additional risk. An epidural, which is considered both an analgesic and an anesthetic, should never be given unless an IV is in place. Medication used to induce or to "speed up" labor can be better controlled when given by IV. An IV is essential for surgical delivery.

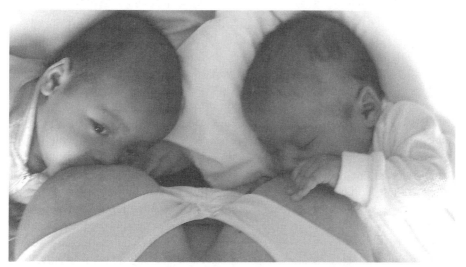

Breastfeeding multiples soon after birth provides benefits to mothers and babies.

Labor Induction and Augmentation (Acceleration)

Induction of labor means that uterine contractions are stimulated artificially before spontaneous, or natural, contractions occur in order to achieve cervical dilatation and birth. Labor augmentation, also called acceleration of labor, is used to speed the progress of spontaneous labor. Both procedures are common during labor with multiple pregnancies. Since labor induction and augmentation are associated with a higher incidence of surgical delivery and fetal distress, neither should be undertaken lightly.

Based on the conclusions of some studies, some obstetric care providers recommend inducing labor for all twin pregnancies by 37 to 38 weeks gestation. The twins in these research samples had better outcomes than those delivered later; however, other research reports conflict with this recommendation in association with uncomplicated twin pregnancies. Although a high number of twin pregnancies result in spontaneous labor and birth before 38 weeks gestation, women whose pregnancies reach 38 weeks may question a recommendation to induce labor. Options to induction may include additional ultrasound or BPP in conjunction with Doppler velocimetry and NST (see Chapter 4) to check on babies' well-being.

Induction may be recommended when there are maternal complications, such as pregnancy-induced hypertension (PIH) or gestational diabetes. Baby-related reasons for induction may include placental insufficiency that is affecting any baby's growth. If you experience premature rupture of membranes (PROM) that is not followed by spontaneous contractions within several hours and begin to run a fever, induction of labor may be suggested. Augmentation may be recommended for a prolonged first stage of labor; however, "prolonged" can be a subjective term.

Maternal nipple stimulation may be all that is needed to induce or augment labor when a woman's cervix already is soft or thin and has begun to dilate. Nipple stimulation is safe and non-invasive, so it is a good procedure to start with. However, do *not* use it without the obstetric care provider's agreement.

Obstetric care providers may suggest artificial rupture of the first baby's membranes as a means to induce or augment labor. Artificial rupture of membranes (AROM) is considered controversial by some care providers, as the amniotic fluid contained within the membranes cushions a baby's head, body, and umbilical cord during labor. (The amniotic sac should never be ruptured intentionally before the first baby is firmly engaged in the pelvis.) Once the membranes have been ruptured, the risk of infection increases, so most care providers want full- or close-to-full-term babies delivered within 24 hours of a rupture of the first baby's membranes.

Oxytocin is the hormone most responsible for spontaneous contractions. To induce or augment (accelerate) labor a synthetic oxytocin, such as pitocin, is used alone or with AROM. Pitocin or similar drugs can cause the uterus to contract too often or for too long, which decreases the amount of oxygen the babies receive and may lead to "fetal distress." If fetal distress is not resolved quickly, an emergency surgical delivery becomes necessary.

The usual procedure for induction or augmentation is to slowly increase the amount of IV pitocin. Women who have had labors both with and without a pitocin drip say contractions can become closer and stronger too quickly and peak more abruptly, which makes it difficult to keep pace and adjust breathing techniques.

Labor Monitoring

Both you and your babies will be monitored throughout labor. If you are admitted to the hospital during the early phase of first-stage labor, a nurse or midwife will time your contractions and feel for the intensity of one or two about every hour. Vaginal examination is performed intermittently to monitor the progress of cervical dilatation. How often exams are performed depends on the labor pattern or any sign of a potential problem. The timing of exams may be influenced by medications used for induction or augmentation and for analgesics/anesthetics. Often a woman is examined before a medication is given or after, depending on her response to the drug.

The nurse or midwife will listen to and count each baby's heart rate two or more times an hour. A fetoscope, which looks like a strange stethoscope, or a Doppler, which allows you to listen, too, may be used. You will be asked to lie flat or in a low semi-sitting position until each baby's heart rate is counted. Since this tends to be an uncomfortable position during contractions, most nurses try to count all the babies' heart rates between two contractions. Occasionally, a nurse may need to listen to one baby during the beginning of a contraction or soon after a contraction peaks and the uterus begins to relax.

Electronic Fetal Monitoring

As labor progresses it is likely that electronic fetal monitoring (EFM) of the babies' heart rates will be recommended. There are two forms of EFM: external monitoring and internal monitoring. Both types measure how each baby responds during and between contractions by measuring each one's heart rate and the differences for each from one heartbeat to the next (variability), and a device measures contraction frequency and intensity/strength. The monitoring machine translates the information to create written recordings, or tracings, of your contraction pattern and the corresponding heart rate with heartbeat variability of each baby. The routine use of EFM is controversial, yet many obstetric care providers believe its use is appropriate during labor with multiples because of the increased risks.

If you have had an NST (see Chapter 4), you will be familiar with the external monitor belts and attached devices that fasten around the abdomen. One device, a transducer, picks up uterine contractions and babies' movements. The device on each of the other belts records each baby's heart rate. The number of belts will depend on the number of babies you're carrying, Prior to the transition phase, the last part of first stage labor, intermittent external monitoring may be an option if all of the babies appear to be responding well to labor and you have not received medication. During intermittent monitoring the belts will be attached for 10 to 20 minutes every hour to hour and a half. If labor is to be induced or augmented, you receive analgesic medication, or there is a question about any baby's response to labor, continuous monitoring will be recommended.

External monitoring is a non-invasive technique, but tracings are prone to disruption because your movements and those of any baby can affect the ability of the devices to pick up and record information. However, belts usually can be repositioned easily. Some women report discomfort associated with pressure from the belts during contractions.

Internal monitoring produces a more accurate tracing of the presenting baby's heart rate and beat-to-beat variability. Only the multiple currently engaged in the pelvis can be monitored internally. (External monitoring is done for the other babies.) In addition, insertion of an internal transducer may be recommended when an accurate tracing of contraction intensity is desired.

Internal monitoring devices cannot be applied unless the presenting baby's membranes are ruptured and the cervix is dilated at least 2 cm. During a vaginal exam a thin-wired electrode is attached to the skin on the presenting part, usually the crown/back of the baby's head, which produces a continuous and clearer tracing of that baby's heart rate. It may produce a small scab on the baby's head that carries a slight risk of infection. A slim, flexible plastic transducer may be inserted to monitor contractions.

Applying an internal monitoring device is a more invasive technique and once begun it restricts the laboring woman's movements to the bed or near the bed. It is more likely to be suggested during labor for a multiple pregnancy because of the increased risks, especially if the active labor phase has begun and contractions are

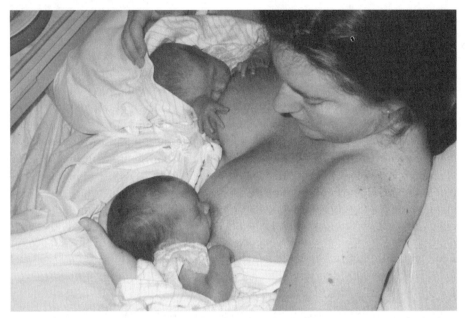

Using the double football hold, this mother breastfeeds her healthy newborns soon after birth.

five or fewer minutes apart with each lasting 40 or more seconds. Care providers may prefer to initiate internal monitoring sooner for induction or augmentation, the administration of analgesic or anesthetic medication, and any sign of fetal distress.

Analgesia/Anesthesia
Unmedicated Birth

Labor hurts. But so do many physical activities. Many exercise workouts are uncomfortable and push one's physical limits yet women continue–not only for the physical benefits but also for what they learn about themselves. If marathoners are celebrated for their achievements, why are women who choose an unmedicated birth treated as pariahs? Unmedicated birth achieves the same personal gains as those learned by coping and transcending other kinds of discomfort or pain, plus babies benefit by not being exposed to sedating drugs.

An unmedicated birth is feasible when full- or close-to-full-term twins (or triplets) meet the criteria for vaginal birth. However, you may have to put up with a few "just in case" interventions because of the increased risks that usually are not associated with labor and birth of a single baby, such as an IV or EFM. You may also have to search during early pregnancy for an obstetric care provider having experience delivering multiples without anesthesia. You can learn alternative methods for coping with the pain of contractions by attending childbirth preparation classes that specialize in teaching coping skills for unmedicated births. (See Resources for information.)

Some obstetric care providers are reluctant to deliver multiples without an anesthetic due to the increased possibility of a complication. There are mothers who report they negotiated with care providers to have epidural tubing put in place during active labor—some with and some without an initial test dose—in case anesthesia later became necessary. This allowed these women to give birth without medication while allowing their care providers to feel prepared for all possibilities.

Analgesia. Medications that relieve pain are called analgesics. Most analgesics given during active labor are some form of narcotic. Women have varied responses to these drugs, which usually are given intramuscularly (IM) or intravenously (IV). Some women report good pain relief after receiving medication. Other women say these drugs had little effect on the actual pain, although many report feeling drowsy between contractions or losing a sense of time passing. Nausea and vomiting are also common side effects of narcotic analgesics.

> **All narcotics affect the babies, because these medications pass through the placenta(s).**

All narcotics affect the babies, because these medications pass through the placenta(s). These medications can contribute to fetal distress, which already is more of a risk for multiples. Also, one or more babies may be sleepy and less responsive at birth. Since it takes a newborn's system longer to eliminate these drugs, a baby's ability to breastfeed can be affected at delivery and for several days after.

Epidural block. A continuous epidural block provides *analgesia* during labor and then serves as an *anesthetic* during a vaginal delivery and episiotomy repair or if a surgical birth becomes necessary. When manipulation of the second (or third) baby is anticipated for breech or transverse positioning, an epidural might be suggested. It may also be used as an anesthetic for a planned surgical birth.

During an epidural block a thin, plastic catheter is inserted in the epidural space of the spinal canal in the lumbar region on the lower half of the back. The anesthetic agent is delivered through the catheter tubing and acts on nerves that branch off the spinal cord, which serve the abdomen, perineum, and legs. In some areas a "one shot" epidural, or one dose of an anesthetic agent, is administered directly into the epidural space for surgical births. An epidural may provide consistent relief or it may work better for some areas of the body than others. Occasionally, an area may remain unaffected by the anesthetic.

Typically a local anesthetic agent, such as bupivacaine (marcaine), xylocaine (lidocaine), or novocaine (procaine) is used. Some of these drugs are short acting and others produce a longer-lasting effect; some reach the placenta(s) in minute amounts and others cross the placenta(s) and into the babies' circulations for long periods. A drop in maternal blood pressure is common with epidurals, so it is monitored closely because a drop can affect the babies' oxygen supply. Allergic reaction to a local anesthetic agent is rare but can occur. Combining a narcotic with a local anesthetic agent in a continuous epidural infusion pump is common in many areas, because care providers can use smaller doses of both types of medication. However, babies are still exposed to two different kinds of medication—each having the potential for different side effects after birth, including possible effects on one or more multiples' ability to breastfeed.

Second Stage Interventions

Second Stage Anesthesia

Anesthetics are given to block the pain associated with giving birth, and for cutting and repairing an episiotomy—an incision made in the perineum (the area between the vagina and rectum) to enlarge the opening of the birth canal/vagina. An episiotomy is more likely to be performed to "speed up" the delivery of a multiple, particularly for a second (or third) baby. Usually anesthesia is given for "assisted" deliveries using forceps or vacuum extraction. Anesthesia is unnecessary when no episiotomy is performed and no assistance is required. Except for continuous epidural, anesthetics generally are given when a baby's presenting part is visible and birth is imminent whether an anesthetic is given for the first or a subsequent multiple. (Many women have delivered multiples without anesthesia for any of the births.)

Local anesthesia: local infiltration and pudendal block. Infiltration of a local anesthetic agent and a pudendal (nerve) block can provide anesthesia for the perineum if an episiotomy becomes necessary during an otherwise unmedicated birth or for delivery in conjunction with narcotic analgesia during labor. With local infiltration an anesthetic agent is delivered directly into the perineal tissue immediately before an episiotomy is cut. Local anesthesia rarely affects babies. However, it sometimes begins to wear off before an episiotomy repair is completed.

A pudendal block is given late in the second stage of labor. It affects the nerves that supply the perineum. In addition to being used for episiotomies, it may also provide anesthesia if low forceps or vacuum extraction is needed for a more rapid delivery of any baby.

Saddle/spinal block. Saddle and spinal blocks are administered just prior to birth by injecting a local anesthetic agent into the spinal fluid, producing numbness from above (spinal) or below (saddle) the waist. A spinal is also an anesthesia option for surgical deliveries. Although the second (or third) multiple is more at risk, care providers may prefer to give a spinal before delivery of the first baby even when anesthesia is not a necessity for that baby.

This anesthetic can also cause a drop in a woman's blood pressure, which can affect babies' oxygen supply. In this case it is more likely to affect the second (or third) baby, since the first baby should be ready for birth when the saddle block is given. You may be told to lie flat for several hours after delivery to prevent a spinal headache.

General anesthesia. Few doctors today routinely put women to sleep to give birth. However, general anesthesia is occasionally used in emergency situations. For instance, it provides rapid anesthesia if a mother is unmedicated and an acute situation arises, requiring the immediate delivery of any baby vaginally or via an emergency surgical birth. General anesthetics may be injected through an IV or inhaled from a mask over a woman's nose and mouth. Often the two methods are combined.

General anesthetic agents cross the placenta(s) and affect babies within minutes. Care providers must be prepared to deliver any baby still in the uterus quickly to prevent or minimize the need for resuscitation. It may take several days for a newborn to eliminate these anesthetic agents, which can affect a baby's ability to breastfeed and interact with his or her mother. Increased maternal bleeding–already more likely after multiple birth–is common due to the muscle relaxation associated with general anesthetic.

"Assisted" Vaginal Delivery

Forceps delivery. Forceps are metal instruments used to expedite the birth of one or more multiples by providing traction that helps guide the head out. Most forceps-assisted births are "low"/"outlet" forceps births, and the forceps are not applied until a baby's head is crowning. Occasionally mid-forceps are used to rotate a baby's head to a more advantageous position–a situation more likely to occur with the second (or third) baby– before guiding that baby's head through the birth canal. Special forceps may be used to help deliver the baby's head during a breech birth of the second (or third) baby.

Forceps may be used when fetal distress occurs during the second stage of labor, and the baby is close, but not quite ready, to be born. Forceps assistance is more often needed after the administration of an epidural block, a spinal or saddle block, and general anesthesia, since anesthesia can interfere with a woman's ability to effectively push to deliver each baby. Occasionally low/outlet forceps are offered to hasten birth if a woman becomes exhausted after a long labor.

Side effects for low/outlet forceps deliveries are usually minimal, although some babies develop a small amount of bruising or swelling in the cheekbone area after forceps application.

Vacuum extraction. Vacuum extraction is similar to forceps assistance except that a "cap" is placed on the crown/back of a baby's head and suction is applied to that area of the head to help guide the baby out of the birth canal. The reasons for using vacuum extraction are similar to those for low/outlet forceps. The area on the baby's head covered by the suction cap may be swollen for a few days or bleeding between the scalp and cranial bone–usually mild–may develop in that area, which may contribute to newborn jaundice.

Third Stage of Labor

The obstetric care provider will be watching for signs that the one large or two (or more) placentas are beginning to separate from the uterine wall even as the last baby's cord is cut. When placental separation begins, you may feel an urge to push if you are unmedicated; you may be asked to push if you've had an epidural or saddle block. The placenta(s) are delivered through the abdominal incision during a surgical delivery. Ask to see your babies' placenta(s) and cords. They have done a truly amazing job looking after two or more babies during your pregnancy.

Greater maternal blood loss or postpartum/postnatal hemorrhage is more common after a multiple birth since the uterus "overstretched" to carry two or more babies, decreasing uterine muscle tone and making it difficult for the uterus to contract effectively to control bleeding. Therefore, you probably will receive IV or IM pitocin to help your uterus contract. Breastfeeding, or pumping your breasts if the babies must spend time in a special care nursery, soon after delivery also contracts the uterus to help minimize bleeding.

What Are They?

> "Twin type" is as much a part of who each multiple is as its gender.

Once all the babies are born, parents of multiples often ask, "What are they?" Unlike parents of single-born infants who may ask this because they want to know their baby's gender, most parents of multiples are wondering whether their babies are identical or fraternal. Of course, asking about each baby's gender often clears up both questions at once. Whatever the combination of identical (monozygotic/MZ) and fraternal (dizygotic/DZ) twinning, wanting to know "twin type" is as much a part of who each multiple is as its gender and it is a valid question to ask.

A single, shared placenta is usually sent to the hospital laboratory for further examination, which includes a microscopic inspection to determine twin type. Because this examination can identify only those identical twins that shared a placenta, it cannot rule out the possibility of identical twinning for same-sex multiples having separate placentas. Also, "wear and tear" damage to the membranes and placental tissue may complicate examination of an apparent single placenta. Blood taken from the umbilical cords can be sent to the hospital's hematology lab to determine the babies' blood type(s) and subtypes, or genetic studies can be done to examine the DNA in each baby's blood or saliva. DNA testing is the most accurate for determining twin type, but it remains the most expensive method. Fortunately, several reliable laboratories have developed kits that parents can send for. The kit includes items needed to swab cells from each multiple's cheek that are returned to the lab for DNA testing. Parents then receive a written report of the results. (See Resources for information about lower-cost DNA zygosity testing.)

KEY POINTS

❑ Labor contractions open the cervix of the uterus for a baby to then be pushed through the birth canal (vagina) and be born.
- For multiple births the cervix opens once and the mother pushes out each baby one at a time.
- Length of labor is about the same for multiple births as for single infant births.
- An unmedicated birth is possible for the vaginal birth of many sets of twins and some triplets.

❑ Multiple pregnancy may affect the labor and birth experience. During labor or delivery, obstetric care providers may be more likely to suggest using:
- Ultrasound to check babies' positions.
- Fetal monitoring to watch each baby's response to labor.
- Medication to block pain in case they need to manipulate a baby during birth, help with delivery of any placenta, or do a cesarean/surgical delivery.
- Medication to induce or augment (speed up) labor.
- "Assisted" delivery using forceps or vacuum extraction.

❑ Medications used for pain relief or to induce or augment/speed up labor can have negative side effects for babies. Side effects may include:
- Fetal distress during labor, which may lead to cesarean/surgical delivery
- "Sleepiness," difficulty latching on, or difficulty continuing to suck during breastfeeding, which may affect any or all multiples and may last for hours to days after their births.

❑ The placenta(s)/afterbirth(s) separate from the uterus and are delivered after the last multiple is born.

❑ Postpartum hemorrhage/excessive bleeding is more common after a multiple birth due to overstretching of the uterus during multiple pregnancy.

❑ Most parents want to know if their multiples are identical or fraternal.
- Lab examination can identify only those identical twins that shared a placenta; it cannot rule out the possibility of identical twinning for same-sex multiples having separate placentas.
- Only DNA testing can "prove" whether same-sex multiples are identical.

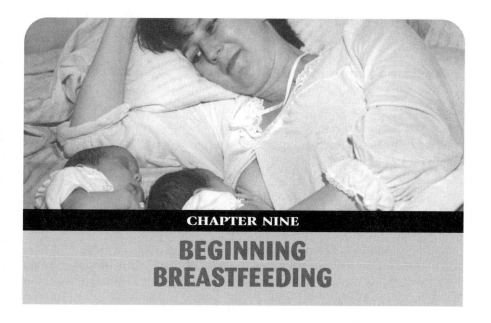

CHAPTER NINE

BEGINNING BREASTFEEDING

The best time to begin breastfeeding healthy, newborn multiples is almost immediately after birth. Multiples born at 36 or more weeks of gestation usually are eager to breastfeed within 30 to 90 minutes of birth. Until one or more is ready to feed, enjoy getting to know your babies. Often the reality of multiples does not actually sink in until you see them together.

Get a good look at each baby and begin putting the new faces with their new names by laying the babies "chests down" on your chest. Take your gown off and clothe them only in diapers for lots of skin contact. If the birthing or recovery room is cool, the babies can wear the knit caps many hospitals provide, and someone can place a blanket or two over all of you. Direct mother-babies body contact helps newborns regulate body temperature, heart and breathing rates, and blood sugar level. Skin contact also lowers stress levels in mothers and infants.

It is easier to tune in to your babies' feeding cues when they are in close bodily contact with you. You will know each is ready to first breastfeed when she roots, or searches with her mouth for food, and puts her hands to her face or mouth. She may begin to squawk to let you know she really means it. These are called feeding cues. Crying is a late feeding cue.

Newborns tend to latch on more easily if they are put to the breast when they demonstrate early feeding cues. When one begins rooting or bringing her hands toward her face, you may notice her inching her way toward the breast to latch on. Ask your midwife, a nurse, or doula to help you position that baby to latch on to the breast. Most new fathers willingly hold the other(s) while mother and one baby begin to learn to work together. Alternate breasts and babies until each has had a turn.

If You Have a Surgical Birth

Breastfeeding one baby at a time within 30 to 90 minutes of a surgical birth is ideal, since the epidural or spinal block keeps you comfortable. If you had an epidural block, you will be able to sit up to breastfeed. Many mothers prefer the "football"/clutch position initially because it avoids contact with the incision. Try cushioning your incision with a pillow if you would rather use the cradle or cross-cradle position to breastfeed.

The midwife or nurse can help you roll to one side to breastfeed if you must lie flat after a spinal block. Pillows or a rolled blanket can be placed at your back to help support you in this position. If you are on your right side, position one baby on her left side facing you. She can lie in the crook of your right arm, or on the bed, to feed at your right breast. When the first baby is finished, prop the second on a pillow facing you slightly lower than, or at the level of, your left breast so he can latch on more easily. A third baby could assume the same position as the first baby and at the right breast again once the second one is satisfied. (Triplets and other higher-order multiples are likelier to be preterm and go directly to the NICU for evaluation after birth.)

Early breastfeeding can be an effective way to minimize postpartum blood loss after giving birth to multiples. Multiple babies overdistend the uterus, interfering with its ability to contract after delivery and causing greater maternal blood loss. Breastfeeding causes and strengthens uterine contractions, which constrict blood vessels at the placental site(s) and enhance uterine involution/shrinking.

During the Hospital Stay

Early, frequent, effective breastfeedings are the best way to let your breasts know to double, triple, quadruple (or more) the amount of milk to be produced. They are also a wonderful way to begin to know the two or more unique persons who have joined your family. If you and your babies cannot be together because they were born early or are affected by another complication(s), see Chapter 10, "Multiples in the Newborn Intensive Care Unit." Beginning to breastfeed when at least one baby can be with you or you are recovering from a pregnancy-related condition is included later in this chapter.

What to Expect the First Few Days

Most healthy babies will be awake, alert, and "cueing" to breastfeed at least several times during the first 24 hours after birth. By their second 24 hours expect them to breastfeed at least 8 and up to 12 times a day–a pattern they probably will continue for several weeks to months. Alert babies will latch on and suck almost continuously, pausing only to take a breath, for at least 5 to 10 minutes from the first feeding.

Breastfeeding each baby on cue from birth lessens the chance of breastfeeding problems later. Unless one or more requires a stay in the NICU, ask that all babies be brought to you for all feedings–day and night–to establish adequate milk production. No matter how many times multiples were seen on ultrasound scans prior to birth, many mothers find

> Multiples born at 36 or more weeks of gestation usually are eager to breastfeed within 30 to 90 minutes of birth.

it difficult to believe more than one baby actually was growing inside them until they see the babies together. This is reality. The time to start handling and feeding all your babies is now.

You may find different feeding positions are more comfortable or work better with the different babies. Don't be concerned if breastfeeding initially seems a bit awkward for all concerned. It takes time for any mother-baby breastfeeding couple to learn to work together, and you must now learn to work as part of two or more different mother-baby breastfeeding partnerships.

The basic mechanics of breastfeeding each multiple are the same as for a single infant, but every baby approaches the mechanics of breastfeeding somewhat differently. Most mothers know when breastfeeding feels "right." If it hurts or you aren't sure that a baby is latched on and feeding properly, ask that a lactation consultant, midwife, or nurse watch each baby breastfeed. The mechanics of effective breastfeeding and typical feeding patterns are discussed in Chapter 13, "Effective Breastfeeding."

Feeding on cue also continues to help your uterus contract and keep bleeding to a minimum, which continues to be particularly beneficial for mothers after a multiple birth. Say "hooray" if you feel menstrual-like cramping soon after a baby begins to breastfeed. These "afterpains" mean your baby's sucking has triggered the release of the hormone oxytocin, which is responsible for the let-down, or the milk-ejection, reflex (MER). This cramping proves that your uterus is contracting and that your baby probably is breastfeeding effectively. You are more likely to feel afterpains if you've given birth before, but first-time mothers often feel them after a multiple birth. (They still occur yet may not be felt by other first-time mothers.) Afterpains usually subside within a few days of giving birth.

Simultaneous Feeding

Breastfeeding two babies at the same time is called *simultaneous feeding*. Some mothers and multiples are ready for simultaneous feedings the day of birth, but often it is several weeks before a mother or her babies are ready. There is no rush.

You can feed each multiple separately at first. Wait to breastfeed two at once until you find it is easy to position and help the individual multiples latch onto the breast one at a time, and until at least one baby can latch on with little help. When

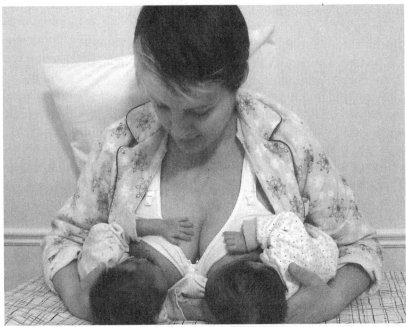

Breastfeeding two at once is not always possible in the early weeks.

you or the babies are still learning, feeding two at once may result in poor technique that can lead to problems, such as sore or cracked nipples, lower milk production, and ineffective breastfeeding for babies.

A lactation consultant, nurse, or midwife can help you learn to position the individual babies for feedings, and she can show you simultaneous feeding positions. You and the babies can practice using different simultaneous feeding positions whether or not the babies are ready for simultaneous feedings. She can also demonstrate ways to handle more than one baby at the same time. Simultaneous breastfeeding is discussed in more depth in Chapter 14, "Coordinating Feedings."

Rooming-In

Rooming-in means that the babies stay with you in your hospital room for all, or most, of the day and night. When you and your newborn multiples are in good condition after birth, full-time rooming-in is the best way to ensure frequent and effective breastfeedings. The more time you and all your multiples spend in each other's company, the more you can get to know them and develop sensitivity to each one's feeding cues. Each baby will benefit from having access to you for frequent feedings.

Partial rooming-in is usually possible during the first day or two after a surgical birth or when you are recovering from a pregnancy-related condition and cannot yet care for your babies full time. If babies can spend only minimal time in your room, still ask that all babies be brought to you for all feedings when possible.

Visitors

Many hospitals now have liberal visiting policies for the postpartum/postnatal unit, and the birth of multiples draws visitors like butterflies to flowers. This can be a blessing or a curse. When visitors support breastfeeding and help hold and cuddle one (or more) while you feed another baby, they are a blessing. If their presence interferes with the newborns' frequent feedings, they are a curse.

Getting to know your babies and making sure they are off to a good breast-feeding start is much more important than introducing multiples to guests. If a baby cues to feed and you are not yet comfortable breastfeeding with others in the room, visitors should be asked to go to the hospital cafeteria for a while or to leave.

Limit visitors to a few helpful ones. You may want to ask someone to stay with you and the babies if your husband is unable to remain around the clock. Rooming-in may be more feasible with a support person to help you–day and night. You might suggest that other friends and relatives postpone their visits until you and the babies have settled in at home–a process that may take days or weeks.

Supplementing or Partial Breastfeeding

Avoid giving any multiple a supplementary bottle of artificial infant milk (AIM), also called infant formula, or a pacifier during your hospital stay unless there is a diagnosed medical reason to do so. (Such reasons are addressed later in this chapter and in Chapter 13, "Effective Breastfeeding.") Also, there usually is no reason to complement, or "top off," with AIM after breastfeeding healthy, term newborns. You will produce more milk sooner if you simply allow all multiples to feed whenever they indicate readiness. Giving any baby something other than mother's breast should always be taken seriously, because of the implications for each multiple's health and long-term feeding behaviors as well as your milk production.

> **Giving any baby something other than mother's breast should always be taken seriously, because of the implications for each multiple's health and long-term feeding behaviors, as well as mother's milk production.**

Sometimes hospital staff think they are doing new mothers of multiples a favor by letting them sleep through a feeding or two, or by bringing one baby alone for a feeding while the other(s) is supplemented. Feeding all the babies for all feedings now means you soon will produce the amount of milk needed for the number of multiples you gave birth to. When one or more is not included in feedings during the first postpartum/postnatal days, you will have to play "catch up" later. Few mothers want to deal with two or more lethargic, sleepy babies who stop "asking" to eat often enough and are losing weight or with two or more hungry, screaming babies who require round-the-clock breastfeeding for several days.

Introducing the babies to artificial bottle nipples/teats and pacifiers can lead to improper sucking behaviors, which some call "nipple confusion." This can result in ineffective breastfeeding for a baby and sore or cracked nipples for mother. Pacifier and bottle-teat use may also interfere with learning to "read" babies' feeding cues and with establishing adequate milk production. Although these problems can be reversed, they easily undermine a mother's confidence and contribute to an over-reliance on supplements, and these practices are associated with early weaning from the breast.

When giving AIM for medical reasons, there are alternative methods for feeding that are more compatible with babies learning effective sucking for breastfeeding. See Chapter 12, "Making Up for a Poor Start," if you think this has already happened.

If you want to ensure continued breastfeeding but are not sure if you want to exclusively breastfeed multiples, wait several weeks before introducing partial breastfeeding if possible. (For more on partial breastfeeding, see Chapter 18, "Full and Partial Breastfeeding.")

Breastfeeding after Surgical Birth

Should your condition interfere with direct breastfeeding, a nurse can apply an electric breast pump to express milk every two to three hours or she may teach a family member or friend to do it.

Many mothers have breastfed multiples after a surgical birth. Generally, mothers say the first 24 to 36 hours after surgery are the most uncomfortable. Incisional tenderness or soreness persists, but decreases, over the first several weeks. (Post-surgical pain medication is discussed below.)

You probably will feel more comfortable breastfeeding after a surgical birth if you use the feeding positions discussed in the first section of this chapter on beginning breastfeeding soon after surgical delivery. If two babies seem ready to breastfeed simultaneously, most mothers recommend the double football (double clutch) position as the most comfortable, since it avoids pressure on the incision. This position is described in Chapter 14, "Coordinating Feedings."

A few older studies reported delays in adequate milk production of a week or more in mothers having surgical births or diabetic conditions. More recent research indicates that such delays tend to be associated with postponed first breastfeeding(s), infrequent breastfeedings, and too frequent supplementation with artificial infant milk (AIM or infant formula).

Other Maternal Conditions Affecting Breastfeeding Initiation

Mothers of multiples are more likely to experience various pregnancy-related conditions. However, such conditions rarely require postponing breastfeeding initiation.

Surgical birth should not interfere with early breastfeeding unless a mother was given a general anesthetic; still breastfeeding often can be initiated within several hours of birth.

Pregnancy-induced hypertension (PIH)/preeclampsia usually resolves within day(s) after delivery. Many mothers affected by PIH receive an IV medication called Magnesium Sulfate for 24 hours after giving birth. This medication has side effects that may include a feeling of detachment from one's body or surroundings, so you are likely to need help with breastfeeding and caring for babies until several hours after the medication is stopped. Occasionally a mother must continue to take blood pressure medication for several days to weeks, but most related medications are compatible with breastfeeding.

Diabetic conditions, whether gestational in nature or chronic, are not a reason for delaying breastfeeding initiation. Although the research information is not clear cut, some mothers report a few-day delay for when milk "comes in" after delivery. Women affected by other conditions associated with insulin resistance, such as polycystic ovarian syndrome (PCOS) have also noticed this delay. Most of these women produce adequate milk for their multiples once copious milk production begins, especially if they are receiving treatment for the condition. Gestational diabetes is more common with multiple pregnancy and PCOS may be one reason for infertility treatment resulting in multiple birth, so it is important to be aware of the possible effects of insulin resistance and be prepared to deal with them.

The effects of surgical delivery, prolonged pregnancy bed rest, and some other pregnancy or birth-related conditions may leave a new mother feeling weak or exhausted and unable to assume full care of her babies immediately after birth. Most mothers experience more discomfort with movement after a surgical birth and many are less mobile during the early recovery phase of such conditions as postpartum/postnatal hemorrhage, PIH, etc. Recovery from surgical birth and other conditions does not affect the basic mechanics of breastfeeding or the fact that each baby still needs to breastfeed effectively 8 to 12 times in 24 hours. If you arrange for someone to stay and help you physically manage multiple newborns while in the hospital, you can have the babies with you (or go to the NICU to be with the babies) as much as possible. This helper may be the babies' father, a relative, or a friend, but you will undoubtedly gain confidence more quickly if it is someone who supports breastfeeding. A postpartum doula also is a good option. (See Resources.) If unable to arrange for such help, ask that a health care worker, such as a nurse stay in your room during breastfeedings to help you with all the babies as often as possible. As you feel better and can do more, ask that all of the babies be brought to you for all feedings if you are not yet up to full or partial rooming-in.

Should your condition interfere with direct breastfeeding for some or all feedings, you can compensate by expressing your milk/colostrum for all missed feedings. Occasionally a mother must focus all her energy on physical recovery for several hours to several days. In those rare instances, a nurse can apply an electric breast pump to express a mother's milk every two to three hours or she may teach

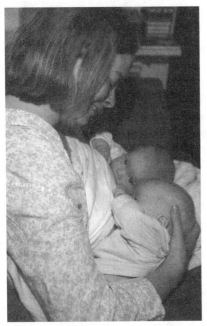

If you are not sure that one or more baby is breastfeeding well, ask for help.

a family member or friend to do it. See "milk expression" later in this chapter for more information.

Pain Medication

You may find a mild analgesic, or pain reliever, helps relieve any perineal tenderness if you received an episiotomy. Medication may also be helpful if "afterpains" become unusually severe or are long lasting. Generally non-narcotic analgesics compatible with breastfeeding are prescribed. Local analgesic or anesthetic sprays and creams prescribed for episiotomy discomfort should not affect your milk. However, your obstetric care provider or a lactation consultant should have references if there is a question about any medication you may need.

Mothers who have had surgical deliveries are more likely to be given narcotic analgesics for the first day or two. However, a new type of post-operative pain medication is becoming available for abdominal surgeries, including surgical births. The new method continuously delivers a small amount, or an infusion, of a local anesthetic through a small catheter into the actual surgical area. This infusion system may be combined with a narcotic analgesic, but it usually results in receiving a lower amount of pain medication. When narcotic analgesics can be decreased, a new mother feels more alert and able to care for her babies.

Breastfeeding triggers the release of hormones that lead to a feeling of relaxation, which may help with pain reduction.

When local anesthetic infusion is not an option, narcotic analgesics are likely to be given during the first post-operative days. Most are considered to be compatible with breastfeeding, and you may be better able to care for and breastfeed your babies when you are more comfortable.

Many mothers and health professionals advise taking pain medication at regular intervals rather than waiting until pain or discomfort becomes severe during the first few days after the surgery. This helps maintain blood levels of the particular medication. Often less medication is taken overall when taking smaller maintenance doses.

Some mothers receive a narcotic analgesic through a patient-controlled analgesia (PCA) pump. The medication is "piggy-backed" into the IV tubing already in place, and it is attached to an automatic timing device. When a new mother becomes uncomfortable, she presses a button to receive more medication. The timing device will not allow overdosing. It generally is used for about 12 to 24 hours after surgery and then a less strong analgesic will be offered instead.

Another method of delivering a narcotic analgesic is to administer a drug, such as Duramorph® through the epidural tubing while in the delivery suite. This medication usually lasts for about 24 hours. Mothers tend to say they felt more alert and able to care for their babies when they received narcotic medication through the epidural; however, nausea and extreme itching are reactions associated with receiving medication via this route.

Some mothers find they are more comfortable and alert after a surgical birth when they receive a stronger nonnarcotic analgesic. Certain nonsteroidal anti-inflammatory (NSAID) drugs may be given by IV or intra-muscular (IM) injections for pain after surgical deliveries. (See Chapter 6, "Getting Ready: Birth Preparations," for information on preparing for birth.)

Generally, narcotics and stronger NSAID medications are prescribed for a limited time after delivery due to related side effects. Most women find a milder analgesic and nonpharmaceutical interventions, such as relaxation techniques, massage, etc., provide adequate pain relief after the first day or two. Skin-to-skin contact with the babies and breastfeeding trigger the release of hormones that lead to a feeling of relaxation, which may help with pain reduction.

When One (or More) Cannot Yet Breastfeed

There are many pregnancy- and birth-related reasons that may interfere with breastfeeding for one (or more) multiple for several hours to several weeks after birth when other(s) breastfeed well. For example, immature body systems may affect one multiple more than another after late preterm delivery at 34 to 37 weeks. Even when babies are full term, each multiple may have been subjected to varying degrees of stress during labor and birth, so their readiness and ability to feed may vary. Also, exposure to analgesic and anesthetic medications during labor may cause one multiple to be too groggy or sleepy to breastfeed effectively for several hours to several days after birth while another seems unaffected. (See Chapter 8, "Happy Birthday.") As a result one can be ready and eager to breastfeed, another may be eager but can't quite coordinate latching on and sucking or staying on long enough, and another simply falls asleep within seconds of coming to the breast. Each multiple is an individual, so each one's responses to life outside the womb, including breastfeeding, will be unique from the start.

> Each multiple is an individual, so each one's responses to life outside the womb, including breastfeeding, will be unique from the start.

The best way to encourage breastfeeding in a sleepy baby or one who is not yet able to latch on and suck effectively is to hold that baby skin-to-skin, her naked chest against mother's naked chest as much and as long as possible. (This is called kangaroo care. See Chapter 10, "Multiples in the Newborn Intensive Care Unit," for more information.)

To increase milk production and provide milk for any baby who is not yet able to breastfeed directly, breastfeed any multiple who is able to do so. In addition to breastfeeding that baby, express milk as often as possible. To save time, use a breast pump to express milk from one breast as a baby feeds on the other. If this requires more coordination than either a mother or her baby are yet ready for, express milk after breastfeeding. Some mothers report they obtain more milk if they pump about an hour after breastfeeding, but the important thing is to express some milk even if the timing does not fit with guidelines for "ideal."

You will want to ensure that any multiple not yet able to breastfeed receives whatever colostrum or milk you express, unless that baby is on IV feeds only. Your colostrum and milk are beneficial in whatever amounts you produce–even if only drops. See the following section and Chapter 11, "Breastfeeding in the NICU," for more specific information about milk expression and alternative methods of feeding that reinforce the mouth behaviors a baby uses when breastfeeding.

Milk Expression

You may produce only drops the first day or two of milk expression. Do not let that discourage you.

If your or any baby's physical condition interferes with breastfeeding 8 to 12 times every 24 hours, you will want to compensate by using some technique of milk expression beginning within 12 to 24 hours of the babies' births when possible. Although most women will still produce adequate milk if milk expression is not initiated during the first 24 hours, the earlier milk expression begins the earlier a mother should expect to produce an increased volume of milk.

Delaying frequent milk expression beyond the first couple of days after birth may contribute to a permanent reduction in milk production following birth. Because there are many factors that influence milk production, the degree of reduction may vary. If even one baby cannot breastfeed or is not breastfeeding effectively, begin milk expression.

There are a variety of techniques for effective milk expression. The most important aspect of any method is that you are able to use it frequently and effectively. In many areas of the world, manual/hand expression is the only method available and mothers have used it for weeks or months to provide milk for preterm or sick newborns. Many women find they can express the thicker colostrum more effectively when using manual/hand expression. Mothers have also used a variety of small pumps to provide their milk for their babies.

Automatic-cycling, full-size, electric breast pumps and double collection kits that enable women to pump both breasts at once have become widely available in the United States and some other countries over the last couple of decades. Double pumping saves time when frequent pumping is a necessity, and research indicates that double pumping results in obtaining higher volumes of milk especially once milk "comes in" after the first few days.

A routine for milk expression should simulate the typical pattern of 8 to 12 daily feedings for a newborn. Determining how much time to dedicate to milk expression will depend on the number of multiples who can effectively breastfeed directly and the number who cannot. You may produce only drops the first day or two of milk expression. Do *not* let that discourage you. If you do not see any increase in milk production within 36 to 48 hours, ask a postpartum/postnatal unit staff member, a lactation consultant, or a La Leche League Leader to review your pumping technique and routine. They will have suggestions for increasing milk production.

Early, frequent, effective breastfeeding or pumping is the best way to ensure double, triple, or quadruple milk production. When you are not certain if one or more babies are breastfeeding often enough or effectively, get help. And don't expect to be an expert immediately. It takes time to get to know two or more babies and differentiate their individual approaches to breastfeeding.

KEY POINTS

❑ Breastfeed healthy, term multiples when they first demonstrate feeding cues, which usually occurs within 30 to 90 minutes of birth.
- Feeding cues include rooting, making sucking motions, bringing hands to face, and crying. But crying is a late feeding cue!

❑ Expect healthy babies to breastfeed at least 8 to 12 times in 24 hours by their second day after birth.
- Full or partial rooming-in makes it easier to breastfeed frequently.
- Having an around-the-clock helper to help hold and position babies for breastfeeding makes rooming-in possible after giving birth to multiples, especially after a surgical delivery.

❑ Feeding two multiples together at once is called simultaneous breastfeeding.
- Most mothers or their babies are not ready to breastfeed simultaneously for several days to several weeks after birth.
- At least one baby should be able to latch on easily and breastfeed effectively before a mother breastfeeds two at once.

❑ Because late preterm birth and increased complications are common with multiple births, often one multiple is able to breastfeed better than the other(s).

❑ Expressing your milk and/or colostrum is essential to establishing and then maintaining milk production when one or more multiples is not yet able to breastfeed effectively.

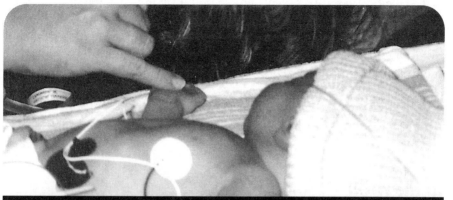

CHAPTER TEN

MULTIPLES IN THE NEWBORN INTENSIVE CARE UNIT

Multiple-birth newborns are several times more likely to spend their first several hours, days, or weeks in a newborn intensive care unit, or NICU (often pronounced "nick-you"). Higher-order multiples are more likely to be born at, or transferred to, regional care centers. These hospitals have the most advanced care and equipment available to handle high-risk pregnancies and extremely preterm or sick babies.

Most multiples requiring a stay in the NICU are there because of their physical conditions after preterm birth. There are other reasons that multiples are more likely than single newborns to be cared for in a NICU. Multiples, including those born at full- or almost full-term, are more often affected by low birth weight, stress during labor or birth, or the effects of pregnancy-related complications. (For information on pregnancy and birth factors associated with NICU stays for multiples, see Chapter 2, "Multiple Pregnancy as High Risk: Fact or Fiction," Chapter 4, "What to Do If..." Chapter 6, "Getting Ready: Birth Preparation," and Chapter 8, "Happy Birthday.")

Any multiple's need for specialized NICU care is likely to interfere with direct breastfeeding, making it necessary for a mother to express/pump her milk for one or more of her babies. Depending on babies' conditions, it may be possible to breastfeed one or more baby for some feedings, or it may be days or weeks before direct breastfeeding of any of the babies is possible. For more information, see Chapter 11, "Breastfeeding in the Newborn Intensive Care Unit."

Not every multiple in a set may require special care or remain in a NICU as long as the other(s), since babies do not mature or recover from physical stress at exactly the same rates. Sometimes only one baby requires special care, especially when the multiples are close to full term at birth. The length of time a baby stays in a NICU varies depending on the reason for special care.

Babies may be discharged once they can maintain stable body temperature and heart and breathing rates in room air. They should also be able to take food well by mouth. Usually a baby must be gaining weight first, but few care providers still insist that all babies reach a certain weight, such as 2200 grams (5 pounds) before discharge.

In the NICU

First Impressions

It may take courage to transform worry into a working relationship with a NICU staff, but your role is as important as theirs.

Entering a NICU for the first time can be an overwhelming and intimidating experience. High-tech equipment that both looks and sounds scary takes up space everywhere. And much of it may be attached to one or more of your babies. Since you are already concerned about your multiples' conditions, their little bodies may look particularly vulnerable with wires and tubes taped or inserted at several spots. The alarms triggered by changes in the babies' physical conditions may only add to your anxiety.

Your vulnerable-looking babies may be "tougher" or in less serious condition than they appear. You may be surprised to learn that some of the fancy-looking equipment and the wires running from them are routinely applied to all babies, such as the probes that monitor a baby's temperature or pulse.

The machines that monitor a baby's breathing and heart rates may initially sound noisy. Alarms frequently sound, but sometimes they are false alarms. For example, a baby's movement may disrupt the message to a machine monitoring breathing, causing an alarm to sound. Once familiar with the different equipment, you may begin to tune out unimportant sounds.

Babies in a NICU need their parents' help to get well and grow, so parents must adapt to this foreign territory in a hurry. It may take courage to transform worry into a working relationship with a NICU staff, but your role is as important as theirs. Most staff members are happy to help you feel more comfortable. Some of these ideas may also help.

- *Ask for explanations.* Learn the names of the equipment and how each item works. Find out what the tubes and wires are for and why each is being used for a particular baby.
- *Learn the NICU language* to help you understand the technology and what certain measurements mean in terms of a baby's condition. Words

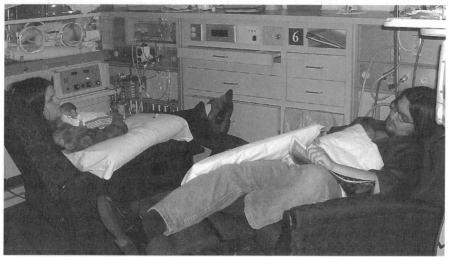

Both mother and father can provide kangaroo care in the NICU.

like "oxygen sats" and "CPAP" are less intimidating once they are explained.

- *Ask for descriptions of the physical signs* that may indicate either improvement or a problem for each baby.
- *Keep a pad of paper and a pen handy.* Write down questions as you think of them. Ask staff members to write down pertinent points when they are explaining something about a baby's condition, so you can go over the notes again at a later time.

Parents' Role

Parents can feel left out or unimportant when a baby's life depends on the technical skills of highly trained neonatologists, neonatal nurses, and other members of the health care team. Do not underestimate your role in your babies' care. You have a profound influence on their physical and emotional progress.

There are many things you can do better than the NICU staff for the babies. Only you can provide your babies with your own milk, and you are the best ones to cuddle your babies kangaroo-style, which positively affects their physical condition. When everyone else is using technical terms to refer to the babies' physical systems, you can remind the staff to look at each baby as a person.

- *Spend as much time as possible in the NICU with your babies.* If your own condition does not yet allow for long visits with them, spend whatever time you can but leave the NICU when you begin to tire. Initially, a 30 to 60 minute visit may sap your energy. Take care of yourself so you can speed your recovery and increase the length of your visits with your babies sooner.

- *Call the NICU frequently–day or night–for updates on the babies' conditions* if you are recovering in a different hospital (and once you are at home). Ask a NICU staff or family member to take a photograph of each baby. Family members may hesitate photographing any baby who is in poor condition. You may have to explain that seeing a photo and understanding the reality of the situation are less frightening than what your imagination dreams up.

- *Multiples are often discharged from a NICU at different times.* This staggered, or phased, discharge may complicate visiting any baby who remains in the NICU once you are busy with at least one newborn at home. It is important to continue to visit any multiple(s) remaining in the hospital as often as you are able. (See "Staggered/Phased Discharge" below.)

- *Remind the staff that each baby is a whole and separate person.* In the high-tech NICU world, this may be a parent's most important task. Ask that everyone call each baby by name; post the babies' names on their incubators or cribs. Share your observations about each baby's unique behaviors and responses with the staff. When you call during the day or night for a report, ask how each baby is responding to the NICU environment or any change in routine. Ask staff members to describe the unique behaviors they see when each baby is fed, bathed, or undergoes some procedure. If any procedure seems to upset a particular baby, work with staff members to find a less stressful way to do the procedure.

- *Talk to your babies* when you are with them, even if they cannot yet be handled or held. Tell each that you love him or her. Staff members will talk to babies, too, but it is your voice each baby heard during the pregnancy. It is your voice each baby recognizes now. Your voice provides continuity in a confusing new world.

  You cannot be with your babies 24 hours a day, but you can record your voice for them. It doesn't matter what you talk about on a tape or CD. Your babies will be able to hear you even when you can't be with them.

- *Touch each baby as soon as conditions allow.* Whether you can only stroke a baby's arm or hold a tiny hand, let each know you are there through touch. As each baby's condition improves, handle and hold your babies as much as possible. The NICU staff can show you the kind of touch and the holds that are more soothing for preterm babies. If equipment monitoring the babies' conditions, helping them breathe, etc., makes you hesitate to hold any, share your concerns with the staff. They will show you how to pick up and cuddle a baby without disturbing crucial equipment.

- *Let the NICU staff know you would like to begin "kangaroo care" once any baby is stable.* During kangaroo care a baby, wearing only a diaper, is placed on the mother's (or father's) bare chest for skin-to-skin contact.

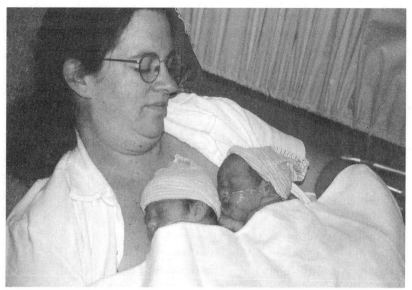

This mother has her premature twins in kangaroo care.

Mother's clothing or a blanket is then placed over both. Each parent may "kangaroo" a baby or one parent may provide kangaroo care for two multiples at once.

Babies become more relaxed during kangaroo care. The skin-to-skin contact with a parent's body helps a preterm baby regulate body temperature as well as cardiac (heart) and respiratory (lungs, breathing) systems. Kangaroo care also enhances babies' brain development and contributes to better weight gains for preterm babies. Not surprisingly, it also helps parents feel more attached to each baby sooner.

> **Kangaroo care helps a preterm baby regulate body temperature as well as cardiac and respiratory systems.**

Ask to initiate kangaroo care with your babies even if it is not routine procedure in your babies' NICU. If there is any hesitation, suggest that the staff do a literature review of the research discussing the benefits of this low-tech, high-touch intervention. Research supports the benefits of kangaroo care for very low birth weight babies and babies still on ventilators.

Many mothers find it is easier to hold these very tiny babies in a modified clutch position, with the baby's head against a parent's breast and the body "wrapped" skin-to-skin around a parent's ribcage, rather than on a parent's bare chest.

- *It is often during kangaroo care that a baby first begins to root for or nuzzle at the breast.* (Described in Chapter 11.) Many mothers have reported obtaining greater amounts of milk during pumping sessions once kangaroo care with their babies had begun–an observation now supported by research.

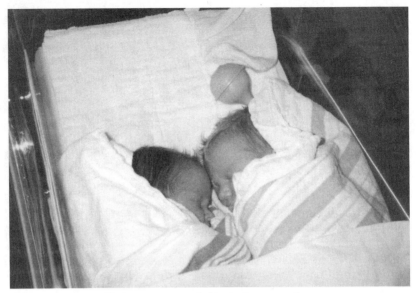

Placing two or more babies in the same crib or
bassinet may decrease their stress levels.

- *Also ask the NICU staff about co-bedding physically stable multiples.* There
  is some evidence that imitating multiples' pre-birth environment, by placing two or more in the same incubator or crib, comforts the babies and
  decreases the stress each experiences. It may help each regulate body systems, and there are some reports that it seems to help multiples develop
  more similar sleep-wake routines–a situation most parents prefer.
- *Ask to have your multiples' incubators or cribs placed side-by-side when
  any baby's condition does not yet allow for co-bedding.* The reality of
  multiples sinks in better when you can see all of them at once. Spending
  time with both/all and developing an attachment with each multiple is easier when they are kept close together.

When Babies Are Sick

You may begin to celebrate as one baby improves but find yourself feeling guilty if another multiple is not yet doing as well.

Do not be surprised if you find you are on an emotional
roller coaster—one that peaks and plunges depending on
daily changes in the babies' conditions. Of course, parents of
multiples may find themselves simultaneously riding two,
three, or more roller coasters that are traveling at different
speeds and peaking or plunging at different times. It may be
difficult to celebrate one baby's progress when another is
still sick. Or you may begin to celebrate as one baby
improves but find yourself feeling guilty if another multiple
is not yet doing as well.

A feeling is neither good nor bad. It simply is. It is possible to feel both happy about one baby's progress and sad about another's condition. Accept all your feelings as valid.

Share your feelings and concerns with staff members. Ask if there is a support group in your area for parents who have, or have had, babies in a NICU. Most of these groups will include many parents of multiples. Talking to someone who has "been there" is often the most helpful thing you can do for yourself.

> **The sicker baby is not avoiding interaction; that baby simply does not have the energy to interact.**

Parent-Infants Attachment

The attachment you begin to form with each newborn multiple creates the foundation for your long-term relationship with each. Certain infant behaviors, such as the ability to make eye contact with a parent, encourage the interaction that helps the attachment process along. Parents tend to respond to a responsive baby, which encourages the baby, and the parent, to interact even more.

A premature or sick baby may not be ready for such interaction. This baby may need all her energy to get well. Because each multiple progresses at her/his own pace, one may begin to interact before the other(s). The sicker baby is not avoiding interaction; that baby simply does not have the energy to interact. Do spend time with a sicker baby. Talking, touching, and cuddling will help both of you feel closer as you wait for the baby to get well.

Many mothers have said they felt more deeply attached, and felt it sooner, to any multiple(s) they handled and interacted with before they felt an attachment to the other(s). Mothers have expressed similar feelings when one multiple requires a stay in a NICU but the mother is able to care for the other(s) in her hospital room or at home. It isn't surprising that a parent might develop a feeling of closeness more quickly with a baby able to be more responsive. However, each multiple depends on the development of a deep attachment with her/his mother (and father). If you feel closer to any and you consistently respond more quickly to that baby than to the other(s), do not feel guilty for this natural response and do not panic. *Do* take immediate action. You may have to work harder on developing a relationship with a less responsive or sicker baby, but there are many concrete actions you can take. (For specific ideas, see Chapter 19, "Enhancing Individuality.")

Getting Ready for Discharge

Parents often feel ambivalent about taking preterm babies home. They worry about caring for tiny or vulnerable babies. Also, babies are being discharged earlier than in the past. They often weigh less than five pounds (2500 gm), and many still require monitoring devices, oxygen, medications, and so on.

You will feel more comfortable taking the babies home if you have spent lots of time in the NICU learning to use any equipment or give any medication that a

Homecoming marks a transition for each multiple and for his or her parents.

baby will need after discharge. Discuss with staff members what to expect as typical feeding routines and how to know if each baby is getting enough. If you are asked to test-weigh a baby before (pre) and after (post) breastfeeding at home, be sure you understand how to use an electronic scale and how to interpret the results. Since most preterm infants are not ready for full breastfeeding at discharge, practice alternative feeding methods for giving additional milk. (See "Alternative feeding methods," in Chapter 12, "Making Up for a Poor Start.")

Some NICUs have rooms where parents can spend the night with one or more babies prior to discharge. If this is available where your multiples are hospitalized, try to take advantage of this practice before bringing home the first baby to be discharged. It can really boost confidence.

Homecoming marks a transition for each multiple and for his or her parents. You may have just gotten used to the NICU routine and now you are faced again with establishing a new routine. After discharge, babies sometimes continue to follow the NICU routine, but some begin to wake more often. This may be due to the transition to home, to attentive parents, or simply to normal infant development.

In case any baby needs to ease into new life at home, you may ask to take a blanket, t-shirt, or some other item that has the scent of the NICU home with each baby. Audio-tape the sounds your babies have become accustomed to hearing in the NICU. Listening to the tape may help soothe one or more fretful babies when first home.

Arrange to have help at home after each baby's discharge. If babies are discharged one by one, you will want to be free to breastfeed any baby now at home, pump your milk as necessary, and visit any multiple(s) still in the NICU. Once all babies are home, it may take a while before everyone learns what to do at breast and before a new routine emerges. You will need extra hands for babies and for other household tasks.

Staggered/Phased Discharge

Multiples rarely mature or recover at exactly the same rates, so one or two may be discharged from the NICU before the other(s). In some ways it may be easier to bring babies home and learn to care for them one or two at a time. However, many mothers find the period between the discharge of the first multiple and the discharge of the last is the most hectic. Each time a baby is discharged, the household routine—no matter how tentative—is disrupted again. Mothers often feel torn between the needs of all the babies—those at home and those in the hospital.

When busy with a baby or two at home, it may become difficult to find time to pump for any multiple(s) in the hospital. Visits to the NICU to see the other multiple(s) become more complicated, which may mean the hospitalized multiple(s) will miss some "practice" breastfeedings. Staggered, or phased, discharge can affect the attachment process. Many say they feel close to a baby who is at home and in their care sooner than the multiple(s) requiring a longer hospital stay.

- Make it a priority to provide your milk for any baby still in the hospital, as this can help you feel closer to that baby. If any baby at home is breast-feeding well, you and that baby can work together to provide milk for the hospitalized multiple. Pump one breast while you breastfeed a baby on the other. This method also may save you time, yet keep you linked with the baby separated from you at the hospital. (Alternate breasts each feeding if only one baby is breastfeeding well.)

- When the baby at the breast is still learning to breastfeed, a mother may find it too difficult to pump while breastfeeding. In this case, pump imme-diately or about an hour after breastfeeding. (More detailed information on pumping your milk is in Chapter 11.)

  ❏ Some mothers prefer this routine even when a baby breastfeeds well, as it allows them to focus on the multiple(s) in the hospital during the pumping sessions. Some place a photo of the hospitalized multiple(s) near the breast pump, or they hold and smell an item, such as a blan-ket, cap, shirt, etc., that has been worn by the hospitalized baby.

- Another priority is to continue to visit any multiple(s) still in the NICU. You and the multiple(s) in the NICU need to have physical contact. Whether you leave the multiple(s) already discharged at home or you take one or more babies with you to the hospital during visits, it will require arranging for some type of child care.

  ❏ If you live nearby, it may be easiest to leave any baby already dis-charged at home with a sitter and visit a baby in the NICU between two breastfeedings for the multiple(s) at home.

  ❏ You may want a sitter to accompany you and the already discharged multiple(s) to the hospital when you are increasing "practice" breast-feedings with a baby in the NICU or if you live some distance from the NICU. To lower the risk of infection, the sitter should care for the dis-charged multiple(s) in a private waiting area where you can go to breastfeed as needed.

  ❏ When the NICU is far from home or care of the discharged multiple(s) limits visits to any baby still in the hospital, maintain close telephone contact with the NICU. Mothers sometimes use a speaker-phone so they can talk to hospital staff while pumping. Some believe milk production improves when they are able to discuss the multiples in the hospital as they pump their milk for those babies.

Take advantage of available technology to keep in touch with the hospitalized multiple(s). With your permission, staff members may be able to email or fax reports on a baby to you at home. As computer technology improves, it may become a stan-dard practice to "watch" a baby in the NICU on the computer or TV screen at home.

It is a red-letter day when you bring the last of the multiples home. Of course, it will again take time for a regular routine to develop. And you may rely on outside help for weeks, months, and even years. Still, most parents find it is less stressful to finally have everyone in one place.

KEY POINTS

❑ One or more of twins and other multiples are more likely to spend time in a newborn intensive care unit (NICU) due to the increase of preterm birth, low birth weight, and stress during labor or birth.

❑ The sights and sounds of a NICU can be overwhelming–or downright scary–but your babies are depending on you to get comfortable there so you can help them.

❑ Talk to and touch your babies. Let the NICU staff know you would like to do "kangaroo care"–skin-to-skin contact–with your babies as soon as possible.

❑ Few preterm babies are fully breastfeeding when they leave the NICU for home. It takes patience and persistence on a mother's part, but most of these babies can eventually breastfeed well.

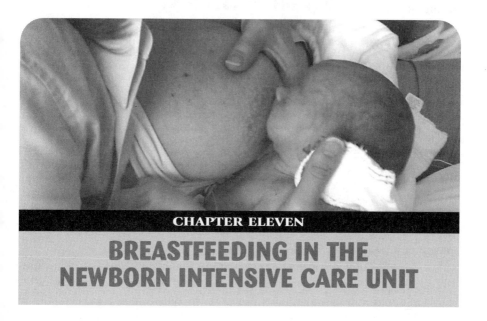

CHAPTER ELEVEN

BREASTFEEDING IN THE NEWBORN INTENSIVE CARE UNIT

Initiating breastfeeding may have to be postponed when multiples are preterm or sick at birth. A baby's maturity and general health help determine readiness for oral, or "by mouth," feedings. One multiple may be ready to begin breastfeeding days or weeks before the other(s). Just as full-term babies differ in their approaches and abilities to breastfeed initially, preterm babies do too. While waiting for each baby to begin breastfeeding, a new mother must depend on other means to establish and maintain milk production.

Your Milk for Your Babies

The milk you express/pump is an invaluable gift to your babies, as it provides them with protection from many diseases and health conditions. The components of human milk are adaptive. Preterm milk is different than full-term milk; it is uniquely suited to preterm babies' immature body systems.

Because your body makes your milk for your babies—no matter when they are born—it is more digestible, and therefore, easier on their cardiac (heart), respiratory (breathing), gastrointestinal (digestive tract), and urinary (kidneys) systems. This means the babies do not have to use as much energy to digest their food, which saves their energy for getting well and growing.

Preterm babies who receive their mothers' own milk have fewer infections, and they are less likely to develop a severe intestinal condition called "necrotizing enterocolitis" (NEC).

Failing to initiate milk expression for several days after birth or failing to pump often enough may have a negative long-term effect on the amount of milk a mother is able to produce.

Expressing Your Milk

To provide your babies with antibody-rich colostrum and to tell your body to gear up for a high rate of milk production, begin to express your milk as soon after the babies' births as possible. Ideally, you begin within six to 12 hours of your babies' births. If your physical condition makes it difficult to express milk initially, a nurse can apply a breast pump or she can teach a family member how to do it.

If you do not begin to express/pump until the second postpartum day, it may take longer for your milk volume to increase or "come in." Usually, more frequent pumping makes up for any time lost during an initial brief delay, but failing to initiate milk expression for several days after birth or failing to pump often enough may have a negative long-term effect on the amount of milk a mother is able to produce.

Do not panic if your circumstances result in a longer delay before beginning to express/pump milk, but do start pumping your breasts as soon as possible. The impact of a longer delay varies, but it is impossible to know which mothers will be more affected. Still, even when production is affected significantly, mothers can provide some milk for their babies, and some mother's milk is better for babies than no mother's milk.

Most mothers obtain more milk when they use a full size hospital-grade, self-cycling, electric breast pump with a double collection kit to establish, increase, and then maintain adequate milk production for preterm or sick multiples. The self-cycling feature automatically creates and releases suction the way a baby does during breastfeeding, and is gentler on a mother's nipples. The "double kit" lets you pump both breasts at once, which saves time and is associated with producing greater amounts, or volume, of milk over each 24-hour period.

The studies that found double/simultaneous pumping resulted in obtaining greater volumes of milk were conducted after mothers' milk had "come in." Some mothers find it easier to learn to use the breast pump if they pump one breast at a time for the first 1 or 2 days after birth. It is better to do single-sided pumping than to postpone or avoid early pumping sessions. However, switch to double-pumping of both breasts at once within 2 or 3 days, or as soon as you notice signs that your milk has "come in."

Not all automatic-cycling, electric breast pumps are created equal. Most breast pumps available for purchase are *not* true full size, hospital-grade breast pumps.

- Many of the portable electric breast pumps available for purchase were designed for use by working mothers, not mothers with preterm or hospitalized newborns. They may appear to be a less expensive alternative than rental pumps, but they were not designed for full-time pumping when

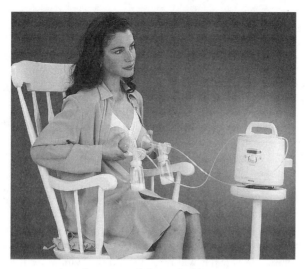

A mother using a full size double pump.

babies are unable to breastfeed. They have not been proven effective in establishing full milk production and then maintaining it for days, or for many weeks, before babies can nurse at the breast.

- Pumping sessions usually take longer with the purchase pumps, even the better ones, and single-sided breast pumping is the only option with many smaller breast pumps. A full size, hospital-grade breast pump is likely to lead to obtaining more milk, more quickly.

  ❑ Renting this type of breast pump may seem to be a major expense when the family budget already is stretched with the arrival of multiples. However, the cost for renting a full size, hospital-grade, automatic-cycling breast pump and purchasing a double collection kit is much less per month than the cost of infant formula for multiples.

  ❑ Health insurance companies often reimburse for this equipment when used to produce milk for preterm or sick babies. Contact your health insurance carrier to ask what information is required to cover this expense.

  ❑ The postpartum or NICU staff, a lactation consultant, or a local La Leche League Leader should know where to rent breast pumps in your area.

Developing a Pumping Routine

The best breast-pumping routine is one that simulates a full-term newborn's typical breastfeeding routine. Most newborns breastfeed at least 8, and as often as 12 to 14, times in 24 hours. Most breastfeedings last about 10 to 40 minutes, and the total

Colostrum is valuable in any amount. Do not pour even a drop down a drain thinking you have expressed too little.

amount of time a baby breastfeeds averages about 140 minutes over the course of 24 hours. Few newborns have more than one 4 to 5 hour span between feedings in 24 hours.

To imitate a full-term newborn's breastfeeding routine, pump your breasts at least 8 to 10 times during each 24 hours, for a minimum daily total of 100, and up to 150, minutes. The milk-making hormones and your breasts need frequent reminders that you are serious about producing milk for all of your babies, so pump every 2 to 3 hours for most of each 24-hour period. Each pumping session is likely to take about 10 to 20 minutes, but continue to pump up to 30 minutes if milk still flows steadily beyond this time. Once your milk has "come in," pump until you obtain no more milk for 1 to 2 minutes.

- The first two weeks after birth appears to be a *critical period* for letting your breasts know what will be expected of them. More frequent pumping during this period is associated with better milk production at two weeks postpartum and also long term. Pump at least 8 times (and 10 if possible) in 24 hours even if the babies are given only small amounts at this time.

- Because colostrum is "thicker" and in less quantity, it is common to obtain only drops or small amounts of milk during pumping sessions in the first few days after birth. Still, at least 8 pumping sessions in 24 hours should be the goal.

- Fewer than 8 daily pumping sessions, especially during the critical period in the weeks immediately after birth, can result in lower milk production both short term and later.

- One 4 to 5 hour span without pumping in order to get uninterrupted sleep may help you recover from birth, particularly a surgical birth. Avoid taking more than one such "break" each day, especially during the first several weeks when your body is establishing milk production. Most new mothers find they do not have to set an alarm; most wake on their own by 4 to 5 hours. Take advantage of any "natural" wake-up to pump.

You, of course, have multiple newborns and will want to produce more milk than is needed for a single baby.

- Mothers usually produce plenty of milk for multiples as long as they continue to pump 8 to 10 times for a total of 120 to 150 minutes in 24 hours, using a hospital-grade, self-cycling pump with a double collection kit.

- Mothers sometimes add an extra one or two pumping sessions when the babies begin to take more during feedings. Within a day or two, the additional pumping sessions usually translate into increased milk production if the mother has already been pumping 8 to 10 times in 24 hours.

- Some mothers add a pumping session to "stay ahead" of babies' caloric requirements or to achieve the milk production needed for hindmilk feedings of one or more. (Hindmilk feedings are discussed later in the chapter.) Settling in once all multiples are home is easier if a mother does not have to also increase milk production at that point.

- A few mothers are actually able to drop a pumping session after the first few weeks because they consistently produce more than 1000 ml (33 oz) in 24 hours. (*Always* talk to a lactation consultant or knowledgeable staff person before changing a productive pumping routine.)

Pumping every 2 to 3 hours may seem like a lot of time spent collecting milk. There are ways to make it more convenient.

- Develop a regular pumping routine, but adapt it to fit your particular situation. Pumping at regular 2 to 3 hour intervals works best for some mothers. Other mothers may "cluster" several sessions–pumping every 1 to 2 hours for part of the day and then less frequently at another part of the day. For instance, it is possible to take a 4 to 5 hour break from pumping at night, but only if a mother pumps more frequently than every 3 hours during the day.
- Although it is not necessary to rigidly follow a schedule when pumping, many mothers report they produce more milk, and produce it faster, when they pump at approximately the same times each day. They say once their body clock adapts to the routine, their milk lets down more quickly and more efficiently.
- If time is an issue for a particular session, pumping for several minutes is still better than missing a session. But do not cut too many sessions short or production will decrease.
- If you do miss a "scheduled" pumping session, pump as soon as you are able. Pump again at the next regularly scheduled time.

Pumping Technique

Developing a pumping session ritual can save time. For instance, claim a convenient and comfortable spot to use as your "pump place" and use it whenever possible.

- Assemble all the pump equipment first; then prepare your breasts for pumping by doing **breast massage.** Breast massage is easy and quick, and research has shown that it results in obtaining more milk over a 24-hour period. (See page 101.)
- Center the flanges/breast shields over your nipples and areola.
- Apply the pump and continue to pump until the steady flow slows to a drip only once every few seconds. (When you first apply the pump, expect to wait a minute or two before milk begins to spray or drip steadily.)
- Turn the pump to "off" and take a brief break to massage your breasts again.

- Reapply the pump, expecting a slight wait before seeing a steady flow, and continue to pump until you see no more milk dripping into the container for 1 to 2 minutes.
- If using single-sided pumping during the first 1 to 3 days after birth, *pump each breast twice* by pumping the right breast for several minutes, pumping the left breast for several minutes, and then repeating at the right breast and then the left. However, *switch to double-pumping* if possible once you are getting a steady flow of milk.
- Many mothers find it helps to look at a photo of the babies, listen to a tape of them crying or making other baby noises, smell a blanket or cap that one of the babies has used, or call to talk to the staff in the NICU as they pump.

Some mothers develop sore or cracked nipples while pumping. Because recent research indicates a link between pumping and breast infections, never ignore sore or cracked nipples. If you become sore:

- First, review your technique. Make sure your nipples are centered within the flanges, so there is no friction on nipple tips during the suction phase of the cycle. Be sure you are not inadvertently shifting the flanges when you become distracted during pumping.
- Ask a lactation consultant to check the fit of the collection kit flanges, which may not be the correct size for your particular breasts. Certain collection kits now allow for changing flange size. In addition to relieving soreness, mothers often find they obtain more milk once a more appropriate sized flange is used.
- Be sure to use a breast pump designed for establishing production and long-term use. Other types can result in sore nipples, as they may require higher suction levels, take longer to remove adequate milk, or create too much suction because they do not have a self-cycling mechanism.
- Some mothers apply a small amount of ultra-purified lanolin to nipples and areola after each pumping session when soreness is an issue. If an area appears to be "scraped" or cracked, ask a lactation consultant or physician to check for infection in order to determine whether a medicated ointment or cream may be more appropriate.

Set a timer or an alarm clock during the day to remind you of when to pump. (Set it during the night only if you find you are not waking on your own within 4 to 5 hours.) You may need a watch with an alarm feature to remind you to pump during visits to the NICU.

- Reset the alarm for the next session as soon as you turn it off for the current one. Life with multiples is complicated enough without having to remember when to pump.

Breast Massage

- Place both hands on either side of one breast, starting at the chest wall or rib cage, and then compress or "squeeze" the breast gently but firmly, while moving the hands down the breast toward the areola. Move the location of your hands slightly and repeat until all areas of one breast, and then the other, have been massaged.
- Or make one hand into a fist and, starting at the chest wall or rib cage, roll the fist down over the breast toward the areola. Repeat the movement until all areas of each breast have been massaged. Use the technique that works best and feels more comfortable.
- Massaging/compressing the breast during pumping can help remove more milk. It can be done during double pumping by making the "peace sign" by spreading your index (second) and middle (third) fingers apart and then, with palms of the hands toward the breasts, slide those fingers over the cup-like pieces of the kit that fit over each breast, which may be called flanges or breast shields, to hold them in place over each breast. Use your thumbs to massage downward toward the areola, moving them to different areas of the breasts as you are able.
- If using single-sided pumping during the first 1 to 3 days after birth, always massage the breast you are currently pumping.

Record pumping sessions over each 24 hours by noting the time and the amount obtained from each breast on a single-sheet, daily checklist chart. Mothers often think they are pumping more frequently than they actually are, and a chart is a concrete reminder of whether you are pumping enough to establish and maintain milk production.

Time-saving strategies can make long-term pumping seem more "doable."
- Many mothers recommend wearing a bra that allows for "hands-free" pumping, so they can accomplish other tasks while pumping. Some mothers purchase a bra designed for "hands-free" pumping; others create one from a well-fitted "regular" bra. It is important that any hands-free bra "hold" flanges in place properly or the pump cannot work. Also, variation in breast shape or size may affect a mother's ability to create or use such a bra. (See Resources for more information.)
- Buy a second collection kit or purchase extra flanges/breast shields. It may save time if you can thoroughly clean several pairs at once.
- Nighttime pumping sessions disturb sleep less when you assemble the pump pieces before going to bed. Then the only thing for you to do during the night is place the flanges over your breasts and turn the machine to "on."

- You may avoid getting out of bed if you place the pump near your bed. (Hospital-grade electric pumps are usually quiet to operate, so the pump is unlikely to disturb your partner or any baby in the room with you.)
- To refrigerate bottles of milk without getting up, place them in an insulated cooler with adequately sized freezer cold/ice pack(s). Cover the cooler with a tight-fitting lid to maintain the temperature, and place the cooler next to the pump. Milk can be transferred to the refrigerator/freezer when you, or a family member, get up. (If pumping for a baby less than 32 weeks gestation, you may be told to bring in frozen milk so you will probably want to freeze milk immediately after pumping.) Use the cooler to keep milk cold/frozen when you transport it to the hospital.
- If you have another child, you probably will need someone in your home to help with her care. Otherwise, it will be difficult to pump frequently enough and also visit the babies in the NICU.

Pumping in the NICU

Take the breast pump collection kit with you to the NICU, so you are able to pump during visits with the babies. Breast pumps may be available in the NICU or you may have to go to a designated "pumping room." Since mothers do not like to take time away from the babies to go to another room, pumping sessions may be missed unnecessarily. *Missed sessions decrease milk production!*

If breast pumps are available in another part of the hospital, ask to have a breast pump moved to the NICU. If pumps are fastened in place and cannot be moved, bring the pump from home to the hospital so you don't have to leave the babies. (Let someone carry it for you, and put a label with your name on this pump.)

Being able to see the babies during pumping sessions can have a positive effect on the let-down, or milk-ejection, reflex.

Ask the staff to inform you when a change in any baby's feeding routine is likely. As each baby's condition improves, an increase in human milk intake may be anticipated. You can adapt your pumping routine if you are aware of expected changes.

If after a few weeks of pumping you are producing far more milk than your babies take and are expected to take for a while, you may be able to decrease the time spent pumping. However, speak with a lactation consultant before making any changes in an obviously successful pumping routine.

How Much Milk?

Mothers often want to know how much milk they should expect to obtain at each pumping session. The amount produced varies from mother to mother and from session to session, which is one reason some mothers must pump more, and some less, than others.

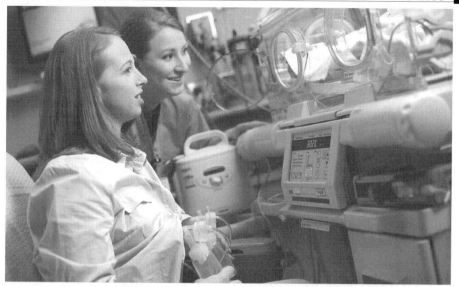

Some mothers get more milk when they are able to pump in the NICU where they can see their babies.

Only small amounts of colostrum are produced for the first few days after birth. However, colostrum is especially high in illness-fighting antibodies, so save every drop of this "liquid gold" for the babies.

No matter how little is obtained from a single pumping session, it can be drawn up in a syringe to be fed to the babies. Many mothers find they obtain more colostrum by using manual (hand) expression of milk until the milk "comes in." (See Appendix for information on Hand-Expression.)

Once the milk "comes in," most mothers pump from one to several ounces each session. Generally, they are able to keep up with their multiples' caloric requirements.

If pumping at least 8 to 10 times in 24 hours with a full-size, hospital-grade electric rental pump and using a double collection kit, the average amount a mother can expect to produce is:

- Day 1 to 5 postpartum: drops to 90 ml (3 oz) in 24 hours. (Plentiful milk "comes in" at about 3 to 5 days postpartum, unless temporarily affected by pregnancy or birth complications.)
- Day 5 to 10: more than 300 to 500 ml (10 to 16.5 oz) in 24 hours. (Pregnancy or birth complications may still affect milk production.)
- By 2 weeks after birth: more than 500 to 750 ml (16.5 to 24 oz) in 24 hours; optimal production is 750 to 1000 ml (24 to 33 oz) in 24 hours. (Pregnancy or birth complications may still affect milk production for certain mothers.)

A mother's physical condition may delay the increased milk volume associated with milk "coming in" in some situations. Do not worry if you have been pumping regularly for several days but are not yet seeing large volumes of milk. It may be related to your prenatal or postpartum health. Usually milk production will improve by 10 days postpartum if you pump at least 8 to 10 times every 24 hours. Milk production may fluctuate when a mother must pump for several weeks.

- Production will drop if you miss or delay pumping sessions, so review your routine. Add 1 to 2 sessions to increase milk production.
- Even slight swelling in the "interstitial" breast tissue surrounding the milk-making cells and related milk ducts may interfere with milk flow during pumping sessions. It may help to move fluid back and away from the areola where the flanges/breast shields of the pump kit are placed. The technique to do this is called *Reverse Pressure Softening (RPS)* or "areolar compression." Its effect lasts only minutes, so be ready to apply the pump immediately afterward. (See Appendix for a detailed description of Reverse Pressure Softening.)

If you have established a regular, frequent pumping routine but you are not seeing an increase in the milk you obtain by 7 to 10 days postpartum, be sure to talk with a lactation consultant. She should be familiar with certain physical conditions that sometimes affect milk production and possible interventions to discuss with your physician.

- Only a small percentage of women have *insufficient glandular (milk-making) tissue* in the breast, although breast surgery, particularly *breast reduction,* may disrupt the milk-making tissue and lower milk production.
- *Thyroid conditions* and *Polycystic Ovarian Syndrome* (PCOS) sometimes affect milk production; however, certain medications used to treat these conditions may reverse or diminish the impact on milk production.
- *Diabetic conditions appear to delay milk "coming in" by a few days* for some women, but they generally do not have a long-term effect and affected mothers usually have no difficulty producing adequate milk by 5 to 10 days postpartum.
- *Severe hemorrhage,* especially if a mother went into shock, may result in decreased milk production.
- If any small fragment of placenta(s) remains in the uterus (*retained placenta*), milk production may be low until the fragments are passed or removed.

The impact of *the mind-body connection* as it concerns milk production is not completely understood. However, there is some evidence that milk production may be influenced briefly when a baby's condition is not stable. Is it any wonder then that milk production could be affected temporarily for some mothers of multiples who are concerned about the health of two or more babies?

Check breast pump equipment for a possible mechanical problem if you have increased the amount of pumping for several days without seeing an increase in milk volume.

- The collection kit flanges may be the wrong size for a particular mother.
- Machine parts can break down or wear out.
- An individual mother may find one breast pump works better for her than another. The agency that rented the pump, NICU staff, or a lactation consultant should be able to help you find a pump that works well for you.
- A galactogogue, a medication that appears to aid milk production, may be prescribed for a short time when production is not improving after several days of increased pumping. Many mothers report better milk production with the use of one or more galactogogues, but these medications can NOT replace regular, frequent milk removal and the use of an appropriate breast pump. Most known pharmaceutical/medication galactogogues were produced for other physical conditions and most have side effects, so they are not prescribed routinely. Speak to your health care provider, a dietitian, or a lactation consultant before taking anything that is considered a galactogogue. Also consult them if a prescribed galactogogue is not helping and you want to try a different one.
  - ❏ A number of herbs are believed to be galactogogues. Herbs are also a form of medication, and they can have side effects. Many do not have good scientific research to support their safety and/or effectiveness.
  - ❏ Some mothers find it helpful to "rotate" different galactogogues. One type may work for 2 to 3 weeks and then milk production seems to drop again. If a different galactogogue is introduced, production then improves. The first galactogogue may be effective if reintroduced later in the rotation.
  - ❏ Other mothers report better results when they combine galactogues–often they take lower amounts. Some herbal galactogogues are packaged in combination.
- If a delay or a drop in plentiful milk production interferes with pumping sessions, continue to pump 8 to 10 times in 24 hours, but avoid looking at the milk as it drips into the bottles; place paper or foil around the bottles if necessary.
- Some mothers phone the NICU staff or a friend to distract them while pumping.
- Visualization is a tool that can be relaxing and improve milk flow. For one scenario, close your eyes after applying the pump and "see" yourself sitting next to a babbling brook. As you follow the water downstream, you notice a waterfall. Watch the water tumble over the falls. As you become more relaxed, the water flowing over the falls turns to milk. (Mothers sometimes report their milk lets down as the waterfall becomes white. If you prefer, substitute a fountain or the waves on a beach that roll in and then back

out for the waterfall.)

- If you feel as if you are about to cry when you sit down to pump, do it. Do not hold tears inside. The increased tension can cause a headache. There is nothing wrong with crying. When tears start falling, milk sometimes lets down and starts falling too.
- Sometimes mothers are unable to produce enough milk to meet all of the babies' caloric requirements each day. Perhaps a family situation does not lend itself to the 8 to 10 (or more) daily pumping sessions usually needed to keep up with multiples' growing appetites. Occasionally, a mother pumps frequently, the equipment is working well, but milk production does not appear to respond.
  - ❏ When milk production is low, or lower than the babies' combined intakes, the sickest baby is often given the most human milk. The other(s) receive the remaining human milk and then are supplemented with infant formula.
  - ❏ Occasionally, banked human milk is available for a sick baby. Banked human milk is scarce because of the low number of milk banks in most countries. (See Resources.)

Storing and Handling Expressed Human Milk

Most NICUs have a procedure for pumping and storing the milk you collect for your babies. *Follow the hospital's instructions.* Ask the staff if the hospital can provide appropriate sterile storage containers. Often you will be given bottles that can be attached to the breast pump, so milk can be expressed directly into the containers.

Your hands and the pieces of the breast pump collection kit that come in contact with your milk should be clean before you begin a pumping session. Follow any guidelines provide by the NICU for cleaning and daily sterilizing of these pieces.

Label containers before placing the milk in the refrigerator. The date and time the milk was expressed should always be included and list any medications you have been taking. (If the NICU staff already has a list of your medications, be sure to keep it updated.) Ask the NICU staff what other information they want included and whether you need to add anything to labels when bringing milk in for multiple babies. Often a NICU provides the labels it wants used.

Generally, mothers are instructed to refrigerate the colostrum or mature milk that will be fed to the babies within 48 hours and then freeze the remaining milk. If babies are not yet being fed milk or they are less than 32 weeks gestation, you probably will be told to freeze the expressed colostrum or mature milk immediately. (Freezing milk kills a virus many mothers carry. This virus in milk does not cause problems for babies after 32 weeks gestation.) Once thawed, human milk must be fed to the babies within 24 hours. It should not be refrozen if unused.

Because of increased antibody activity, fresh refrigerated human milk usually is preferred to frozen when it's available. However, frozen human milk retains most of its antibody action after thawing and, of course, it still is nutritionally superior and more digestible than any other food available for preterm or sick babies.

To keep milk cold or frozen during transport between your home and the hospital, use an insulated cooler lined with enough frozen cold/ice pack(s) to avoid any warming. Usually, frozen milk does not begin to thaw unless you are traveling a great distance. The NICU staff should show you where to refrigerate or freeze your labeled milk once at the hospital.

Feeding Expressed Human Milk

Colostrum was designed to be babies' first food, and many NICUs choose to follow Nature's sequence by offering colostrum as preterm or sick babies' first milk feedings. *Colostrum is valuable in any amount. Do not pour even a drop down a drain thinking you have expressed too little.* Those few drops are extremely valuable because the antibodies are present in high amounts in colostrum. Whether fresh or frozen, it is the perfect first food for your babies. Although only a small quantity may be expressed during a pumping session, any amount can be drawn up in a syringe and fed to babies when any is ready for enteral (gastrointestinal tract) feedings.

The NICU neonatologists, nurses, and dietitians will determine when each baby is ready for milk feedings and how much each should be given. If there is not enough milk for each baby at every feeding, you should be involved in any discussion of how to "divide" your milk. As noted earlier, a sicker multiple often is given more human milk than the other(s).

Preterm human milk is not the same as human milk produced for full-term babies. Nature adapted human milk to suit the needs of babies who arrive early. However, Nature could not anticipate the tremendous advances that have occurred in the care and subsequent survival of very early (less than 30 weeks gestation) and very low birth weight (VLBW) (less than 3.3 lb, 1500 gm) preterm babies during the last few decades. The small stomachs and immature body systems of VLBW babies may not be able to handle the volume of human milk required for their rapid growth needs when they first begin milk feedings. Because of this, a *human milk fortifier* (HMF) may be added to a mother's milk to provide extra calories and more of certain vitamins and minerals.

In some cases, offering several daily *hindmilk feedings* eliminates the need for a commercial fortifier for extra calories, although preterm babies may still need fortification with certain vitamins and minerals. Hindmilk is the milk obtained later in a breastfeeding or pumping. Hindmilk is higher in fat than the foremilk–the milk available at the beginning of a feeding/pumping–so it is higher in calories. If weight gain is an issue for any multiple and you have been keeping pace with the amount of milk your babies are taking, ask their neonatologist whether providing hindmilk for some feedings may be beneficial. The basics for obtaining hindmilk for feedings include:

- Attaching collection containers labeled "foremilk" prior to pumping.
- Pumping into the "foremilk" containers for about two minutes beyond the time you notice milk spraying/dripping steadily with "let down."
- Stopping the pumping session to change to collection containers labeled "hindmilk."
- Resuming the pumping session until a minute or two beyond the time when no drops of milk are seen dripping from your breasts.
- Saving both foremilk and hindmilk by refrigerating or freezing, according to the instructions from the NICU.
- If pumping hindmilk for one baby but not for the other(s), you have several options;
  - ❑ Change bottles only on one side; leave the other bottle alone. Be careful to label bottles correctly.
  - ❑ Always separate pumping into "foremilk" and "hindmilk" minutes. The NICU staff can then add foremilk to hindmilk for any multiple on regular milk feedings.
  - ❑ Alternate pumping sessions–"separating" milk into fore/hindmilk during some sessions and pumping straight through without changing collection bottles at other pumpings.

Hindmilk feedings may be used until a baby shows a steady weight gain and "regular" human milk can provide the appropriate calories to meet a baby's growth requirements. If your babies are growing at different rates, you may be asked to separate milk for hindmilk feeding of one multiple and to bring in regular milk for the other(s).

The frozen foremilk will eventually be used. You may find it helpful if complementing feedings when weight gain is no longer an issue, or you may add it to some of your babies' early solid foods, etc.

Beginning Breastfeeding

Ideally, each baby's first experience of sucking will be at your breast. Be sure the NICU staff understands your breastfeeding goals and that you want to avoid, or at least minimize, infant feeding practices that might interfere with breastfeeding.

Working with NICU Staff

Some NICUs have a specific progression plan for helping babies transition to breastfeeding. Staff members at these NICUs are trained to support mothers and babies as they learn to work together to breastfeed. Even when a NICU does not have a well-established plan, most NICU staff members will be willing to support you as you begin to breastfeed your babies.

Different NICU staff teams may coordinate the medical care for each multiple, and the teams may vary somewhat in their approaches–in part due to the babies' differing conditions and in part because there often is more than one way to address a health issue. If different NICU teams care for your babies, you will have to get to know and work with each, which may get confusing at times.

You will want to be certain that each staff team is aware of your goal to form a long-term breastfeeding relationship with each baby. Let them know that you want your breast to provide each multiple's first sucking, or oral feeding, experiences. Many mothers post a "reminder" on a strategic spot on each multiple's incubator or crib, such as "No bottles before mother's breast."

Non-Nutritive Breastfeeding

For a baby to effectively breastfeed, or transfer milk from mother's breast into his mouth, and ultimately his gastrointestinal (GI) tract, a baby must rhythmically coordinate sucking and swallowing with breathing. Babies begin to suck and swallow amniotic fluid during the second trimester of pregnancy, but they cannot coordinate sucking with swallowing until they are about 32 weeks gestation. Then it may be another one to two months before a preterm baby consistently and effortlessly coordinates *suck-swallow-breathe* to take in enough calories at each feeding.

> **Sucking on your emptied breast is an excellent way to introduce non-nutritive sucking during a gavage feeding**

Preterm VLBW babies often show an interest in sucking before they are ready for feedings by mouth. Until that occurs, they are given enteral milk feedings via a thin gavage tube/catheter inserted into the baby's mouth (orogastric) or nose (nasogastric) to its stomach. A baby may be offered a pacifier, or "dummy," during gavage feedings. Pacifier use can interfere with breastfeeding for a full-term, healthy baby. However, studies show that when preterm babies suck on a pacifier during gavage feedings they become more relaxed, their breathing stabilizes, and they gain weight more quickly. When a baby sucks without ingesting any liquid, it is called *non-nutritive sucking.* Babies make more rapid mouth movements during non-nutritive sucking than nutritive sucking.

Sucking on your "empty" breast is an excellent way to introduce each multiple to non-nutritive sucking during a gavage feeding. Once the NICU staff determines that any multiple is ready for non-nutritive sucking, arrange for that multiple's first empty breast experience to be timed with one of your visits to the unit.

To offer an empty breast, pump your breasts completely immediately before a (potential) non-nutritive sucking session. The fresh milk you pump can be used for the next gavage feeding or frozen for a later feeding. Of course, your breasts are never totally empty, but the amount of milk in them will be slight and it will flow much more slowly if you have pumped first. Plus, any remaining milk the baby tastes will be higher-calorie hindmilk droplets.

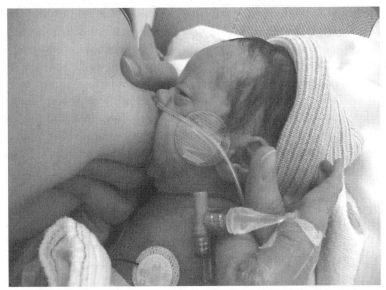

A premature baby can latch onto the breast sooner than you might think.

Preterm babies' first experience with non-nutritive sucking often occurs spontaneously during *kangaroo care* sessions, surprising the mother, the baby, and even the NICU staff! During kangaroo care babies sometimes "seek" the breast and, if close enough, they may begin to nuzzle and lick. Occasionally, a baby takes advantage of the opportunity and latches on. For this reason you may want to empty your breasts before you and a baby begin to enjoy a kangaroo care session.

Once any multiple is able to go to an empty breast, spend as much time in the NICU as possible so she can take full advantage of "at breast," non-nutritive sucking sessions. During these early "practice" breastfeedings, each baby begins to associate the taste and smell of your milk with your breast. However, don't be surprised if one multiple latches on as if she has been doing it forever while another needs days or weeks to "get" it.

Nutritive Breastfeeding

The NICU staff will watch for the signs that indicate each multiple is developing an ability to coordinate sucking and swallowing with breathing. Each baby's first nutritive sucking experience ideally occurs at the breast. Babies who are ready for oral feedings of liquid food are ready to begin drinking, rather than just tasting, during breastfeeding.

It used to be thought that breastfeeding was more difficult or stressful for preterm babies than bottle-feeding. Several studies have shown that preterm babies actually have fewer episodes of cardiopulmonary (heart or breathing pattern) distress during breastfeeding. Some newer research indicates that breastfeeding may also help preterm babies develop rhythmic suck-swallow-breathe coordination more quickly.

However, just as multiples vary in their ability to latch onto the breast, they will also vary in the ability to actually breastfeed (remove milk) while coordinating sucking-swallowing-breathing. It can be very frustrating when one is moving forward in his ability to breastfeed while another seems to be going nowhere–or even backward.

Consider all of these early breastfeedings as practice to help maintain perspective. Applaud the "know it all" multiple who zooms ahead but don't become discouraged or develop unrealistic expectations about a multiple who needs more time to learn. When a multiple has difficulty latching on or removing milk during direct breastfeeding, there are some strategies that may help.

- Placing a thin, silicone *nipple shield* over a mother's nipple/areola has been found to help many preterm babies latch onto the breast better or remove milk from the breast more effectively. (Some preterm babies latch on well but the shield may still help these babies remove more milk during breastfeeding.)
- Preterm babies often have difficulty controlling the faster flow when the milk lets down, so many mothers pump their breasts for a few minutes before they start to breastfeed these early learners. Pumping through the initial let-down:
  - ❑ Slows the flow of milk.
  - ❑ Means milk is readily available when the baby goes to breast.
  - ❑ Provides baby with more higher-fat hindmilk.
- As each baby learns to coordinate the actions of suck-swallow-breathe, a mother begins to breastfeed without pumping first. Some babies still may have difficulty controlling the initial forceful flow of the let-down and need to be taken off the breast until the flow slows. That is all right. Although it sometimes takes several weeks or months, each baby will learn to handle the flow with let-down as he matures.
- Since mothers do not have ounce/milliliter markers on their breasts to show how much a baby has taken during breastfeeding, *test-weighing* can provide that information. Using a sensitive electronic scale that picks up differences of one to two grams, a NICU staff member can weigh a baby immediately before a breastfeeding. The staff member weighs him again immediately afterward without changing any item of the baby's clothing. The difference between the pre- and post-feeding weights is the amount the baby took during the feeding.

Increasing Breastfeeding

Preterm or sick babies rarely are fully breastfed when they are discharged from the NICU. It takes patience and persistence to work on improving breastfeeding with two or more babies. Allow time to gain confidence in your ability to produce enough milk and in each baby's ability to breastfeed correctly.

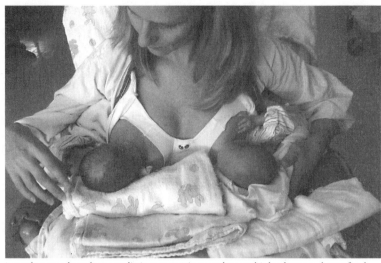

A mother needs to have realistic expectations as her multiples learn to breastfeed.

When preterm or sick babies first come home, a mother usually wants concrete evidence that each baby is getting enough milk. Test-weighing the babies for daily breastfeedings lets you know how well each baby is removing milk. Just as the NICU staff may have test-weighed your babies during their hospitalization, you can do this at home by renting a sensitive electronic scale to weigh each baby immediately before and after a breastfeeding. By subtracting the pre-feeding weight from the post-feeding weight, you can determine exactly how much milk a baby received during a feeding. Test-weights should help you know when you can safely begin to decrease supplementary feedings.

Once each baby is gaining weight steadily, you may still want to weigh babies daily and then weekly. As babies' abilities to breastfeed improve and you gain confidence, "measure" breastfeeding by monitoring babies' diaper counts and weight gain as noted in Chapter 13, "Effective Breastfeeding." Before long, you will find weight checks during routine pediatric examinations are all that are necessary. (Information about renting an electronic scale is in Resources.)

Any amount of breastfeeding, or the bottle-feeding of human milk, is valuable.

Juggling breastfeedings, pumping sessions, and alternative feedings can leave a mother feeling overwhelmed and exhausted. You will feel more in charge if you have someone help with babies' supplementary feedings or hold babies while you use a breast pump. See Chapter 12, "Making Up for a Poor Start," for a discussion of alternative feeding methods and ideas for coping until babies make the transition to being mainly or fully breastfed.

Multiples' ability to breastfeed will vary from baby to baby and from day to day. Do not become discouraged. Do what you can to keep breastfeeding, which also may vary from day to day! It may take time, but if you and the babies keep practicing, eventually each will figure out how to breastfeed well. A couple of true stories illustrate how this can work.

Case A: A set of quadruplets was born at 31 weeks gestation and they were discharged one or two at a time between what would have been their 34th to 36th week of gestation. All four had significant difficulty breastfeeding at the time of discharge. Although their mother had help much of each day, she still found it hard to care for four babies, give them "practice" breastfeedings, and pump her breasts often. However, she remembered the breastfeeding relationship she had with her older child, so she kept putting each to breast two to three times a day. Usually she pumped at least once or twice a day, but some days she had no time to pump at all. About three months after the quads' births she began to breastfeed one baby almost fully because infant formula was upsetting his system. Milk production increased, so she began breastfeeding the other three babies more often. At a year one quad weaned, but the other three continued to breastfeed beyond their second birthday.

Case B: Both babies of a set of twins born at 35 weeks required a stay in the NICU because of breathing difficulties at birth. One baby was discharged at one week and the other came home at two weeks. Their mother pumped and for the next two weeks both twins were fully fed with human milk. Both babies were put to breast several times a day, and one or both would seem to make progress one day only to slide backward the next. By four weeks the mother was discouraged and exhausted. She did not think she could continue to pump, work at breastfeeding, and handle double bottle-feedings for much longer. After paying a lactation consultant to observe each baby at breast and make suggestions to improve technique, she decided to discontinue all bottles for one baby at a time closely watching baby's wet diapers and stools. (Both babies were gaining weight appropriately.)

First she discontinued bottles for the baby having the most difficulty breastfeeding. Over one weekend that baby was offered only the breast. Between feedings the mother increased skin contact with this baby, and by Monday morning this twin was fully breastfed. (This is sometimes called a "babymoon." For more on this concept, see "For Effective Breastfeeders" in Chapter 12.) Dad meanwhile had been caring for the other twin. He now took over the care of the fully breastfeeding baby, except for the baby's feedings, so the mother could continue the progress made with the first baby yet concentrate on the twin who had been under dad's care for the weekend. Both babies were fully breastfed by the next morning, and they continued to be fully breastfed until they started taking solid foods between six and seven months.

Full and Partial Breastfeeding

Many breastfeeding "teams" eventually make the transition to full breastfeeding even after days or weeks in a NICU. However, full breastfeeding is not always possible and sometimes it is not desired because of an ongoing feeding difficulty for one or more babies or due to a family situation. Any amount of breastfeeding, or the bottle-feeding of human milk, still is valuable. (For a more complete discussion of these options, read Chapter 18, "Full and Partial Breastfeeding.")

One of the greatest challenges of breastfeeding multiples is that a high percentage of these babies initially require a stay in a hospital NICU. Nonetheless, many mothers and their multiples have gone on to breastfeed—fully or partially—for months or years. Mothers succeed by expressing their milk frequently to establish lactation, practicing breastfeeding until each baby gets it "right," and persisting even when difficulties last days or weeks.

KEY POINTS

- ❑ Your milk is a special gift that only you can give your babies. Begin pumping the day they are born or as soon as possible. Using a full size, hospital-grade, electric breast pump with a double collection kit that lets you pump both breasts at once, pump your breasts **at least** 8 times and 10 or more times per day if possible.
- • Rent a full size, hospital-grade pump for use at home after discharge from the hospital. Chart when you pump and how much you obtain on an easy-to-read sheet of paper to make sure you are pumping often and long enough.
- • Milk should "come in" by about 3 to 5 days postpartum and most mothers begin obtaining about 20 to 33 oz (600 to 1000 ml) of milk by 10 to 14 days postpartum if pumping often enough with a full size hospital-grade breast pump.
- • Certain health conditions may affect the amount of milk produced. Talk to a lactation consultant if you are pumping 8 to 10 times but obtaining less than 16 to 17 oz (500 ml) in 24 hours by one to two weeks after giving birth.
- ❑ It takes time for preterm or sick babies to learn to breastfeed effectively. Few preterm babies are fully breastfeeding when discharged from the NICU. It may take patience and persistence, but most of these babies will eventually breastfeed well.

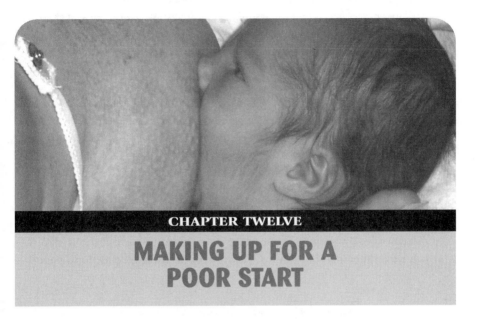

CHAPTER TWELVE

MAKING UP FOR A POOR START

Newborn multiples often get off to a poor breastfeeding start because of pregnancy or birth-related complications. Many are born early, and a week or two can make a big difference in babies' ability to breastfeed well. Even full-term, healthy multiples sometimes get off to a poor breastfeeding start if any experience stress before birth, early feedings are delayed, or only one baby is brought to breastfeed at each feeding while the other(s) is given a bottle to "let mother rest." If this has already happened, you and your babies can make up for lost time.

Babies *can* learn to breastfeed (remove milk) better. Mothers *can* increase milk production. Believe in your body's ability to make milk for your multiples, and believe in their ability to learn to breastfeed well. It takes motivation for any mother to improve milk production for a single baby, much less for multiples. But you and your babies can do it together.

Keeping Babies Healthy While Increasing Milk Production

When a slow breastfeeding start means you must work to increase milk production, babies' hydration and weight gain may be a concern whether each baby breastfeeds well or any baby is having difficulty. Read the section in Chapter 9, "Beginning Breastfeeding," so you will know the signs that the babies are doing well.

- When babies breastfeed well and diaper counts are within the normal number, you should feel reassured about milk production. However, you may want to weigh each baby once or twice a week until you feel confident that each is gaining weight appropriately. To get accurate weights, use the same scale, weigh each baby in the nude, and check weights at about the same time of day.

- You may want to check weight more frequently for any baby who is having difficulty breastfeeding. Certain electronic digital scales allow you to figure how much a baby receives during a single feeding. To use this type of scale, weigh a baby before a feeding (pre-feeding), "lock" in the weight, and weigh the baby again after feeding (post-feeding). The scale subtracts the "pre-feeding" from the "post-feeding" weight and lists the difference in ounces or grams. This is the amount the baby took in during breastfeeding. Leaders and lactation consultants refer to this as "test-weighing." This type of scale also provides more reliable information about day-to-day weight differences for any baby who must be weighed daily for a period of time.

Frequent weighing is not necessary for most newborns, but when any baby's nutritional intake or weight is in question, the use of an electronic digital scale may help guide decisions about the need to supplement any baby and whether breast pumping is needed. This type of scale can be rented through some breast pump rental stations. (See Resources—"Equipment.")

For Effective Breastfeeders

The best treatment for a poor beginning is to take an effectively breastfeeding baby to bed for several days of almost round-the-clock breastfeeding.

The information in this section refers only to any multiple able to latch on and breastfeed effectively. For these babies, the best treatment for a poor breastfeeding beginning is to take them to bed for several days of almost round-the-clock breastfeeding, which some have dubbed a "babymoon." Let each baby breastfeed whenever she indicates readiness, usually about 10 to 14 times in 24 hours, and you probably will find you are bursting with milk within a few days. Once milk production increases to meet the babies' needs, most babies will settle into the more usual 8 to 12 breastfeedings in 24 hours.

- Most mothers take only one multiple at a time on a babymoon, even when two have begun to breastfeed more effectively, because it is more manageable. However, they continue to breastfeed the other multiple(s) at least a few times each day. When the babymooning multiple resumes a typical breastfeeding pattern, babymoon with another one.

If milk production needs a boost but taking one or more babies to bed for a few days is not a realistic option, try these suggestions:

- Breastfeed each baby 10 to 12 times a day, simultaneously or separately. (This feeding increase may also be done with one baby at a time.) Because babies are likely to become hungrier sooner when milk production is not yet what it needs to be, babies usually are happy to go along with the extra feedings.
- Or increase "feedings" by expressing/pumping your breasts. Some mothers save time by pumping one breast while feeding a baby on the other; other mothers pump immediately or about an hour after a feeding.
- Keep track of each baby's wet/stool diaper count and each one's weight to know whether any baby may need additional milk in the form of expressed human milk or infant formula and about how much to offer. If your goal is to fully breastfeed, develop a plan with your babies' pediatric care provider so that you offer a baby no more supplement than is necessary to produce a good diaper count and an adequate weight gain. (See Chapter 13, "Effective Breastfeeding.")
- If any baby needs additional milk while production catches up with baby's breastfeeding ability, it is rarely necessary to offer it after every breastfeeding. Offering a little extra once or twice a day may be enough. Giving other milk, especially infant formula, too often interferes with a mother's milk production. Babies digest infant formula differently, so they often "request" fewer breastfeedings. This lowers milk production unless you also pump, which leads to juggling breastfeeding, other feedings, and pumping sessions. It is easy to become overwhelmed and lose confidence when trying to do it all.
  - ❏ Using a tube system at breast may be the ideal way to offer additional milk to any effectively breastfeeding baby. Its use may actually save you time once you and any baby get used to it. (See "Alternative Feeding Methods" below.)
- If any multiple is receiving more than 1 ounce (30 ml) of additional milk, gradually decrease the amount of any supplement given at a feeding by 1/2 to 1 ounce (15 to 30 ml) every few days. Expect the babies to breastfeed an extra time or two in 24 hours. Their diaper counts might dip or their rates of weight gain may slow for a few days each time you do this. When babies go back to their usual routines, their diaper counts pick up and they again gain at least a half ounce (15 g) a day, you probably are ready to subtract another 1/2 to 1 ounce (15 to 30 ml) from each feeding.

When One (or More) Has a Feeding Difficulty

It can be doubly or triply (or more) frustrating to work through a problem with that multiple(s) while also caring for the other(s).

Newborn babies are not all born with the same level of breastfeeding proficiency. The ability to latch on and breastfeed well may vary a little or a lot among multiples. If you think any baby is not breastfeeding effectively, read the section on "difficulty latching on or sucking" in Chapter 15, "Breastfeeding Difficulties in Young Babies."

When one or more newborns has difficulty breastfeeding, it can be doubly or triply (or more) frustrating to work through a problem with that multiple(s) while also caring for the other(s). The sheer number of babies may mean it takes longer to work with an individual baby experiencing difficulty, which may add to the frustration level.

Relax. Do what you can for today. Take it one day at a time, and expect some breastfeedings–and some days–to go better than others. With patience and persistence the magic moment will come when each multiple figures out what must be done to get that good milk from your warm breast.

- As often as possible, breastfeed the one having difficulty but consider it "practice" and limit breastfeeding to five to 15 minutes before offering expressed milk or some infant formula. (Depending on family circumstances, "as often as possible" may vary from every feeding to only a few feedings a day.) However, when the baby seems to finally get it, keep going!
- Move on to an alternative feeding method if the baby cannot latch on after several attempts, keeps falling asleep within a minute or two of latching on, or if either you or the baby becomes frustrated. When you and the baby have been working at breastfeeding for about 15 minutes and it still doesn't feel right, offer that baby something else.
- Long periods at the breast do *not* teach the baby to breastfeed if his mouth is not yet able to do it effectively; a baby's sucking becomes less organized over time during a particular feeding–not more or better organized. And long practice sessions take away from the time a mother needs to remove milk via pumping.
- Offer this baby the breast *whenever* he demonstrates early feeding cues, such as rooting, licking, or putting hands to face or mouth.
- *Increase skin-to-skin contact* with this baby as much as possible. Take the baby's and your shirts off. Lie down or sit with the baby's bare chest directly against your bare chest. (Cover both of you with a sheet or light blanket if desired.) The baby will get to know the comfortable feel and smell of the breast without the "pressure to perform." (The other multiple[s] will like this, too! There is no such thing as "too much" skin contact between a mother and each of her babies!)

❑ Placing baby's bare chest against your bare chest between feedings lets the baby learn that your breast is a pleasant place to be; it has helped many babies "wake up and smell the milk" better. Skin-to-skin contact is a high-touch, low-tech strategy that really helps babies progress to effective breastfeeding.

❑ Some babies begin to breastfeed better when on mother's chest in a tub of water maintained at skin-temperature (about 99° F, 37.2° C for infants). Place the baby chest-to-chest and allow him to seek the breast without much assistance from you. *Caution.* Ask the babies' health care provider before taking a preterm baby in the tub with you, and always take *only one* baby in the tub at a time.

• Breastfeed a multiple having difficulty along with another multiple who breastfeeds well. The baby with effective sucking will stimulate a good let-down (milk-ejection) reflex, which sometimes forces a "weaker" multiple to move his mouth correctly to swallow milk. You could also use an electric breast pump at one breast while simultaneously feeding the baby having difficulty. At best, the baby may finally figure out how to use her mouth to handle the flow of milk. At worst, she will sputter and let go of the breast.

• Sometimes a difficulty either latching onto or feeding directly from the breast is overcome by the mother covering her nipple with a thin, silicone *nipple shield.* Eventually, the nipple shield is removed at some point during a feeding. However, a few babies continue to breastfeed only when the shield is in place.

❑ When a multiple having difficulty begins to breastfeed through a nipple shield, a mother often feels hopeful about long-term breastfeeding for this baby–and she should. It is a big step forward. However, nipple shield use can have drawbacks.

❑ Watch for signs of a decrease in milk production. Although milk usually transfers well through a thin, silicone nipple shield when a baby is breastfeeding effectively, a mother should continue to pump until the baby "proves" he is breastfeeding well by suckling for at least 10 to 30 minutes, having appropriate diaper counts, and gaining sufficient weight.

❑ Taking test-weights over a few days, as described above in "Keeping Babies Healthy While Increasing Milk Production" is a way to know more precisely how effectively a baby is breastfeeding through a shield.

❑ Some babies seem to become dependent on a shield for breastfeeding and refuse to breastfeed without it, which can be, but is not always, a problem.

❑ Stay in contact with an LLL Leader or a lactation consultant if using a nipple shield for any baby.

Compensatory Milk Expression

How often you pump should depend on each baby's ability to get nourishment at the breast, your family situation, and whether your goal is full or partial breastfeeding.

Milk production is affected when any baby cannot suck effectively, since this baby is not removing milk well. Therefore, continue to express your milk until all babies are breastfeeding well. (See the first section "For Effective Breastfeeders" above.) You will also want to pump if milk production is currently low due to a pregnancy or birth complication you experienced.

• Renting a full-size, hospital-grade electric breast pump is usually the most effective (removal of more milk) and efficient (quickest) option for expressing milk.*

• Using a double collection kit to pump both breasts at once saves time and research shows it results in better milk production.

• Even the best portable electric breast pumps with double collection kits were not designed to help "bring in" (establish) milk production in the weeks immediately after birth. They also were not meant for the around-the-clock pumping needed to maintain milk production for babies not yet able to effectively breastfeed. Use a pump designed for the job you need it to do.

• Some mothers pump one breast while one multiple effectively breastfeeds on the other. (A double collection kit can be adjusted for pumping only one breast.) As when using the double collection kit, this may save time and result in better milk production.

• Some mothers pump immediately after all, or several, daily feedings. Other mothers pump about an hour after a feeding. Almost any milk expression routine will work if a mother is consistent.

• How often you pump should depend on each baby's ability to get nourishment at the breast, your family situation, and whether your goal is full or partial breastfeeding. If your goal is to fully nourish your babies with your milk for several weeks or months, a combination of babies' effective breastfeeding and a pump will need to remove milk from both breasts at least 10 times and up to 16 times a day. This translates to a total of at least 140 minutes spent with each effectively breastfeeding baby or for pumping sessions. To establish or maintain adequate milk production for partial breastfeeding, milk should be removed from your breasts at least 8 times a day for a total of at least 100 to 120 minutes.

---

* Any rental fee is quickly made up by what it would cost to purchase infant formula for multiples. In addition, many insurance companies reimburse for breast pump rental if an explanatory letter from the pediatric care provider accompanies the reimbursement claim. (See Chapter 11, "Breastfeeding in the Newborn Intensive Care Unit," for general guidelines about using a breast pump.)

- Most mothers find pumping sessions last about 10 to 20 minutes. Pump one to two minutes past the point when you obtain no milk and then stop. If you often obtain a fair amount of milk beyond a 20-minute session, speak to a lactation consultant before cutting back on the number or length of sessions.
- If you do not have time for a complete pumping session, a few minutes spent pumping is better than skipping a session completely.
- If your goal is to fully breastfeed your babies but for now you can only meet the feeding/pumping quota for partial breastfeeding, give yourself a break. Meet the goal for partial breastfeeding now. When you are able, increase the number of (effective) breastfeeding or pumping sessions. Most mothers find milk production increases within days of adding extra breastfeeding or pumping sessions.

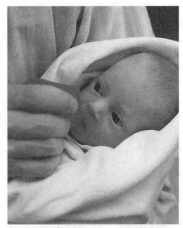

Cup-feeding a tiny baby.

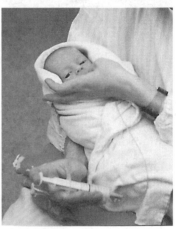

Syringe-feeding with tube taped to mother's finger.

You may be able to reduce the number of pumping sessions or spend less total time pumping once one or more multiples is breastfeeding well. However, *you should continue to pump every day as long as any baby continues to have difficulty breastfeeding.* Your body still needs the reminder that it is making milk for multiple babies.

Alternative Feeding Methods

Any baby not yet able to get the nourishment he needs through direct breastfeeding can be fed your milk, or an infant formula, by another method for some or all feedings. Ideally, your milk is available for alternative feedings, but it is not always possible to achieve the

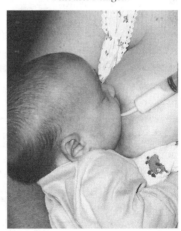

Syringe-feeding at the breast.

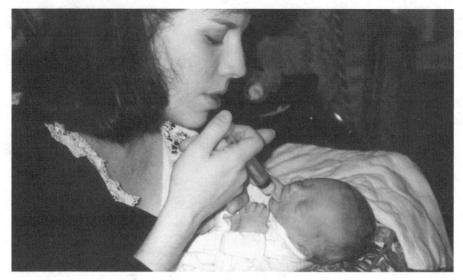

Feeding with a syringe.

If any baby needs additional milk until production catches up with baby's breastfeeding ability, it is rarely necessary to offer it after every breastfeeding.

ideal when providing for multiple babies. When plentiful milk production is delayed or you are unable to pump as often as needed, another source of nutrition has to be used until milk production improves. Once an initial breastfeeding difficulty is resolved, it may take extra time to increase milk production so there is enough for multiples. Ask your babies' health care provider about supplements if there is not enough of your expressed milk for all alternative feedings.

There are many methods for feeding expressed human milk or formula to the babies. However, some methods are less likely to interfere with the oral (mouth) behaviors babies use during effective breastfeeding. Most mothers prefer a feeding method that does not compound a feeding difficulty a baby already has. They also do not want to use a method that may create a new problem. Ideally, an alternative feeding method reinforces the oral behaviors the baby will use for effective breastfeeding.

There are exceptions. If you have to get nourishment into a baby who is in danger of becoming dehydrated or one whose weight gain is severely compromised, you must use whichever method gets food into the baby. You can introduce a different feeding method once the baby is hydrated and gaining weight.

Work with a La Leche League Leader or a lactation consultant if you must use an alternative feeding method. Many mothers are unfamiliar with all the alternatives and several methods require a demonstration for correct use. The incorrect use of any method, including bottle-feeding, may create physical stress for a baby.

Mothers of multiples have used one or more of the following options when any of their babies were not yet breastfeeding well.

Commercial or "homemade" devices for delivering nourishment while a baby sucks on a thin tube taped at breast or to a parent's finger.
- "At breast" devices can be an excellent way to provide supplemental nourishment to the baby who seems to have the basic idea, or for the baby who breastfeeds effectively but whose mother is not yet producing enough milk. The baby gets extra calories while "telling" the breast to make more milk. (These devices do *not* "teach" a baby how to breastfeed.) One commercial device includes two tubes—one for each breast, which may be ideal when two effectively breastfeeding multiples need supplementary fluids. Sources for commercial "at breast" tube feeding devices are listed under "Equipment" in Resources. Homemade devices consist of a thin tube, such as an infant feeding tube found in a hospital, which is attached to a syringe or dipped in a bottle/container filled with mother's milk or formula.
- Finger-feeding devices may be used for a baby who can suck but is not yet breastfeeding well. Baby receives nourishment while sucking on the thin tube taped to mother's or a feeding helper's (very clean) finger. As the baby sucks on the finger, milk is drawn through the tube and swallowed. Some devices allow the person feeding the baby to deliver a small amount of milk if baby stops sucking on the finger as a "reminder" to keep eating.

Direct feeding devices that deliver milk directly into a baby's mouth.
- Devices used for direct feeding include a spoon, medicine dropper, syringe, or cup. Although most of these devices are readily available, it is important to let a baby set the pace of feedings when using any of these devices.
- Spoons and medicine droppers may be available in most households but neither holds much liquid. Both work well but using them may become tedious. Some mothers use a hollow medicine spoon that will hold more, or they fill several droppers and line them up before beginning a feeding. Another drawback of a medicine dropper is that the bulb end can be difficult to keep clean.
- Syringes come in various sizes—from about 1 ml to more than 20 ml (2/3 oz). Feeding/oral and periodontal syringes are available in pharmacies or medical supply shops. If you cannot buy them over the counter in your area, your baby's pediatric care provider may be able to "prescribe" them for you or they can be ordered online.
- When using a dropper, medicine spoon, or syringe, direct a drop or two of milk into the buccal space of the lower jaw—the space between the gum and the lower lip/cheek. Adapt the pace of the feeding to the baby's

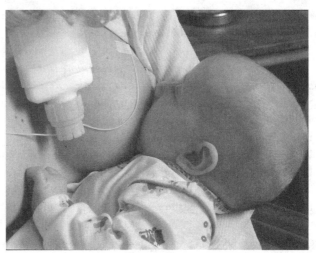

Using an at-breast nursing supplementer (SNS).

responses. Once a baby figures out the milk is coming, the baby indicates readiness for a faster feeding pace. You will quickly learn how much to offer at a time.

- Cup-feeding of newborns is not common in Western cultures. However, it is used to feed liquids to larger preterm or sick newborns in many countries, and research has shown it is a safe feeding option. A small glass or flexible plastic cup, such as a medicine cup or shot glass is used for cup feedings. (Check the rim of the cup to avoid rough edges before cup-feeding a baby.)

  ❑ The idea is for a baby to sip or lap the fluid in the cup with its tongue, so only awake, alert babies should be cup-fed. Studies show that spillage may be a problem, which may be an issue if keeping track of the amount a baby takes is important.

Using bottles

- Feeding babies with bottles using artificial nipples (teats), especially in the first several weeks after birth, is associated with a greater number of breastfeeding problems and early weaning. However, some amount of bottle-feeding may be difficult to avoid when supplementing multiples for one or more weeks. Sometimes bottle-feeding is introduced as a step in the development of appropriate sucking behavior for a particular multiple.

- If a baby receives a fast flow of liquid through a bottle nipple (teat), she must adjust her tongue and jaw movements in order to control the flow of liquid in her mouth and throat so she can take a breath. Learning mouth (oral) movements that are different from those used for breastfeeding can interfere with an ability to latch on deeply to the breast or suckle effectively at the breast.

- If breastfeeding is the goal but bottle-feeding is used for any supplementation, then reinforce breastfeeding oral behaviors during bottle-feeding as much as possible by using a slow-flow (stage 1/newborn) brand of nipples (teats) to minimize the interference with breastfeeding oral behaviors.
- Unfortunately, the term "slow-flow" on the label does not guarantee a slow flow rate, so test the flow from a nipple (teat) before each use. Check for: 1) leakage where the teat fits on the bottle, 2) the time between drops when the bottle is held at an angle, and 3) the "heaviness" of the stream when the liquid-filled teat is compressed/squeezed between your fingers. There should be no leakage and at least 2 to 3 seconds between drops when the bottle is held at an angle. When the teat is compressed, the stream through the teat hole should look very "thin." If the flow rate is too rapid or the stream is too heavy/thick, choose another teat or try a different brand.
- Watch the baby during bottle-feedings. Signs that a baby is having difficulty controlling the flow through the teat include 1) a lot of drooling out of the mouth while feeding, 2) jaw clenching/biting down, 3) sputtering, and 4) coughing or gagging. A baby who gulps liquid and finishes a bottle-feeding in fewer than 5 minutes is probably getting too much, too quickly. Again, choose another teat or try a different brand to slow things down.

No Method Is Perfect

There is no "best" alternative feeding method. Some methods work better in one situation, or for one baby, than another. And just as alternative feeding methods may

---

Guidelines for Bottle-Feeding the Breastfed Baby

You (or a feeding helper) should:
- Place baby in an almost upright (sitting to semi-sitting) position with one hand supporting baby's neck and shoulders.
- Gently touch the tip of baby's nose with the bottle teat before stroking down from baby's nose and over her upper lip to stimulate the rooting reflex, which encourages baby's mouth to open wide. Let baby "latch on" to the bottle teat as you want baby to latch onto your breast.
- Baby is likely to pause after a few minutes of feeding. Take advantage of this natural pause to give baby a sense of the ebb and flow that occurs during breastfeeding by stopping the feeding and perhaps even angling the bottle down for 20 to 30 seconds until baby indicates readiness to resume the feeding. Do not immediately jiggle the bottle teat in baby's mouth to "remind" her to resume feeding.
- Bottle-feedings should not be rushed. If the average newborn spends 10 to 30 minutes "emptying" the first breast when breastfeeding, nature may be trying to tell parents something. Take another look at bottle-teat flow rate when baby empties a 60 to 120 ml (2 to 4 oz) bottle in less than 10 minutes.

enable you and any of your multiples to work through a breastfeeding difficulty, they may also prolong a feeding problem or create a new problem.

In addition to the different tongue and jaw movements a baby may use with alternative feeding methods, other feeding methods may prolong or create a breast-feeding problem because:

- The breastfed baby must wait for the let-down reflex; other feeding methods offer a baby *instant gratification*.
    - ❑ To avoid or lessen the issue of instant gratification, some mothers find it helpful to pump for a minute or two just prior to breastfeeding to hasten the let-down reflex.
    - ❑ This pumping may also help any multiple who has difficulty controlling the flow during let-down or for a baby who might benefit from more hindmilk.
- The breastfed baby must open wide and stick out her tongue if she is to latch on and feed correctly; a baby barely has to open her mouth when fed by most other methods.
    - ❑ Encourage baby to start with a wide open mouth when using an alternative feeding method. Stroke from the tip of baby's nose down over the top lip to stimulate the rooting reflex, which encourages a baby to open wide.
    - ❑ Once open wide, wait for baby to extend, or stick out, her tongue before offering the spoon, syringe, bottle, etc.

Additional Tips

Let family and friends help manage babies for other types of feedings.

Unless you are supplementing with a feeding-tube device taped to your breast, let family and friends help manage babies for other types of feedings. Their assistance will free you for "practice" breastfeedings with each baby, pumping to maintain adequate milk production, and more skin-to-skin contact with babies between feedings or pumping sessions. Extra skin-to-skin contact with you is particularly important for any multiple who is fed by a helper more often than the other(s).

Offer available human milk before offering any artificial infant formula. When there is not enough expressed milk to fully feed every baby, mothers of multiples sometimes have to make hard decisions about which baby will get how much. A baby who has been sick or one who has more difficulty digesting infant formula may need more of the expressed human milk than the other(s).

To avoid wasting any of your milk, do not mix expressed milk with infant formula. Also, you may want to keep its taste and scent separate. Offer your milk first and then follow it if necessary with the artificial formula. (See Chapter 18, "Full and Partial Breastfeeding.")

As Each Baby Improves

It may seem that one or more of your babies will never figure out how to breastfeed. However, patience and persistence almost always pay off. You will probably find that each
baby makes sudden breastfeeding progress, levels off,
makes progress, levels off, makes progress, and so on.

It is almost always possible to make up for lost time when multiples or their mother get off to a slow start.

When any multiple seems able to latch on, even if it
takes several tries, and remains awake and interested in
suckling for 5 or more minutes, it may be time to move to
the suggestions for "For Effective Breastfeeders" at the beginning of the chapter.
Consider taking a "babymoon" with one multiple at a time when diaper counts and
weight gain have been appropriate for at least several days to a week and you have
no real concerns about milk production.

A few babies balk if they have been receiving the instant gratification of other
kinds of feedings and then are expected (and ready) to trigger a let-down. Most of
them figure out what to do within a day or two if mother consistently breastfeeds
without offering another alternative. A "reluctant" baby sometimes learns more
quickly if breastfed simultaneously with another multiple. One baby stimulates a let-
down for both. After a few effective simultaneous feedings, most babies get used to
a pause between first latching onto the breast and the increased flow with let-down.

It seems unfair that the mother of multiples, the mother most in need of a good
breastfeeding beginning, is the least likely to get a good start. Although life is not
always fair, it is almost always possible to make up for lost time when multiples or
their mother get off to a slow start. When it is not possible to completely make up
for a slow start, it is possible to combine feeding methods. Partial breastfeeding is
definitely better than no breastfeeding (or mother's milk) at all!

Contact a La Leche League Leader or a lactation consultant to help you. She will
have ideas to help you save time and maintain perspective.

KEY POINTS

❏ Breastfeeding often gets off to a slow start with multiples because preterm delivery or other pregnancy-birth complications are more common.

❏ To make up for a poor start once any baby is able to latch on and suckle well, breastfeed that baby around-the-clock (or more than 10 times in 24 hours) for several days.
  • If there is a need to increase milk production, a feeding tube device at breast allows one or two babies to receive extra calories while each breastfeeds.

  • It may not be necessary to supplement every feeding. Babies' diapers and weight gains are the guide. As milk production improves, gradually cut back on any supplements.

❏ Until all babies breastfeed (remove milk directly from the breast) well:
  • Offer 5 to 15 minute "practice" breastfeeds.

  • Then offer–or let someone else offer–pumped/expressed milk or formula; some feeding methods are less likely to interfere with breastfeeding than others.

❏ Pump your breasts using a rented, hospital-grade electric breast pump and a double collection kit with properly fitted breast flanges/shields until all babies breastfeed well; less frequent pumping may be possible as babies' breastfeeding improves.

❏ It may take time, but most multiples eventually do breastfeed effectively when their mother continues to let all multiples "practice" breastfeeding and remains patient but persistent.

❏ Stay in touch with an LLL Leader or a lactation consultant for both emotional support and hints for the changing breastfeeding situation until all babies can breastfeed well.

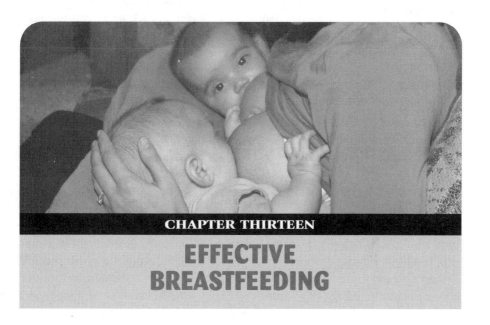

CHAPTER THIRTEEN

EFFECTIVE BREASTFEEDING

It takes time to learn to recognize and adapt to the different, yet normal, approaches of two, three, four, or more babies. Many of the questions LLL Leaders get from worried mothers of multiples are about perceived rather than actual breastfeeding problems. Understanding how milk is produced, what infant behaviors and feeding patterns are considered normal, and how to coordinate multiples' frequent breastfeedings may increase your confidence during the early learning period with your newborns.

Establishing and Maintaining Lactation

Making Enough Milk for Two, Three, or More

When you are lactating, or producing milk, demand for the product (your milk) determines the amount your body makes. Milk is produced within each breast in cells that cluster to form numerous balloon-shaped alveoli. One such cluster is called an alveolus. These cells take nutrients from your blood to make milk that is then secreted into the lumen, which looks similar to the inside of a balloon, of each alveolus. The milk stored in the lumen empties into small milk ducts, which in turn empty into larger ducts that transport milk to an even larger mammary duct that eventually opens at the nipple tip.

An alveolus is essentially a milk-making factory and the lumen its warehouse.

There are about 15 to 25 lobes, or groupings containing numerous milk-making alveoli, in each breast that ultimately empty into the mammary ducts that open at the nipple tip. It is through these openings, or nipple pores, that milk is released during "let-down," which is also referred to as the milk-ejection reflex (MER). Milk ejection occurs when a baby's sucking triggers the release of the hormone oxytocin, which causes muscle cells around the alveoli to contract, forcing milk stored in the alveolar lumen into the ducts and eventually out through nipple pores.

When a baby breastfeeds effectively, the breasts are "told" to produce more milk in two ways: 1. The hormone prolactin is released, which stimulates the alveolar cells to make milk, and 2. The removal of available milk from the alveolar lumen signals the milk-making cells of that alveolus to increase production.

An alveolus is essentially a milk-making factory and the lumen its warehouse. When the milk is removed from this "warehouse" during breastfeeding (or pumping), biochemical messengers inform the "factory" that the product is in demand and to step up production. However, if milk builds up in the warehouse because of infrequent breastfeeding (or pumping) or a baby's ineffective sucking, messengers let the factory know that demand for the product is down and the factory slows production. If no milk is removed for several days, the alveoli "factory" begins to close down.

When multiple newborns breastfeed effectively, they kick the factory into high gear. The more often multiple babies breastfeed, the more milk the "factory" makes. The "factory" usually can produce enough for all multiples as long as their mother trusts her babies by putting them to breast whenever they "ask"/cue to feed, or she expresses her milk frequently because one or more is not yet feeding effectively or is not yet able to breastfeed.

Feeding Behaviors
Getting It "Right"

You must look for normal feeding behaviors when breastfeeding each multiple yet also recognize normal variations in their individual patterns.

A baby latches onto the breast effectively by using the lower jaw and tongue to draw the entire nipple and a mouthful of areola into its mouth. To do this correctly, a baby's mouth must gape wide open. Stroke the baby's upper lip with your nipple or a finger to stimulate a reflex that will cause him to open wide and stick his tongue over his lower gum. As this occurs, bring the baby deeply onto the breast in one motion. When latched on properly, the baby will look as if he has a mouth full of areola, the angle at the corner of baby's mouth will be wide, and the tip of his nose and his entire chin will touch your breast. When properly latched on, the baby's

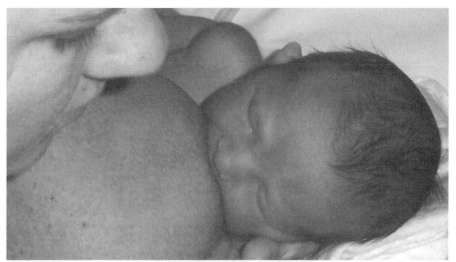

When a baby is breastfeeding effectively, he takes a large mouthful of breast tissue.

tongue and palate do not come into contact with the nipple tip, so effective breast-feeding should not hurt your nipples.

As the baby sucks, his lower jaw and tongue compress the areola up against his hard palate. His tongue works with a wave-like motion from the front to the back of his mouth and then releases, creating the suction that draws the milk through the pores in the nipple tip. When a baby is suckling effectively, you will see most of the "action" in his lower jaw and throat and you will notice his jaw moving up and down at a rhythm of about one suck per second. A drawing in/dimpling at the cheeks, a lot of movement/fluttering of the upper lip, or a suck rhythm that remains at more than one suck per second after the first one to two minutes of breastfeeding is seen with less effective or ineffective breastfeeding/milk removal. For illustrations of effective latch-on, see Chapter 16.

Typical Feeding Patterns for Effective Breastfeeding

There is a range of "normal" feeding behaviors within each feeding itself, and within a 24-hour period, for an individual baby, yet certain behaviors almost always are present during effective breastfeeding. Since you will be working with two or more new learners, you must look for these behaviors when breastfeeding each multiple yet also recognize normal variations in their individual patterns.

Each baby who is breastfeeding effectively generally:

- Wakes and cues for at least 8, up to about 12, daily breastfeedings by the second 24 hours after birth.

Some babies cue for and do well with eight feedings a day; others require 10 to 12, and occasionally up to 14, feedings daily.

- Assumes a nutritive sucking pattern (with let-down/MER) in a rhythm of about one suck per second, pausing for a breath every several sucks, within one to two minutes of beginning to breastfeed.
- Remains awake and sustains almost continuous sucking for at least the first 5 to 10 minutes.
- Detaches from/lets go of the breast without mother's help after 10 to 30 minutes of feeding (actual suckling) at the first breast.
- Demonstrates satisfaction (a full tummy) by relaxing as the feeding progresses, until sleepy or asleep by the time of self-detachment from the breast.

Typical variations for each multiple occur in the total number of 8 to 12 feedings each baby desires in a 24 hour period and in the total time taken for an individual feeding. Some babies cue for and do well with eight feedings a day; others require 10 to 12, and occasionally up to 14, feedings daily.

Most newborns breastfeed for at least 20 to 30 minutes on the first breast, others feed a little longer, and some are satisfied after 10 to 15 minutes. Any baby may sometimes "ask" for more after the first breast for some feedings yet act satisfied after feeding on one breast for others. He might take 30 minutes to feed for one feeding and self-detach after 10 minutes for another.

A few newborns, and many older, more efficient breastfeeders, act as though they are going through a fast-food, drive-through window and gobble all they want in one 5 to 10 minute cycle of sucking. Most newborns feed for five to six minutes, pause and perhaps snooze for a few minutes while still latched on, and then resume feeding through another cycle or two (or even more) within a 20 to 30 minute feeding before self-detaching from the first breast. These "gourmet" babies seem to enjoy the ambiance of the "restaurant" and space enthusiastic suckling so their meal arrives like different courses.

The challenge of multiples is that one may be a gobbler and another a gourmet. One may be happy with seven to nine daily breastfeedings, but another may need at least 12 feedings every day. One may breastfeed at regular two to three hour intervals; another "clusters" several feedings into a couple of hours here, then spaces a feeding three to five hours apart there.

The feeding styles of the multiples described above are both within the "normal" range, but it can become confusing when keeping track of two or more babies having different styles. Any individual style may be considered a normal variation as long as each baby breastfeeds effectively and continues to grow and develop. However, it may be reassuring to measure if all of the babies are getting enough when breastfeeding.

Mothers have breastfed for thousands of years without worrying that their breasts were not equipped with ounce (oz) or ml markers. They simply watched what came out at a baby's other end. Any baby producing enough daily wet diapers (voids) and bowel movements (stools) generally is getting enough of his mother's milk.

In the first few days after birth a baby may wet only two to four diapers in a 24-hour period. These early wet diapers may be barely damp and the urine may look darker and more concentrated. As your milk "comes in," you will notice wet diapers increasing in number and in the degree of saturation throughout the first week. By the end of the first week each multiple should produce at least six soaking wet diapers in 24 hours. Each also should pass at least two to three stools/bowel movements during their first few days, but by the end of the first week through at least the first four to six weeks expect each to pass three to five or more loose, mustard-yellow, seedy stools if getting only your milk. (Expect a couple of large stools and a few small ones.)

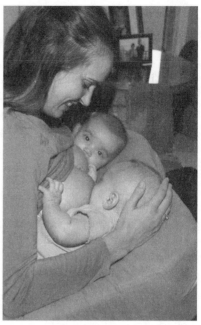

A nursing pillow helps this mother feed both babies at once.

If the babies latch on and breastfeed well, but you still feel concerned about their intakes of your milk, weigh each baby nude one or more times a week. Always use the same scale to be certain that the weight gains are accurate. When their diaper counts are appropriate, you should see each baby gain at least 1/2 to one ounce (15 to 30 gm) a day, or 4 to 7 ounces (120 to 210 gm) a week, by 24 hours of when your milk "comes in" at two to four days after their birth. You may need to take daily weights, or weigh one or more before and after some feedings, if any are having difficulty breastfeeding or are not gaining appropriate weight. A more sensitive scale is available for rent in these situations. (See Chapter 15, "Breastfeeding Difficulties in Young Babies.")

Keeping Track

Making sure that two or more new learners are breastfeeding often enough and having appropriate diaper counts in the first weeks can be confusing. To feel reassured and gain a sense of each baby's breastfeeding pattern, monitor each baby's feedings, wet diapers, and stools on a simple, checklist style 24-hour chart. (A sample is included in the Appendix).

Make enough copies of the chart to last for several days to several weeks. (This is a good task for Daddy.) Writing babies' names on charts is one way to identify each one's chart, or print the chart on different-colored papers and then

> To gain a sense of each baby's breastfeeding pattern, monitor each baby's feedings, wet diapers, and stools on a simple checklist-style chart.

assign each multiple a specific color. When things get hectic–an everyday occurrence with young multiples—it may be easier to identify a color than search for a name. Date each chart and note the babies' weekly (or daily) weights when taken.

You may toss the charts in the trash once each baby has established a weight gain and you feel confident that each is breastfeeding effectively. At times it may be necessary to maintain a chart for one but not for another. Some mothers continue to monitor their multiples' daily feedings and urine and stool output. They find that charting helps them recognize their babies' emerging feeding and wake-sleep patterns. The charts provide a visible reminder that the babies' feeding styles and daily routines are improving from week to week.

Frequency Days: Sudden "Demand" for Extra Feedings

> Most adults vary the number of times and the amount they eat from day to day. Babies are no different.

Just when you thought a bit of order was emerging from the chaos, your babies suddenly demand several extra breastfeedings a day. They may also seem fussier. Any semblance of a daily routine flies right out the window. You worry that you are losing your milk and wonder if your body can really make enough milk for multiples.

Never fear. It is not unusual for babies who have been breastfeeding well to suddenly want to breastfeed several more times in a day. The most likely cause is a frequency day. When each baby "asks" to eat more often for several days, it is often because of a growth spurt. Most adults vary the number of times and the amount they eat from day to day. Babies are no different. Within several days most babies return to fewer daily feedings. It is not unusual for one or more to actually feed a little less often than she did prior to the frequency spurt.

Anticipating Frequency Spurts

Babies generally experience about three frequency spurts before four months. The first one occurs at about 10 to 21 days, another at some time between four to six weeks, and again at about three months. A fourth may occur around six months of age. Preterm babies may not experience frequency spurts on this schedule, but they can be expected to have several such spurts in the early months.

Multiples' frequency spurts tend to last longer than the two to three day period that is common for a single infant. When two or more multiples go through a frequency spurt simultaneously, the time may stretch to four to seven days. If multiples "piggy-back" frequency spurts, one experiences the typical two to three day increase in feedings while the other(s) breastfeed as usual. As the frequency spurt ends for one baby, who now resumes a routine of fewer feedings, another multiple begins a frequency spurt and increases the number of feedings for a few more days.

Getting through Frequency Days and Spurts

Frequency spurts often take mothers of multiples by surprise. When busy accommodating two or more babies who suddenly want to eat more often, they don't have time to realize they are in the midst of a frequency day or spurt until it is over. A mother may think she's "losing" her milk and consider supplementing her babies' diet if a frequency spurt is not recognized for what it is. However, this is not the time to supplement or offer solid food.

> **Do not try to impose an inflexible feeding schedule, since this may interfere with milk production.**

You cannot go wrong when you let each baby be your guide. Breastfeed each baby when each cues to feed. Do not try to impose an inflexible feeding schedule, since this may interfere with milk production.

Stop and examine your situation any time a baby suddenly wants to breastfeed more frequently or whenever you find yourself wondering whether you are making enough milk. Mothers often say that just the realization that one is in the midst of a frequency spurt or day can help to weather this temporary challenge.

Even when a mother recognizes that her babies are in the midst of a frequency spurt, she may wonder after several days if she will get through it. "Survival" seems less of an issue if someone is available to help hold babies or to take over household tasks. Since the timing of frequency spurts can be anticipated to some extent, plan for help in advance. That way all you have to do is shout "frequency spurt" into the phone and help will come running.

> **A mother may think she's "losing" her milk and consider supplementing her babies' diet if a frequency spurt is not recognized for what it is.**

Thus far, every mother of multiples has survived her babies' frequency spurts, although few ever forget them. Fortunately, most spurts are followed by a period of relative calm for mother and babies. (Frequency spurts for older babies are discussed in Chapter 28, "Breastfeeding, Starting Solids, and Weaning.")

Most women can make enough milk for several babies, since milk production is based on milk removal. Multiple babies breastfeeding multiple times each day results in milk production for that number of multiples. Although normal babies' feeding patterns vary, most babies breastfeed about 8 to 12 times a day. When they breastfeed effectively, it is reflected in their diapers. Charting the number of feedings and the diaper count for each baby can help assure that all babies are getting enough milk. If you are ever not certain whether one or more babies is breastfeeding correctly, read Chapter 15, "Breastfeeding Difficulties in Young Babies," and call an LLL Leader or a lactation consultant for help and encouragement.

KEY POINTS

❑ Milk production depends on milk removal/"emptying" from the breast by breastfeeding or pumping/expressing milk.
  • The more milk removed, the more milk the breast makes.

  • When milk is not removed or not enough is removed, the breast slows production and makes less.

❑ When breastfeeding well, expect that in 24 hours each multiple will:
  • Breastfeed 8 to 12 times.

  • Soak 6 or more diapers with pale yellow urine.

  • Pass 3 to 5 or more loose, yellow stools/bowel movements of varying size.

  • Gain more than 1/2 oz (15 gm).

❑ You may want to keep track of each baby's feedings and diaper counts on a simple checklist chart until each is gaining weight well.

❑ Between birth and six months babies have several "frequency spurts" when they want to breastfeed more than 12 times in 24 hours.
  • The best way to deal with a frequency spurt is to continue to let each baby breastfeed based on feeding cues, even when that means additional feedings.

  • These spurts last only a few days.

❑ If you ever wonder whether your multiples are breastfeeding effectively, read Chapter 15 and contact a La Leche League Leader or a lactation consultant in your area.

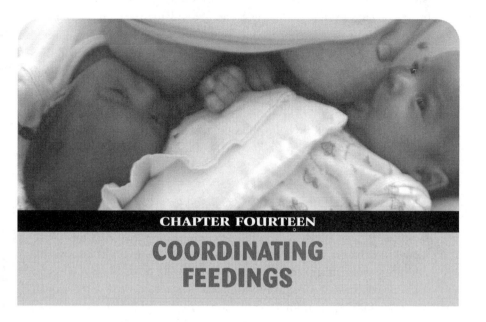

CHAPTER FOURTEEN

COORDINATING FEEDINGS

The breastfeeding "learning period" often lasts longer with multiples–for both babies and mother. A mother and her single newborn usually learn how to work as a breastfeeding "couple" within three to six weeks. Don't be concerned if it feels as though you and your babies are still using a learner permit at three to six months! When you have double, triple, or quadruple the number of babies, it only makes sense that it may take double, triple, or quadruple the time to learn to work as two or more breastfeeding couples.

Coordinating breastfeeding with multiples is the easy part–virtually anything works. You may be amazed at the adaptability of your fantastic female body! As long as each baby latches on and sucks well (effectively removes milk), all you have to do is respond to each one's feeding cues by offering the breast. (If any baby is not yet breastfeeding effectively, see Chapter 12 "Making Up for a Poor Start.")

Feeding Rotation

Mothers of multiples tend to use a variation of one of the three feeding rotations explained below. Some mothers never change how they rotate their multiples at the breast, but most adapt the "plan" in response to babies' growth and their own milk production. Since almost anything works, develop a feeding rotation plan that suits you and meets your babies' needs. The most common feeding rotations plans are to:

1. **Alternate babies and breasts for every feeding.** For instance, Baby A [and quad C] begins feeding on the right breast, and Baby B [and quad D] begins on the left. The opposite, or second, breast is offered to any baby indicating interest after self-detachment from the first breast, even when another multiple has already fed on the opposite side or is not yet ready to feed. At the next feeding, Baby A [and quad C] begins on the left breast and Baby B [and quad D] begins on the right. If Baby A fed from both breasts before Baby B fed at all, Baby B will probably indicate readiness to feed first at the subsequent feeding. Likewise, quads C and D are likely to wake first for the next feeding.

   - A variation of this plan is to *offer the fullest breast to the first baby to indicate readiness* for a feeding. Mothers of odd-numbered multiples, such as triplets or quintuplets, often continue to use some variation of this plan until their babies wean. Many mothers use a variation of this plan for the first few weeks after birth, especially if one or all babies do not breastfeed effectively or when one (or more) indicates a need to feed at the second breast. Once lactation (milk production) is well established, some multiples overfeed if given both breasts during a single feeding. When this occurs, many mothers move to rotation plan 2 or 3.

2. **Alternate babies and breasts every 24 hours.** Feed Baby A (and C) on the right breast and Baby B (and D) on the left today, and switch who feeds on which breast tomorrow. (If any baby cues to feed again soon after "finishing," she would go back on the same breast.) Most mothers like this plan because each baby affects milk production in both breasts, yet it is easy to keep track of who ate where and when. Mothers with triplets sometimes adapt the plan by rotating breasts and babies every 8 to 12 hours.

3. **Assign a specific breast to each of even-numbered multiples.** Each breast then adapts to that multiple's intake. Although assigning a breast to each may sound the least complicated, and it has worked well for many mothers, it may have the most drawbacks. Therefore, it may be best to reserve this option unless one or more infants shows a strong preference for a particular breast.

   - Mothers may experience significant differences in breast sizes for a few months when their babies' food intakes differ. Although this problem is merely cosmetic when babies are gaining weight adequately, it may also be a sign of decreased milk production in one breast if any multiple breastfeeds ineffectively.

- Once used to a particular breast, some babies will refuse to feed from both breasts if another baby is unable or unwilling to breastfeed for a period of time, such as for one multiple's nursing strike. (Nursing strikes appear to be more common with multiples. See "Nursing Strikes" in Chapter 28.)
  - ❏ If assigning each baby a breast works best for you, alternate feeding positions on occasion. This provides the babies with the stimulation and sense of alternating breasts.

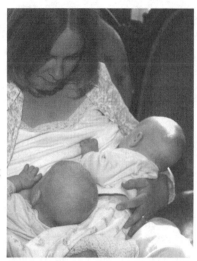

These babies are nursing in the parallel or layered hold. (See descriptions of positions later in this chapter.)

- Consider assigning each a breast if any multiple *frequently* has difficulty handling the milk-ejection reflex (letdown), is uncomfortably gassy, passes frothy stools, or shows other strong signs of intestinal discomfort. Infant regulation of milk production in a single breast sometimes diminishes these symptoms for the affected multiple.

Feeding Routine vs. Schedule

Unrestricted "on cue," sometimes referred to as "demand," breastfeeding is best during the early weeks after birth. It is not unusual for one multiple to need to breastfeed more often than another. Always responding to the babies' feeding cues by offering the breast helps establish sufficient milk production for multiples.

Respecting multiples' cues can help you develop a sense of each baby as an individual with a distinct feeding pattern and sleep-wake cycle. Putting babies off in an effort to lengthen the time between feedings or develop a schedule can result in insufficient milk production and babies who do not gain enough weight.

> Respecting multiples' cues can help you develop a sense of each baby as an individual with a distinct feeding pattern and sleep-wake cycle.

Mothers of monozygotic (identical) multiples tend to find their babies fall into a similar feeding routine without their help. This makes sense since body clocks have a genetic component. When body clocks have babies awake and hungry at about the same times, simultaneous feedings can help (see below). It is not surprising that dizygotic (fraternal) multiples may develop similar or quite different routines, since they share only half of their genetic material. If your babies fall into the "different routines" category:

- Try waking one and feeding him along with the other to save time.

- Breastfeed one alone, and then immediately wake and feed another.
- Some mothers combine unrestricted "on cue" feeding with these more "scheduled" feedings. For instance, a mother may feed "on cue" during the night, but wake one to feed with or after another during the day. Another mother might feed in response to each baby's cues during the day but wake both at once during the night. The part of the day when babies are fed on cue and the part that is more scheduled depends on what works best for an individual mother and her babies.
- There are pros and cons to disrupting a baby's body clock. Feeding babies together, or one after another, may result in extra minutes for yourself and other family members. Yet it also means you must always deal with at least two babies at once, which can seem overwhelming. This routine also increases the possibility of interfering with the body clock of a baby who is ready to lengthen the time between feedings or sleep longer at night. On the other hand, feeding babies separately provides the opportunity to hold one baby and gaze into his face, a luxury you will enjoy, but it also means you may be constantly caring for a baby if one tends to wake just as another falls asleep.
- Some babies do not seem to be bothered if awakened to eat with, or just after, another. Others protest any manipulation of their natural routines. Some may be easy to wake during early infancy yet object to this as they get older. And others cannot tolerate changes to their natural feeding patterns when they are tiny, but handle them just fine several weeks or months later.
- If manipulating feeding routines is not working, give yourself and the babies a break. You only create extra work and feel more frustration when you persist in wanting to do something that does not seem to be working. If the babies' routines do not evolve into one that also works for you, you can try again later.
- Mothers of triplets, quadruplets, or more may have to breastfeed on a schedule with babies fed every three hours for part or all of the day and night. (Some mothers of higher-order multiples breastfeed "on cue" for part of the day or night.) If one baby is not content to wait three hours, a mother may breastfeed that baby earlier when she is able, or she may complement a feeding with her expressed milk or infant formula. (See Chapter 18, "Full and Partial Breastfeeding.")

Simultaneous "Twogether" Feedings

Feeding two multiples at once saves time and babies' tears when two are hungry or need attention at once. Some mothers breastfeed simultaneously at every feeding. Other mothers always feed their multiples separately. They may enjoy the individual time with each baby, find it easier to manage, or have babies with very different routines. Most mothers combine simultaneous and separate feedings. As with other aspects of breastfeeding, the beauty of feeding multiples simultaneously is in its ability to adapt to meet multiples' changing needs.

Some health professionals think mothers make more milk if they breastfeed multiples simultaneously. They base this belief on research that mothers produce more milk if they pump both breasts at once when using a breast pump. However, many mothers have breastfed multiples individually for all, or most, feedings and produced more than enough milk to completely feed all of them. The important issue in effectively breastfeeding multiples is to respond to the babies' individual feeding cues, which usually means breastfeeding each at least 8 to 12 times in 24 hours.

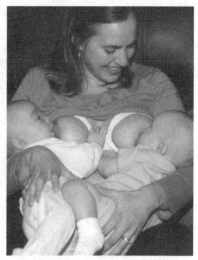

These babies are demonstrating the "V" hold, a variation of the double cradle hold.

Your babies may have strong opinions about any decision to breastfeed two of them together. Some babies seem to resist simultaneous feedings, yet other multiples refuse to breastfeed unless they hear or touch another who is feeding on the opposite breast.

- Wait until at least one baby is able to latch on easily and suckle (remove milk) well before breastfeeding two at once. Occasionally, simultaneous breastfeeding begins the first day, since some babies latch on and breastfeed quite well from birth. Many multiples continue to need a bit of help during breastfeeding for several days, weeks, or months.

> **You are alone with the baby you currently have eye contact with.**

  ❏ It is more difficult to physically manage simultaneous feedings than feeding one. When two babies still need guidance to latch on deeply, trying to feed them together can result in sore or damaged nipples for the mother.
  ❏ It is more difficult to monitor whether each baby is suckling well during simultaneous feeds, and poor weight gain for one or both babies could occur.
- Often a mother needs time to feel comfortable and learn to coordinate each baby alone before breastfeeding two at once. If babies latch on well but you are not yet ready, wait awhile. There is no reason to rush.
- If simultaneous feeding was previously helpful but is not currently working for you or the babies, introduce more individual breastfeeding. You can always try simultaneous feedings again later.

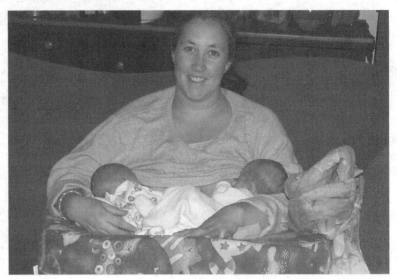

These babies are in the double cradle or crisscross hold.

- Simultaneous feedings are very helpful for multiples with similar body clocks. It is difficult to enjoy feeding Baby A if Baby B is breaking your heart with cries of hunger. Of course, rushing poor Baby A through her feeding may then lead to feelings of guilt while feeding Baby B.

  ❑ If you or your babies are not yet ready for simultaneous breastfeeding, but two (or more) are hungry at the same time, rotate babies onto and off the breast every few minutes until everyone is satisfied. Also, mother's touch often calms a crying baby who is waiting to be fed. (See Chapter 20, "Comforting a Fussy Baby," for ideas.)

  ❑ Ask for help with simultaneous feeding when two babies are hungry and either is still learning to breastfeed well. An extra pair of hands to support Baby A after he latches on allows you to concentrate on helping Baby B get started. If one or both has difficulty staying latched on, it may be helpful for someone to support one or both babies' heads in place for a few minutes or for the entire feeding. (Babies' heads can be supported by placing fingers on their neck, at the base of their heads. Some babies object to a hand on the back of their heads by pulling off of the breast.)

  > **The important issue in effectively breastfeeding multiples is to respond to the babies' individual feeding cues.**

- Mothers often express concern that they are not able to spend individual time with each baby during simultaneous breastfeeding, but that is not really true. Since it is impossible to interact with more than one baby at a time, anyway, spend some individual time with each.

❏ You are alone with whichever baby you currently have eye contact with. Spend a few minutes talking just to that baby. Then make eye contact and talk to the other.

❏ Simultaneous feeding may actually help you get to know each baby better, since you no longer feel as though you must rush breastfeeding one to feed another. Everyone can enjoy the time together.

Getting Comfortable

It usually takes time to learn to physically manage simultaneous feeding. Experiment with different chairs (or a sofa), pillows, and feeding positions until you find an arrangement that works best for you.

• Always position babies in a way that brings them to the breast–not you (your breasts) to them. Leaning over babies or placing yourself in an awkward position is not conducive to comfort during 8 to 12 daily simultaneous breastfeedings.

• If you are feeding *triplets or more,* particular two-baby combinations may work together better than others. Also, a certain feeding position may work for one combination of babies while a different position works best for another combination.

• Most mothers recommend a roomy sofa or chair with a stool or ottoman for propping feet up. *An upholstered recliner may be ideal.* When adjusted to a semi-reclining position, gravity helps hold the babies in place and a footrest is built in.

• Sitting on a bean-bag type chair that molds to the body or sitting on the floor while leaning back against a wall or sofa are comfortable positions for some mothers.

• Experiment with various sizes and types of pillows, placing them across your lap and under your arms. Pillows should help you relax during feedings by supporting your head, back, or legs to relieve muscle tension. They also become "extra arms" that can prop, support, and hold babies in position.

❏ Some mothers prefer using bed pillows that "cradle" the babies. With each baby on a separate pillow, a mother can pull the second baby to her once the first baby is latched on. A baby who has drifted to sleep is less likely to be disrupted if mother can move the pillow he is on slightly away from her body, but where she can still see and touch him, until the second baby finishes breastfeeding. (You may want to work with bed or sofa pillows already available at home before investing in a commercial breastfeeding pillow.)

❏ Many mothers swear by "nursing pillows" designed specifically for breastfeeding twins. To feed two babies at once, you will need a breastfeeding pillow with a wide shelf that wraps around the waist and under the arms. (Smaller, contoured pillows were designed for feeding only one baby.) Many recommend a pillow having a belt that fastens in back, although a few mothers feel "trapped" with a belted breastfeeding pillow. A firmer pillow will support babies' heads better. Some brands have a gentle slope to "hold" babies near mother's body, but these pillows also have a flat underside, which some mothers prefer.

❑ A few mothers combine a breastfeeding pillow to "hold" the babies in place with bed pillows under their arms or at their backs to relieve tension.

Simultaneous Feeding Positions

There are three basic simultaneous positions used when sitting. Most other position descriptions are variations of these.

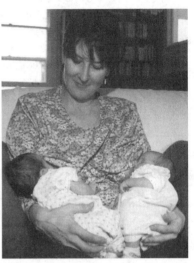

1. *Double-cradle or crisscross hold.* Place one baby in the crook of each arm in the traditional cradle hold. Crisscross their bodies on a pillow along your abdomen or in your lap.

A variation of the double-cradle is the *V hold.* With knees flexed and legs slightly propped, place each baby in the cradle hold with one of their bodies lying along each of your thighs–their knees or feet meet to form a V. Once babies are a few months old, some mothers adapt this position to breastfeed two babies while lying in bed.

An example of the double cradle or "V" hold with smaller babies

The double-cradle is a "hands on" position. This position may be more difficult to manage initially, especially when either baby has difficulty latching on, since it leaves a mother with no free hands. Mothers tend to use it more often as babies get older and gain head control or once two babies latch on without help.

2. *Double-clutch or double football hold.* Hold each baby in the clutch position with a baby's body tucked under each of your arms and each arm supported on a pillow. You can support a baby's neck and shoulders in each of your hands or place their heads and upper bodies on firm pillows.

A variation of this position is to hold each baby's head as for the clutch hold, but position each of their bodies on a pillow almost at a right (90°) angle, or perpendicular, from yours. Check the babies' ear-to-hip alignment to make sure both are in a good position to suck, swallow, and breathe. (You should be able to draw a straight line from the tip of a baby's ear to her hip.)

Mothers often prefer this position after a surgical delivery to avoid pressure on the incision. Babies having difficulty latching on may be easier to manage in this position, because your hands are free to help guide them. It is also possible to read a story to older children, eat a snack, or look something up in this book when hands are free.

However, this position is the least "hands on," and it is possible to literally prop your breasts and ignore the babies. If that happens often, it defeats one of the main advantages of breastfeeding multiples.

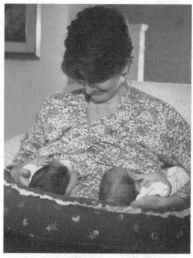

The double football or clutch hold.

3. *Combination cradle-clutch hold.* Position the first baby in the crook of your arm in the cradle hold. Then place the second baby in the clutch (football) position. To leave the dominant hand free, right-handed mothers would hold the first baby in the cradle of the left arm and position the second baby in the clutch hold at the right breast.

Left-handed mothers would simply reverse this.

Always position babies in a way that brings them to the breast– not you (your breasts) to them.

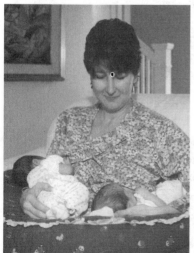

The combination cradle-clutch (or football) hold.

A common variation of this hold is called the *parallel, or layered, hold,* in which the first baby begins feeding in the traditional cradle hold. The second baby is positioned with her head "gently" resting on the first baby's abdomen or legs, and her body tucked under your arm or supported on a pillow at a right angle.

Many mothers claim this is their favorite position during infancy. It is "hands on" yet still gives them a free hand. It is more easily mastered than some positions, even when one or more babies is have difficulty latching on. Many mothers find discreet breastfeeding is possible using this position.

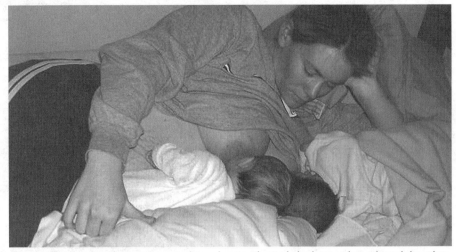

This mother has found a way to nurse lying down with one baby lying at her side and the other angled in the opposite direction. (Feet toward mother's head.)

Additional Positions

There are several less used simultaneous feeding positions, and you might find one is more comfortable for you and your babies.

- *Double saddle or double straddle position.* Seat a baby on each of your thighs facing you. Hold the back of each one's head in each of your hands and support their backs/torso areas with your forearms. Each baby straddles one of your thighs with her legs, as if sitting on a saddle. If you lean back, the babies would lean forward during the feeding. Or you can lean forward while supporting the babies in a more upright position. This position is used more often with older babies; however, there are mothers with babies less than three months old who find it a comfortable position.

> Ask for help with simultaneous feeding when two babies are hungry, but either is still learning to breastfeed well.

- *Double prone position.* Lean back in a recliner or on pillows until you feel well supported in a semi-sitting or supine–flat on your back–position. Lay the babies on their tummies/abdomens so they face your breasts. Their abdomens and legs are lying parallel along, and facing, your abdomen but with their heads turned slightly toward the middle of your chest, so each keeps her nose (airway) clear for breathing.

Mothers with larger breasts sometimes find a baby can latch on more easily in this position, as some of the breast may "disappear" when mother is lying back.

- *Double- or single-kneel position.* As babies grow in length and gain more head and upper body control, some mothers manage simultaneous night feedings by placing one or both babies in a kneeling position at the side(s) of the body. Help a baby to "kneel" on the bed facing the side of your body. The baby then leans forward to latch on with her upper body supported by your chest wall. Both babies can be placed in this position or it can be used in combination with one baby in a side-lying position. If one baby is in a more exaggerated side-lying position, so that you also are rolled to the side to face that baby, the kneeling baby may become more of a "standing" baby!

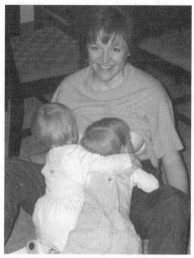

The double-straddle position works well for older babies.

- *Elbow-prop position.* In this position you are prone–lying on your abdomen–propped up by your elbows. The babies lie on their backs underneath you. (Their feet could point in any direction that works!) This probably is the least-used simultaneous feeding position; however, some mothers set up a mattress on the floor and use this position so that babies can remain where they are if they drift off to sleep. Other mothers report they found this position beneficial when treating a plugged duct.

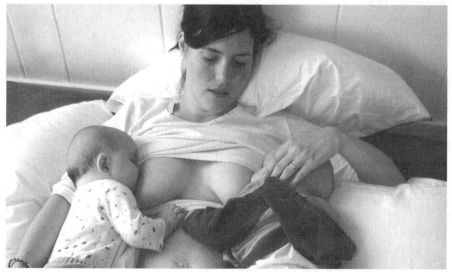

This mother has her babies in the double prone position.

Other Hints

Who latches on first? While learning to breastfeed simulta-neously, most mothers find it easier to put the more profi-cient "latcher" to breast first. The mother then uses her free hand(s) to work with the baby needing more help. Yet some mothers report the opposite; they say it is easier to help the less-skilled baby latch on when they have two free hands and an empty lap. When the more proficient baby knows what to do, all they really have to do is pull that baby over and help him get into position. Since different methods work for different mother-babies trios, experiment until you find what works best for you and your babies.

> It is fairly easy to breastfeed one baby "invisibly," but two create more of a show—some mothers would call it a circus!

Burping

Burping often is less of a concern for breastfed babies. The newborn who feeds smoothly, taking in very little air during feedings, may not need to burp. A gulper, however, may be happier after a good belch.

Wait for a baby to self-detach from the breast. Positioning for burping then depends on which simultaneous feeding position is being used. When using the double-cradle position, move your arm to help Baby A lean forward and cup that baby's chin in the hand of the arm still cradling Baby B. This frees the arm and hand that had been cradling Baby A so you can pat his back. Moving a baby up onto your shoulder to burp may be easier from the cradle-clutch combination, double-football, straddle, or prone positions.

Discreet Feeding

Discreet simultaneous breastfeeding may seem an oxymoron but many a mother of multiples has found a way! The cradle-clutch combination and double-clutch posi-tions lend themselves more to discreet feeding with very young babies, but many mothers feed older multiples discreetly using the double-cradle. Breastfeeding with both babies in slings that help cover mother's body is another way some achieve discreet simultaneous feeding.

Once able to feed two discreetly, you still may feel rather conspicuous. It is fair-ly easy to breastfeed one baby "invisibly," but two create more of a show—some mothers would call it a circus! So breastfeed babies separately or together, whichev-er is more comfortable for all concerned, when at the homes of others or in a pub-lic place.

KEY POINTS

❑ Almost any "rotation" plan works when breastfeeding multiples as long as it respects your individual babies' feeding cues for approximately 8 to 12 feedings every 24 hours. The three common rotations are:
  1. Offer each multiple both breasts at every feeding. (When used, it is often for only the first few weeks after birth.)
  2. Assign each baby a single breast for 24 hours, switching every 24 hours.
  3. Assign each baby a single breast for all breastfeedings.

❑ Simultaneous breastfeeding, or feeding two babies at once, saves time if at least one baby is able to latch on easily and suck (remove milk) well at breast. There is no rush to feed two at once until the babies–and you–are ready.

❑ Pillows can become "extra arms" when feeding two at once, so try different kinds of pillows on your lap and under your arms to help you get comfortable. Many mothers use a nursing pillow made especially for simultaneous breastfeeding; avoid pillows that are intended for breastfeeding only one baby.

❑ The three most common simultaneous breastfeeding positions are:
  1. Double-cradle: With each baby's head "cradled" in the crook (in the bent elbow area) of your arm, crisscross their bodies over your tummy or down toward your legs.
  2. Double-clutch (double-football): While supporting a baby's neck and shoulders in each of your hands, tuck each one's body and feet under each of your arms, along your rib cage on either side of your chest.
  3. Cradle-clutch combination: Place the first baby in the cradle and then place the second baby in the clutch (football) position.
  Positions 1 and 3 let you cuddle the babies more during feedings, but position 2 may be easier when learning to breastfeed two at once.

❑ Breastfeeding discreetly, or in a way that others cannot tell you are breastfeeding, can be more difficult with simultaneous feeding. However, many mothers have done it using position 3 and some with position 2. It may be possible to discreetly breastfeed two at once using position 1 after babies are a bit older.

❑ Because two same-age babies tend to attract attention, discreet simultaneous breastfeeding may be difficult even after you and your babies have figured out a good way to do it!

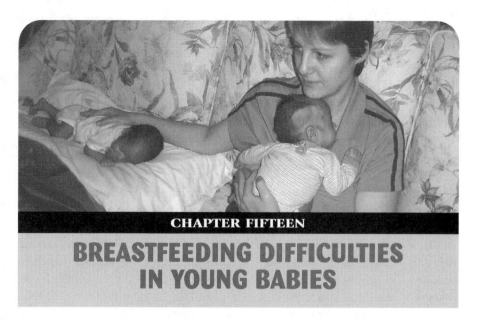

CHAPTER FIFTEEN

BREASTFEEDING DIFFICULTIES IN YOUNG BABIES

Odds are fairly high that at least one baby of a multiple set will experience some difficulty breastfeeding. Sheer numbers account for some of the odds. The more babies one has the greater likelihood that one or two will need extra time to "get the hang of it." Sometimes there is no real difficulty, but one or two are not as adept as the other(s). In addition, multiple-birth babies are more likely to be affected by pregnancy and birth complications, procedures, or medications associated with breastfeeding difficulties.

Multiples *are more likely to be born early,* which means their nervous systems may not yet be mature enough to coordinate the oral (mouth) behaviors needed for breastfeeding. Pregnancy, labor, and birth complications, procedures, or medications may temporarily affect a part of a baby's nervous system or the physical structures involved in breastfeeding. This may create a delay in early, frequent breastfeeding or result in the introduction of supplementary feedings with the introduction of oral objects, such as artificial nipples (teats), pacifiers, or feeding devices in a baby's mouth. If a baby must use his mouth differently with the bottle teat/nipple, feeding device, or pacifier than during breastfeeding, then latching on to the breast or actual breastfeeding may become more difficult.

Many so-called "breastfeeding" difficulties are actually "having multiples" difficulties. Often an aspect of the adjustment process is labeled a breastfeeding difficulty when breastfeeding is going well. For instance, figuring out the distinct breastfeeding styles of two or more unique individual babies may seem to be the prob-

Issues related to parenting multiples in general can easily become thought of as breastfeeding problems.

lem when it really is more an issue of getting to know and caring for two or more different little persons. Since each breastfed multiple can be expected to eat 8 to 12 times in 24 hours, issues related to parenting multiples in general can easily be thought of as breastfeeding problems in particular.

Many breastfeeding problems can be avoided when a mother understands how milk is made, the mechanics of infant latch-on, and typical infant breastfeeding patterns. (See Chapter 13, "Effective Breastfeeding.") If a problem should arise, ask yourself whether it is a true breastfeeding problem or whether breastfeeding has somehow gotten confused with an "adjusting to multiples" issue.

Don't lump the babies together. A difficulty with one multiple is a difficulty with one particular baby. When faced with the care of multiple babies, it is easy to think the entire "team" has a problem when it is just one who needs some help.

Try to determine where a problem actually lies–is it your problem, a problem with one (or more) of the babies, or is it related to someone/something outside of your breastfeeding team? Ask yourself how you would feel and what approach you might have taken had you given birth to a single baby and this problem occurred.

Often only one multiple has a particular difficulty; however, it is possible for two babies to have the same difficulty. Or two babies could have a difficulty, yet each baby's difficulty may be with a different aspect of breastfeeding. No wonder mothers of multiples can feel confused!

Common baby-related difficulties are addressed in this chapter. Most baby problems are related to either an issue with basic breastfeeding management or some difficulty a baby is having with latching on or suckling well. In either case, the baby is not able to obtain as much of your milk as he needs.

Work with your babies' health care provider. Also, contact an experienced La Leche League (LLL) Leader or a lactation consultant *today.* She can help you look at the babies' individual breastfeeding behaviors and patterns to see where a difficulty might lie. She also can help you develop a realistic plan to begin to deal with the problem. Most importantly, she will listen when you need to express concerns or vent frustration. While others may ask why you want to continue breastfeeding multiples, she will provide the praise and moral support you deserve.

It may take both patience and persistence to work with any baby who is experiencing a breastfeeding difficulty, especially when you have multiple babies to care for. However, most breastfeeding problems can be resolved, and breastfeeding your babies is worth the time and effort you put into solving any difficulties.

Difficulty Latching On or Sucking

Mothers usually know when any multiple is not yet breastfeeding "right." Some signs that a baby is not breastfeeding effectively are obvious while others are more subtle. Review the following list of "warning flags." However, if you do not find your multiple's difficulty on this list and you still are concerned, trust your instincts and seek more help.

A baby may be having difficulty if he consistently exhibits any of the following behaviors:

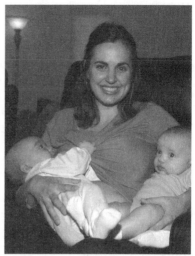

One baby may want to nurse more often but another baby still wants to be close to mother.

1. Breastfeeds fewer than 8 times, or more than 14 times, in 24 hours.

2. Has difficulty latching on to the breast, which may include clamping or "biting" down during latch-on, attempting but being unable to grasp the breast, "pushing away" from the breast, or being unable to "stay on" after latching on.

3. Dimples (sucks in) his cheeks, makes clicking sounds, or purses his lips often during his feedings.

4. Often drifts to sleep after feeding for only a minute or two; rarely breastfeeds 5 to 10 minutes on the first breast without frequent reminders to suck or falling off the breast.

5. Frequently feeds for *longer than* 40 minutes without self-detaching, so that feedings last 50 to 60 minutes or longer. Or she may fuss or cry and act hungry again within minutes of ending many of her feedings.

6. Passes fewer than 3 to 4 loose, seedy, mustard-yellow bowel movements a day during the first 4 to 6 weeks after birth.

7. Does not experience a daily increase in the number of wet diapers during the first few days after birth, or is not producing *at least* 5 to 6 soaking wet diapers every 24 hours by 5 to 7 days after birth.

8. Does not begin to gain at least 1/2 oz (15 gm) a day by the end of the first week after birth.

A mother is more likely to experience *sore or cracked nipples* when a baby is not latching on correctly or breastfeeding effectively. *Inadequate milk production* is likely to occur if any multiple is not removing milk well, because the breasts are not being "told" to make enough milk. *Severe engorgement, a plugged duct, or mastitis* may also be related to a baby's inability to breastfeed well. *Any nipple or breast problem* is a sign that a baby's breastfeeding behaviors should be closely examined. (See Chapter 16, "When Mother Has a Breastfeeding Difficulty.")

Do yourself a favor; get help as soon as a breastfeeding difficulty develops.

Continued difficulty latching on, "weak" or uncoordinated (disorganized) suck-ing, and drifting to sleep soon after beginning to breastfeed are common after preterm birth, and sometimes occur with infant distress during labor or delivery or after the use of medications or procedures during labor or birth. There may also be differences in the maturity of each multiple's brain and nervous system. One baby may not yet be able to coordinate the mouth movements used for breastfeeding as well as the other(s). A baby might have a physical problem that interferes with the ability to latch on or suck, such as a short frenulum (tongue-tie).

Problem-Solving Ideas

When faced with the care of multiple babies, it is easy to think the entire "team" has a problem when it is just one who needs some help.

Get help if you think any baby is not breastfeeding correct-ly even if someone told you that this baby appeared to be breastfeeding well. No one can see into a baby's mouth and watch him breastfeed. You know what you are feeling. You are the one monitoring each multiple's daily feedings and diaper counts.

Someone knowledgeable about the structures in a baby's mouth and breastfeeding management, such as a pediatric care provider, a lactation consultant, or an experienced LLL Leader should inspect the baby's mouth and watch him breastfeed. If a minor prob-lem with breastfeeding mechanics is the culprit, a simple change in technique may make all the difference. For situations requiring more than a "quick fix," an experi-enced breastfeeding support person will have ideas for resolving or coping with it.

If a baby's maturity, pregnancy or birth complications, or labor and birth med-ications have affected his ability to suck, it may take several days or several weeks for the baby to learn to breastfeed correctly. The baby will learn, but in the mean-time you can:

- Offer the breast when the baby demonstrates early feeding cues, such as "seeking" the breast, rooting, making sucking movements, bringing hands to face/mouth.
  - ❑ When a baby is having difficulty at the breast, feeding behaviors become less organized as his cues escalate to hard crying.
- Do not worry if the baby cannot latch on or breastfeed long enough for this feeding–or the next, or the one after that. Unless there is another health condition affecting feeding, most babies do learn to breastfeed if a mother continues to offer the breast.
- If a baby "resists" or seems to pull away from the breast, experiment with breastfeeding positions until you find one that seems more comfortable for the baby. Support only the baby's neck and shoulders so that the baby can turn or adjust his head and does not feel "pushed" into the breast. Some babies react by pulling away if there is any pressure on the back of their head. Try the side-lying position for a baby having a "pull away" difficulty.

- A sleepy baby may cue to breastfeed fewer than 8 times a day. If you notice the sleepy baby moving arms or legs or making facial and eye movements, stimulate the baby to wake him to breastfeed.
  - ❏ Unwrap blankets that might be keeping him too warm, and undress the baby to put him to breast skin-to-skin. (You can drape a light blanket over his body if drafts are a concern.) Change his diaper if he drifts off to sleep within a couple of minutes of beginning to breastfeed.
  - ❏ The sleepy baby may breastfeed better if you massage your breast and squeeze (compress) milk into his mouth when he pauses during a breastfeeding.
- Read the section "When One (Or More) Has a Feeding Difficulty" in Chapter 12, "Making Up for a Poor Start." Many of the strategies in that section of the chapter apply to the sleepy baby, including the information about skin-to-skin contact, "practice" breastfeedings, breast pump use to increase or maintain milk production, alternative feeding methods, monitoring diaper counts, and progression to more direct breastfeeding.
- If a baby latches on but the let-down, or milk-ejection, reflex overwhelms him, take the baby off the breast until the flow of milk slows.
  - ❏ You also could offer an emptier breast by feeding this baby after another multiple breastfeeds. Or pump just until the let-down and then let the baby latch on after the flow has slowed a bit.
- Feed a multiple having difficulty simultaneously with one who breastfeeds well. Sometimes the one having difficulty figures out what to do in response to the flow of milk triggered by the better breastfeeder. (The worst that may happen is the one having difficulty will sputter and release the breast.)
- Continue to pump your milk to ensure that milk is effectively removed often enough and thoroughly enough until all babies are breastfeeding well. How often you pump may depend on a baby's problem, how well the other(s) breastfeed, and the amount of help you have at home. The more help you have, the more time you will have both to work with a baby still learning to breastfeed well and to pump milk for any supplemental feedings.
- If a deviation in the physical structure of a baby's mouth is suspected and may be causing the baby to use incorrect breastfeeding mechanics/mouth movements, have that baby examined as soon as possible by an appropriate health care provider. If treatment is delayed, it may take longer for a baby's breastfeeding mechanics to improve.
- On days when you wonder whether a particular multiple will ever breastfeed well, call an LLL Leader or a lactation consultant. She will give you a pep talk and help you maintain perspective. (For more detail and additional ideas, read Chapter 13, "Effective Breastfeeding," Chapter 12, "Making Up for a Poor Start," and Chapter 18, "Full and Partial Breastfeeding.")

Minor Feeding Difficulties

Some babies experience difficulty for the first week or two whenever they first latch on or begin to feed, yet after a few attempts and several minutes they do latch on and breastfeed effectively. Mothers of these babies often say they feel nipple soreness or pain when the baby first goes to the breast, but their discomfort eases after the first few minutes of feeding. These babies usually have diaper counts and weight gains that are within normal limits.

If you experience this type of problem with one or more multiples, it may be related to breastfeeding mechanics. Often a simple fine-tuning of positioning or latch-on technique will "cure" the problem. See Chapter 16 for a review of these techniques. Call an LLL Leader or a lactation consultant if you still have difficulty correcting the mechanics after looking at the illustrations. She may be able to offer suggestions over the phone, or she may want to see you and that baby to work on technique.

Frequency Spurts: Sudden "Demand" for Extra Feedings

It may not seem so at the time, but young babies' sudden "demand" for more frequent breastfeeding usually is not a problem. When any baby who has been breastfeeding well suddenly asks to eat several additional times in a day, suspect a "frequency spurt." Frequency spurts are discussed in greater detail in Chapter 13, "Effective Breastfeeding," since they appear to be a normal aspect of breastfeeding.

Weight Gain Issues

New mothers often express concern about their babies' weight gains, especially when breastfeeding for the first time. It often takes a while for a new mother of single baby to gain confidence that her body will produce enough milk for her baby to grow properly. Confidence may take even longer to acquire when breastfeeding multiples. However, each baby will let you know how she is doing through her breastfeeding pattern and her diaper count. (See Chapter 13, "Effective Breastfeeding.")

Babies with typical feeding patterns and adequate diaper counts usually gain at least 1/2 ounce (15 gm) a day, or at least four ounces (112 gm) a week, and most gain an ounce (28 to 30 gm) or more a day (6 to 8 ounces/200 gm a week) for the first several months. Weight gain tends to taper down after several months. Breastfed babies continue to gain steadily but at a slower rate.

A few young babies gain less than four ounces some weeks. However, their diaper counts are appropriate and they maintain a steady, albeit slower, rate of gain. Although this baby may need to be monitored more closely, a slow but steady pattern may be normal for some babies. It is important to differentiate between the normal, slow-gaining baby and the baby with a true weight gain problem.

It can be fascinating to watch the growth patterns of dizygotic (fraternal) multiples. Although they are getting the same milk, they often grow and develop at very different rates. Sometimes one gains several pounds a month, yet another barely falls within the normal range. However, both may be perfectly healthy; they simply have different genes for body build.

> **It is important to differentiate between the normal, slow-gaining baby and the baby with a true weight gain problem.**

There are times, though, when one (or more) truly is not gaining the weight he should. A problem with weight gain may occur during the newborn period or it may arise later. When any baby is not gaining adequate weight, review the information in this chapter about "difficulty latching on or sucking" and examine the baby's breastfeeding routine.

- *Is this multiple truly breastfeeding at least 8 times in 24 hours?* If so, is that often enough for this particular baby? (Different multiples may require different numbers of feedings for appropriate growth.) Are you trying to develop a schedule by stretching the time between feedings? Is it possible that this baby often gets "put off" because you have to care for the other(s)?

- *Are you certain that this baby's breastfeeding technique is correct?* When a baby is unable to suckle correctly, she may be unable to take in enough milk for growth. Does latch-on seem to take a lot of time or does this baby frequently have difficulty latching on? Does she have trouble staying latched on? Does she quickly drift off to sleep after latching on?

- *Do many of her feedings take longer than 40 minutes?* Does she often fuss or act hungry again within minutes of "finishing" a feeding? Does she typically breastfeed more than 12 times a day? (Many babies feed more often during occasional frequency spurts.)

- *Does this baby have enough wet and soiled diapers?* Frequently, a decrease or an inadequate number of daily soiled diapers is one of the first signs that a baby is not getting the calories needed for weight gain. When the number of wet diapers decreases, it may be a sign that a baby is not getting enough fluid as well.

- *Does the baby use a pacifier?* Pacifier use can interfere with the daily number of breastfeedings, especially if used to stretch the time between feedings. Pacifier use may affect some babies' ability to suck correctly when at the breast.

- *Is this baby receiving supplementary water?* Water has no calories. It may help hydrate a baby, but it does not contribute to weight gain. Plus, it can confuse your ability to interpret the wet diaper count. Human milk, or complementary infant formula, contains calories and enough water to keep babies hydrated.

- *Are you taking care of yourself?* A baby's feeding pattern or his incorrect breastfeeding behavior is at the heart of most infant weight gain problems. However, milk production in a mother of multiples may be somewhat more sensitive to a mother's poor diet, extreme fatigue, minor illnesses, etc. These things may also affect your fatigue level and subsequent ability to respond to your babies' cues.

  Get help if you think any baby is not breastfeeding correctly even if someone told you that this baby appeared to be breastfeeding well.

  ❏ Have you been feeling sluggish, blue, or depressed? Is your appetite poor? Have you had trouble sleeping when the babies sleep? If you answer "yes" to any of these questions, you may need a health care provider to check for a postpartum thyroid condition or a postpartum mood disorder. Thyroid conditions can directly affect milk production, and mood disorders may affect a mother's response to her babies' cues.

  ❏ Do you have polycystic ovarian syndrome (PCOS) and, if so, are you being treated? One aspect of PCOS is insulin resistance, which appears to affect milk production if left untreated.

Solving the Problem

You will want to work closely with the babies' health care provider and a lactation consultant or experienced breastfeeding support leader when any multiple's weight gain is inadequate. Read Chapter 12, "Making Up for a Poor Start." The following suggestions can help when coping with a baby who seems to breastfeed well but is not gaining adequate weight.

- Put this baby to breast whenever the baby demonstrates feeding cues. (These cues are described earlier in this chapter and in Chapter 9, "Beginning Breastfeeding.")

  ❏ If a multiple who is not gaining enough weight does not wake on his own for more than 8 daily feedings, watch for the baby to begin to move his extremities and make facial grimaces. These are signs that he has reached a light sleep state and can be awakened more easily to breastfeed.

  ❏ Do not offer a pacifier to this baby; offer this baby the breast.

- Monitor this baby's daily feedings and diaper counts on a chart. (See Appendix.)

- Weigh the baby as often as the pediatric care provider suggests. Different types of scales and their usefulness are discussed in Chapter 11, "Breastfeeding in the Newborn Intensive Care Unit," and Chapter 12, "Making Up for a Poor Start."

  ❏ As noted in those chapters, accurate electronic scales are available for rent. This type of scale works well for daily weights but it is particularly helpful for determining precisely how much milk a multiple is taking in during breastfeeding.

❑ You may be expected to bring the baby to the pediatric care provider's office more often until an adequate weight gain is established. Let the provider know if it will be a hardship to make frequent office visits for weight checks. Some pediatric care providers or community lactation consultants make home visits to monitor a baby's weight.

• Supplement this baby's feedings with your pumped milk as needed or an infant formula when your milk is not available. A discussion of supplementary feeding, and which feeding method may be more appropriate depending on a particular baby's ability to breastfeed effectively, is included in Chapter 12. Pump your breasts as needed to increase (or maintain) milk production whether a weight gain problem is believed to be related to a sucking difficulty, the baby has not been breastfeeding often enough, or the reason is unknown.

• As a baby's weight improves, ask the baby's care provider and an LLL Leader or a lactation consultant to help you develop a plan for safely decreasing or eliminating supplemental feedings while adding breastfeedings, monitoring diapers, and so on.

Many breastfeeding problems can be resolved quickly and some take more time. The information in this chapter may help you identify and begin working on a problem, but you may need help to sort through it. Do yourself a favor; get help as soon as a breastfeeding difficulty develops. Contact the babies' health care provider, but don't wait to reach the end of your particular rope before you call an experienced LLL Leader or a lactation consultant. Having her help may save you and your babies a lot of time and trouble.

> **Many breastfeeding problems can be resolved quickly and some take more time.**

KEY POINTS

❑ Giving birth to multiple infants means there is more chance that one (or more) may have some sort of difficulty breastfeeding, especially when multiples are born early or experienced stress during pregnancy, labor, or birth.

❑ Even when breastfeeding is really going well, having two, three, or more times the usual number of babies to care for may sometimes cause a mother to think there is a problem with breastfeeding.

❑ Most breastfeeding difficulties are related to mismanagement of the breastfeeding process, a baby with a problem latching on, or a baby who is unable to suckle effectively in order to remove enough milk.

❑ When two or more multiples have difficulty breastfeeding, they may share the same difficulty or each may have trouble with different aspects of breastfeeding. This can be very confusing for their mother!

❑ If any multiple is not having enough stool/wet diapers or not gaining enough weight, or if breastfeeding is hurting your nipples/breasts, this baby probably is not breastfeeding effectively.

- Trust yourself if you think something is not quite right with breastfeeding for one or more babies. You know yourself and your babies better than anyone else. If you are concerned, that is a good reason to get more help and information.

- In addition to calling your babies' pediatric health care provider, get help immediately from a knowledgeable/experienced breastfeeding support person, such as a La Leche League Leader, or from a certified lactation consultant (IBCLC). She will have ideas for your particular situation.

❑ Most breastfeeding difficulties can be solved, and quick improvement is possible for many issues *if* you get help as soon as a difficulty develops.

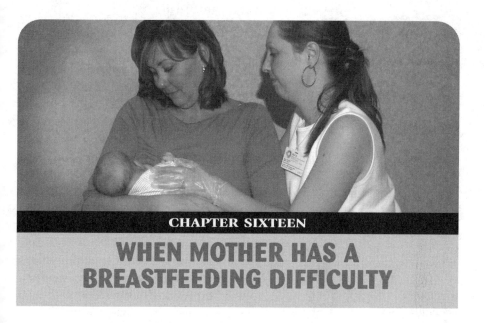

CHAPTER SIXTEEN

WHEN MOTHER HAS A BREASTFEEDING DIFFICULTY

A new mother is not more prone to breastfeeding difficulties simply because she has multiple babies to feed. However, the presence of two or more babies with differing breastfeeding abilities or styles multiplies the likelihood that a baby will experience some difficulty. A mother and her babies work together when they are breastfeeding. If breastfeeding is not quite "right" yet for a baby, the mother often experiences a problem, too.

This chapter deals with difficulties that can affect you–the mother. Baby-related difficulties are discussed in the previous chapter. The information in this chapter is meant to complement, not take the place of, the support of an experienced LLL Leader or a board-certified lactation consultant. She can help you get to the root of the problem, individualize a plan for solving it, and help you decide if it is something that should be reported to your care provider.

Sore Nipples

Sore or cracked nipples usually tell a mother that there is a "mechanical" problem with some aspect of breastfeeding. "Mechanics" refers to how parts work together, so breastfeeding mechanics refers to how the breast and the baby's mouth fit and work together. When any baby does not latch on correctly or cannot suckle effectively, the action of the baby's mouth can irritate the nipple tip or bruise sensitive breast tissue. Slight irritation may produce some redness and a feeling of soreness;

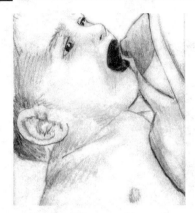

Baby needs to open his mouth very wide.

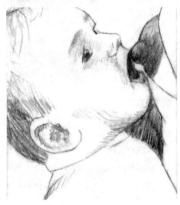

Latching on chin first helps baby get a large mouthful of breast tissue.

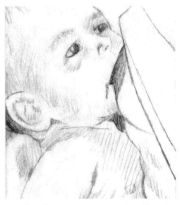

When baby is latched on well, his chin touches the breast and his mouth covers all or most of the mother's areola.

Babies are usually more willing to work at fine-tuning their latch-on and feeding technique when they are not ravenously hungry.

greater irritation can lead to nipple cracks or fissures. Most nipple soreness is short-lived if it is dealt with immediately.

The best way to prevent sore nipples is to get off to a good breastfeeding start when your babies are born. (See Chapter 9, "Beginning Breastfeeding, and Chapter 13, "Effective Breastfeeding.") Ask a nurse or a lactation consultant to help you initially as each baby latches on and begins to breastfeed. A little nipple tenderness when a baby first latches on is not unusual during the first week. (If you've experienced tenderness at certain times in the menstrual cycle, it may feel similar to that.) However, it should not be so painful you want to "bite a bullet" during any part of a feeding, and you should not see any redness, scraped nipple or areolar skin, creasing or a stripe across the nipple tip, or nipple cracking.

Although it may sound contradictory, frequent feedings are beneficial when nipples are tender or sore. Babies are usually more willing to work at fine-tuning their latch-on and feeding technique when they are not ravenously hungry. Waiting to put hungry babies to the breast can lead to nipple damage, as it may be more difficult for them to latch on to overfull breasts. Also, extremely hungry babies may be less "gentle" when they latch on.

A baby's mouth must open, or gape wide, in order for him to latch on deeply and get a good mouthful of breast tissue. Failing to open wide may cause a baby to get only the tip of the nipple or may cause him to "inch" his way onto your breast, which may damage nipple and areolar skin.

If your nipples become sore, you develop any redness, creasing, or cracking, or nipple tenderness persists beyond two weeks, something is not quite right. Do not simply grin and bear it. Take a closer look at the breastfeeding mechanics with each multiple. (Also see Chapter 13, "Effective Breastfeeding.")

1. Is any baby having difficulty latching on to the breast or are any not breast-feeding well once they are latched on? Does it hurt as a baby latches on or during actual breastfeeding? Does it feel the same or different with each multiple? A lactation consultant, LLL Leader, or health professional can tell you whether the latch-on or feeding behaviors look appropriate, but only you know whether it feels right.

2. Is each baby positioned so that she is in good alignment to coordinate suck-ing, swallowing, and breathing? When a baby is in good alignment, you can draw an imaginary straight line from baby's ear through the upper arm to the hip.

3. Could the "hold" you use to support your breast during latch-on interfere with a baby's ability to latch on deeply? When busy assisting a baby with latch-on, a mother may not notice if she covers part of the areola with her fingers, which can make it impossible for baby to latch on deeply.

4. Is any baby latching on before his mouth is open wide as in a gape or yawn? All babies, including preterm babies, can open wide. Some babies open wide immediately and some gradually open wider and wider before opening wide enough for a deep latch-on.

5. Does the baby get deeply on the breast in one motion, or is he "nibbling" his way up the areola, until he finally achieves a correct, deep latch-on? You want to help a baby latch on deeply in one smooth motion.

6. Are you trying to help two babies latch on so you can feed them simultane-ously? Feeding two at once takes more skill on both the mother's and at least one baby's part. Incorrect latch-on techniques may be reinforced when distracted by and assisting two hungry babies at once.

Often a minor "mechanical" issue is the root of the problem, which means many, or most, sore nipple problems are easy to resolve. Once the mechanics are corrected, you may be amazed at how quickly sore nipples heal. While you and your babies correct the mechanics, you may want to try some coping ideas that have worked for other mothers.

- Some mothers do Reverse Pressure Softening (RPS) or express a little milk before a baby latches on to "soften" the areola and hasten the let-down (milk-ejection) reflex. (A description of RPS may be found in the Appendix.)

- Avoid simultaneous feedings until at least one of the participating babies consistently latches on easily and correctly.
- If one baby latches on and breastfeeds without causing discomfort, assign that baby to the sorer side. (If concerned that the baby causing discomfort will create a similar problem on the less sore nipple, alternate babies and breasts but let the better breastfeeder feed twice on the sorer breast for every one breastfeed for the other baby.)
- Do not shorten feeding time. Continue to let babies breastfeed until each self-detaches, which usually occurs within 10 to 30 minutes for the effectively breastfeeding baby. Limiting feeding time can interfere with a baby's nutritional and caloric intake, since milk with higher fat content is "delivered" later in each feeding. If soreness persists throughout an entire feeding, it is a signal to get help from someone qualified in breastfeeding problem management.
- Some mothers express a little milk onto their nipples after a feeding; it is believed that the immunological properties of the milk promote healing.
- Some studies support the use of applying an ultra purified lanolin product to the nipples after feeding to both soothe and heal irritated tissue. Avoid other creams, oils, or lotions. (Lansinoh Brand Lanolin for Breastfeeding Mothers® should not cause a reaction for those with an allergy to sheep or wool, but if you have this allergy and you are using a different brand of purified lanolin, test for a reaction by applying a small amount of the purified lanolin to the inside bend of your elbow before using it on your nipples.) Do not air- or blow-dry nipples or expose nipples to a heat lamp. These treatments dry the skin, causing unnecessary scabbing and further damage.
- Some mothers find the use of hydrogel pads designed for use on damaged nipples is another soothing treatment. Hydrogel pads that can be rinsed when removed are the safest to use since they have not been found to increase the incidence of infections. Read and follow directions carefully.
- Because nipple tissue damage may invite infection, keep nipples clean. At least once a day wash nipples with a non-antibacterial, non-perfumed soap and then rinse well.

If a structure in any multiple's mouth differs even slightly from "normal," it may affect breastfeeding mechanics and cause persistent nipple pain and damage. Tongue-tie is an example of a "baby issue" in which a difference or deviation can affect a baby's ability to move or use that structure to latch on or maintain suckling. Because the baby cannot use the tongue correctly, nipple damage may follow. A mother-related structural issue may be an extremely inverted nipple that a baby has difficulty latching onto or that gets "caught" in a baby's mouth in a way that creates soreness for a mother. For these kinds of situations it may be necessary to fix the structural problem before nipples can completely heal.

Thrush

Suspect a fungal (yeast/ thrush) infection if nipples or areola feel itchy or if they suddenly look very "shiny" or "flaky." Fungal infections may be associated with a burning pain of the nipple/areola or with a burning sensation felt deep within the breast, which may occur during or between feedings. Some mothers complain of cracking on the side of or at the base of the nipple, where the nipple shaft meets the areola.

Mothers of multiples may be more susceptible to fungal infections, because they are more likely to have been treated with antibiotics for a pregnancy- or birth-related procedure or complication. If any multiple-birth newborns were affected by complications requiring antibiotic treatment, they would be more susceptible to oral thrush that can be passed to mother's nipples during breastfeeding. Antibiotic use is associated with fungal infections because antibiotics kill both disease-producing "bad" bacteria and the "good" bacteria that keep fungus from overgrowing. When "good" bacteria are destroyed, fungus can grow.

A fungal infection is not related to breastfeeding "mechanics." It may cause sore, red, or damaged nipples even when each baby is using correct breastfeeding techniques. A fungal infection may also be the cause of sore, cracked nipples that develop in later months of breastfeeding.

If any multiple develops an oral fungal infection (thrush), it will probably appear as cheesy-white patches in the baby's mouth. A fiery-red diaper rash is also a sign of a fungal infection.

Usually both mother and (all) her babies require treatment with an anti-fungal medication to eliminate it. Be scrupulous about continuing treatment through the recommended period. An LLL Leader or a lactation consultant will be able to give you more in-depth information.

Certain other skin conditions may look similar to a fungal infection. When cracking occurs in nipple tissue, it is possible to develop a bacterial infection. Occasionally a mother affected by psoriasis has developed it on her nipples/areola, and some mothers have experienced dermatitis or eczema in that area. Because these conditions can have a similar appearance, see your health care provider or ask for a referral to a dermatologist for any skin condition of the nipples/areola that does not respond to treatment.

No matter what the cause, persistent nipple soreness or tissue damage that does not respond to the usual kinds of treatment is **always** a sign to contact someone qualified in breastfeeding problem management.

Engorgement

Milk production markedly increases in the amount (volume) produced by the second to sixth day after birth. (Delays in plentiful production are occasionally seen for up to 10 to 14 days in mothers affected by certain health or birth-related conditions.) With the fairly rapid increase in milk volume, a new mother's breasts may feel fuller

If you develop severe engorgement, the most important treatment is to remove the milk!

and heavier, and the skin may be more taut. These pronounced breast changes cause some to say their milk has "come in." The breast fullness many women experience is not due simply to an increased volume of milk. When hormonal changes after birth "tell" a mother's body that the time has come to make a lot of milk, extra fluid from blood and lymph circulatory systems are sent to the breasts to provide the materials that will become human milk. When the flow of these fluids gets ahead of the removal of "stored" milk via breastfeeding or pumping, the "interstitial" breast tissue that surrounds the milk-making alveoli and related milk ducts become congested, causing swelling in the breasts.

A combination of the rapid increase in milk production and the swelling in surrounding breast tissue is referred to as breast engorgement. The degree to which women experience the signs of engorgement varies widely. The breast changes associated with engorgement are very dramatic in some women and hardly noticed by others.

Full breasts should be "emptied" frequently and completely by babies who breastfeed effectively. The idea is to keep milk moving out of the breasts and into the babies, so the extra fluid can be used to make more milk or it can move back into the mother's circulation. This strategy is also the best way to avoid severe engorgement.

Healthy newborn multiples that breastfeed effectively may help a mother avoid severe engorgement. Breast tissue congestion is less likely to occur when multiples breastfeed frequently. If any multiple is not yet able to breastfeed or any baby is not yet breastfeeding effectively, a full size, hospital-grade, electric breast pump can be used every one to three hours to drain full breasts. *Keep the milk moving*–one way or another.

Severe Engorgement

If a mother develops severe engorgement, her breasts become hard and "lumpy"; she may feel as if they are filled with small rocks as far up as the collarbone and under the armpit. Engorged breasts usually feel sore or painful and may look red. The areola may become so "tight" from fluid congestion that a mother's nipples flatten, which can make it difficult for a baby to latch on.

It is not known exactly why some women develop severe engorgement, but it is less likely to occur when effective breastfeeding or pumping has occurred prior to milk "coming in." The increase in the amount of intravenous fluid women receive during labor and delivery is believed to play a role in severe engorgement. Also, women with breast implants may be prone to severe engorgement.

It is important to begin treating severe engorgement as soon as the symptoms develop. For one thing, you will feel comfortable sooner. More importantly, quick treatment may avoid a long-term milk production problem. Also, unresolved severe engorgement may lead to other problems, such as plugged milk ducts or mastitis–an inflammation or infection in the breast tissue surrounding the alveoli and milk ducts.

If you develop severe engorgement, the most important treatment is to remove the milk! Babies who are able to breastfeed effectively are the best milk removers available. If none of the babies breastfeed well yet or none can latch on well due to the engorgement, pump your breasts frequently. Until engorgement resolves, breastfeed or pump every one to three hours. In addition to frequent milk removal, many other treatments have been suggested for severe engorgement. Most have little support from research. Taking an anti-inflammatory medication is an intervention that appears to help. Ask your health care provider which type may be most appropriate in your circumstances.

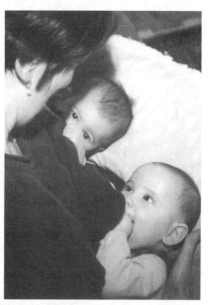

Nothing can compare to the satisfaction of having two pairs of eyes gazing up at you as two babies fill their tummies with your warm sweet milk.

Severe engorgement interventions that may be suggested for use immediately before breastfeeding or pumping include:

1. *Reverse Pressure Softening (RPS), or areolar compression,* a technique used to relieve swelling in the areola area to help soften it and make it stretchier and easier for a baby to latch onto or fit into the collection kit flange/breast shield better. With RPS you use your fingers to exert steady, gentle pressure on your areola next to the base of the nipple tip and inward toward your chest wall. Apply this inward pressure for at least a minute, although it may take longer. (Some mothers use a 3-minute egg timer or use the length of a standard television commercial.) A mother with breast implants should discuss the technique with her health care provider before trying it. See the Appendix for details.

2. *The application of a warm, wet compress or taking a warm shower* to expose the breasts to the flow of water just before breastfeeding or pumping is thought by some to encourage let-down of milk. Because heat is also associated with increasing swelling, it should not be applied for more than a few minutes.

Severe engorgement interventions that may be suggested for use after breastfeeding or pumping to help reduce any swelling include:

1. *Application of cold compresses or ice packs to engorged breasts* for 20 minutes after breastfeeding or pumping. Cold may help reduce swelling in the breasts just as it reduces swelling in any part of the body. When swelling decreases, a mother feels more comfortable and her milk usually flows better during the next breastfeeding or pumping session. Continue to apply cold packs between breastfeeding or pumping sessions for 24 hours or until swelling is no longer a concern.

   ❏ Cold packs should not be placed directly on the skin; place a piece of cloth, such as a towel, sheet, or t-shirt between your skin and a cold pack.

   ❏ Cold packs should be removed after 20 minutes, but you may alternate cold for 20 minutes on, at least 30 minutes off, 20 on, etc

   ❏ Some mothers find a sealed bag of frozen peas, beans, corn, etc., creates a cold pack that "molds" to and surrounds the breast.

2. *Application of cabbage leaf compresses.* The research on the benefits of cabbage compress use is not definitive but the theory is that ordinary, fresh, uncooked green cabbage leaves contain a substance that reduces swelling. It is thought that this substance might reduce milk production if cabbage leaf treatment is used for too long or too often.

   ❏ To make cabbage leaf compresses, wash fresh green cabbage leaves in cool water–some recommend adding a little soap to the cool water and rinsing with cool water–and refrigerate. Washing removes any chemicals or bacteria on the cabbage; cool water is recommended to avoid "cooking" the cabbage, which may decrease the helpful substance in the leaves. Refrigerated leaves usually feel more soothing on hot, engorged breasts but refrigeration is not necessary.

   ❏ Apply green cabbage leaves directly to all engorged areas of the breasts except the nipple. Cabbage compresses can be held in place by wearing them inside your bra. (If you are allergic or sensitive to cabbage, you may not want to use or watch for any itching or a rash and remove immediately.)

   ❏ Some women find they need to devein the cabbage leaves or go over leaves with a rolling pin (or hit them with a meat tenderizing tool) to get the leaves to fit their breasts better.

   ❏ Remove the cabbage once the leaves have "cooked"/wilted. You may then want to apply cold compresses after "resting" breasts for 30 minutes.

   ❏ Most suggest using cabbage leave compresses no more than 2 or 3 times in 24 hours.

3. *"Elevating" the breasts by lying flat on the back or in a recliner chair,* which is thought to help fluids re-enter the general circulation with the help of gravity.

If using a breast pump to remove milk during severe engorgement because your babies cannot yet breastfeed or any baby is unable to latch on, consider the following:

1. A full size, hospital-grade, electric breast pump that you can rent is generally more effective than a purchased breast pump. The action of these rental pumps is also gentler because suction is automatically cycled and released.

2. If the collection kit flanges/breast shields are too small, fluid congestion (engorgement) in the areola may increase, making milk removal more difficult.

3. Use RPS immediately before pumping to reduce swelling in the areola and stimulate milk let-down. (See Appendix.)

4. If milk is not flowing well within several minutes of applying the breast pump, stop and repeat RPS. Then reapply the pump. Stop and repeat RPS, alternating with pumping until milk begins to flow.

5. Pump every 1 to 2 hours until milk begins to flow within minutes of beginning to pump. (Put effectively breastfeeding multiples back to breast as soon as possible; effective breastfeeding is better at removing milk.)

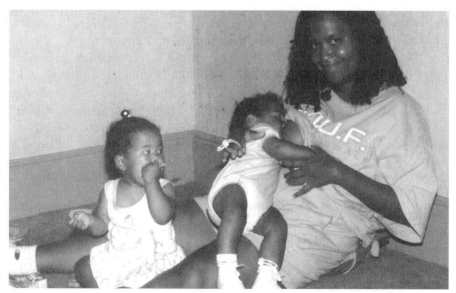

Once you have overcome any problems or challenges in the early weeks, there are many satisfying moments to enjoy.

6. If by the third pumping session (and third hour) you have not begun to get a good flow within 5 minutes of beginning to pump, get help from an LLL Leader, a lactation consultant, or another health care provider. There may be a problem with the equipment, pumping technique, etc.

7. Continue to pump for a minute or two beyond the time you see the last drop being expressed. Pumping usually takes 10 to 30 minutes. Some mothers break for a minute or two after the initial flow noticeably slows. These mothers do RPS a second time, reapply the pump and then continue to pump for a minute or two beyond the time the last drops are expressed.

Contact an LLL Leader, a board-certified lactation consultant, or your health care provider if severe engorgement *does not respond to treatment* within 12 to 18 hours. Certainly, call her before this if you have questions or need encouragement.

Later Engorgement

Full breasts should be "emptied" frequently and completely by babies who breastfeed effectively.

Engorgement may occur whenever any baby or a mother abruptly drops a breastfeeding or when a breastfeeding is "put off" in an attempt to lengthen the time between feedings. A mother of multiples already is producing significantly more milk than the average breastfeeding mother, so she will have more milk building up if a feeding is missed, especially if two (or more) babies suddenly drop a feeding or are encouraged to wait longer between feeds. Because of the greater milk volume, a mother of multiples may be more prone to a plugged duct or mastitis following such engorgement.

The treatment for this type of engorgement is the same as for engorgement during the first week. *Remove the milk.* Put a willing baby to the breast. If you actually want to decrease production, do it slowly so the breasts can adapt to the change gradually. You could hand-express or pump milk briefly–only to the point of relieving fullness–if you begin to feel engorged. *Warning.* Delaying feedings to lengthen the time between feedings may also result in poor infant weight gain and one or more unhappy babies.

Insufficient Milk Production

In surveys of mothers of multiples, the fear of not producing enough milk is usually the greatest reason for weaning the babies. Almost every mother of multiples wonders at some time or another whether she is making enough milk. Although many mothers fully, or exclusively, breastfeed twins, triplets, and even quadruplets, multiples' needs for milk could push a mother's milk-making ability to the limit–or beyond—especially for higher-order multiples. If you ever feel concerned about the amount of milk you are producing for your babies, contact a La Leche League Leader or a lactation consultant to help you figure out whether there is a problem or not.

Perceived Milk Insufficiency

Breastfed babies generally eat more often than artificially fed babies. The total number of breastfeedings for multiple babies' adds up to a lot of feedings each day. Turn back to Chapter 13, "Effective Breastfeeding," to read about typical feeding patterns and the signs that each baby is getting enough milk. If each baby usually is satisfied with 8 to 12 daily feedings, and all have diaper counts and weight gains that are within the normal range, you are making plenty of milk.

Sometimes mothers express concern that they are "losing" their milk once the initial breast fullness or engorgement subsides. The breasts feel soft much of the time. This is not indicative of a production problem as long as babies' diaper counts and weight gains are within the normal range. It usually means the breasts have adapted to each baby's demands and are producing that daily quantity of milk.

> **Almost every mother of multiples wonders at some time or another whether she is making enough milk.**

Friends, relatives, and even some health professionals may question whether a mother can produce enough milk for multiples. They may point to babies' requests for frequent feedings as a sign that one or more babies is not getting enough milk. Do not allow pressure from others to cause you to lose confidence in your body's ability to meet the demands placed upon it. Instead look at your babies' individual feeding patterns, diaper counts, and weight gains.

True Milk Insufficiency

It is thought that only one to two percent of mothers worldwide are physically unable to produce milk. Breast size is not related to a woman's ability to produce milk. Mothers with breasts of all different sizes and shapes have fully breastfed twins and triplets for several months. Women who have experienced difficulty conceiving do not usually have difficulty producing milk.

Although no one has yet studied large numbers of women breastfeeding multiples, especially those with triplets or more, insufficient milk production usually is related to infrequent or inadequate removal of milk rather than a mother's physical inability to produce enough milk. Increasing the number of (effective) breastfeedings or pumping sessions almost always results in increased milk production within several days. If you truly are concerned about adequate milk production, first look at the babies'

> **Don't allow pressure from others to cause you to lose confidence in your body's ability to meet the demands placed upon it.**

feeding patterns, diaper counts, and weight gains.

- Typically, breastfed babies are satisfied with about 8 to 12 daily breastfeedings. If any baby is breastfeeding fewer than 8 times in 24 hours, he may not be removing milk often enough to generate adequate production. Beware of the "good" baby who is sleepy or undemanding.

  A baby who rarely seems satisfied and consistently demands to breastfeed 14 or more times in 24 hours may not be sucking as effectively as needed, so the baby breastfeeds more but milk removal is low. This can also have a negative effect on milk production.

- A baby who is not getting enough milk often has only small-sized or fewer than 3 soiled diapers a day. A decrease in a baby's daily number of stools (bowel movements), especially during the first 4 to 6 weeks after birth, often is the first sign that a baby is not getting enough milk.

- A baby who consistently gains less than one-half ounce (14 to 15 gm) a day, or less than four ounces (112 to 120 gm) a week, during the first three months, is probably not getting enough milk.

What do you do if any baby's diaper count or weight gain indicates you are not making enough milk? First, stay calm. Then figure out whether the problem belongs to the baby or to you.

1. *Most problems with insufficient milk are baby issues.* If at least one baby is gaining weight normally and the other(s) is not, most likely the difficulty is with the multiple(s) who is not gaining. A diaper count and weight gain problem for two or more babies, however, does not automatically mean that the mother is the one with the problem. It is not unusual for all multiples to experience some sucking difficulty in the first weeks, especially when babies are preterm or all experienced some complication. Most baby problems can be fixed. See the previous chapter for ideas to cope when a baby is not getting enough to eat because he cannot remove milk well or is not waking often enough to eat.

2. *Scheduling babies' feedings may result in inadequate milk production.* Sometimes mothers try to lengthen the time between feedings for one or more multiples in order to develop a household routine. Eight daily feedings may be an adequate number of feedings for some babies, but it is not enough for the baby who needs to breastfeed 12 times a day to get enough calories. Imposing rigid feeding restrictions or inflexible schedules on any baby could lead to inadequate weight gain and reduced milk production.

3. *If you depend only on pumping your breasts or combining breastfeeding with pumping to maintain milk production,* look at your pumping routine. Are you using the right equipment for the job? (For a discussion of pumping, see Chapters 11 and 12.) Did you inadvertently drop a pumping session as

you became more involved with your babies' care?

4. *Increasing milk production usually requires a short period of an increase in the number of effective breastfeedings or pumpings* –no matter what the reason for lowered milk production. That is the only way to learn whether your body can make more milk.

Mother Issues

For the small percentage of women who cannot make milk–or who cannot produce adequate milk in spite of effective breastfeeding, most difficulties are associated with either a deviation in breast structure or a health condition that affects the breasts' ability to produce milk.

Structural deviations may have biological, surgical, or traumatic causes. Examples may include:

1. Insufficient glandular (milk-making) tissue to support full milk production. Women with this condition often report they noticed little, or no, breast change during pregnancy or soon after birth. (However, little or no breast change is not a definite sign that a woman will experience a difficulty producing milk!)

2. Severely inverted nipples that cannot be drawn out for feedings. (See "Flat or Inverted Nipples," in this chapter.)

3. The failure of breasts or nipples to mature during puberty.

4. There is some evidence that inadequate milk removal during the early days to weeks postpartum may affect a woman's ability to produce sufficient milk to fully breastfeed during the particular milk-making/lactation period for this baby/babies.

5. A history of breast surgery, such as breast reduction, in which significant breast tissue was removed. Scarring that follows the outer circle of the areola (periareolar) may be associated with disruption of the milk ducts or of the nerves involved with milk production. This scarring is more common with breast reduction procedures but is used for some types of breast augmentation/implant procedures. (See "Related Parenting Books" in Resources.)

6. Occasionally, a breast biopsy, abscess, or severe mastitis damages some structure involved in milk production, however, such damage is usually limited to a small area of one breast.

7. Severe breast injury may damage some breast tissue involved in milk production. When it occurs, it is often to only one breast. Full thickness, third degree burns of the chest may damage breast tissue and other structures involved in milk production or leave severe scarring and adhesions that interfere with milk making. Blunt force trauma, such as an extreme blow to the breast area in an automobile accident could potentially damage breast

tissue or other structures involved in milk production.

8. Cardiac or other surgery in the chest area may disrupt nerves, milk-making tissue, or milk ducts. The effect is usually limited to one breast.

Health conditions with the potential to affect the breasts' ability to produce adequate milk usually have some hormonal basis and may include:

1. Retained placental fragment(s) that result in hormone levels that inhibit the milk from "coming in." Women with retained placental fragment(s) tend to experience little or no change in milk production by postpartum day three to five. In addition, this condition should be suspected when a mother continues to have periods of heavy, bright red bleeding, severe uterine cramping, or an enlarged uterus beyond a week postpartum. Mothers of multiples are more prone to this condition, and removing any fragment(s) usually resolves the milk production problem.

2. Polycystic ovarian syndrome (PCOS). Although most women affected by PCOS make adequate milk, a significant minority experience difficulty of varying degree. Treatment during pregnancy and early lactation for insulin resistance, which is a symptom of PCOS, may improve the ability to produce milk.

3. Thyroid dysfunctions. Undiagnosed and untreated thyroid conditions, particularly low thyroid (hypothyroidism), can affect a mother's ability to produce milk. Pregnancy may alter thyroid function; also, postpartum thyroid conditions appear to occur more often after multiple pregnancy. Proper treatment often results in increased milk production.

Report the "warning flags" noted above to your health care provider, but still feel cautiously optimistic about producing milk and breastfeeding. Many women with such histories do produce plenty of milk; although this may not apply to the mother with multiple babies. However, usually only time will tell whether milk production will be affected.

There are also mothers who report significant *sudden increases in milk production* at two to four months postpartum. In all these reported instances, the mothers had continued to regularly breastfeed or pump their milk on a daily basis in spite of insufficient milk production during the early weeks to months. And the increases, while often significant compared to prior production, often were not enough to fully breastfeed. Still, the increases were great enough to add considerably to the amount of mother's milk their multiples received. Unfortunately, there is not yet a way to know which mothers will experience such an increase after several weeks or months and which will not. All that is known is that when a mother stops breastfeeding or pumping her breasts will get the message to quit producing milk after this particular pregnancy.

When a knowledgeable lactation consultant or LLL Leader have ruled out breastfeeding (or pumping) management as the most likely cause of insufficient milk production, many mothers try an herbal or medication galactogogue to boost milk making. A galactogogue is a natural or synthetic chemical that many have found to aid milk production. Galactogogues do not replace adequate milk removal via breastfeeding or pumping. A single galactogue, a combination, or a rotation of different galactogues has helped many mothers who used them in addition to good milk removal. (See "Related Parenting Books" under "Breastfeeding" in Resources.)

Alternatives

If you are not producing the quantity of milk needed for your multiples, it does not mean you must wean your babies. Consider partial breastfeeding if milk production does not improve significantly after more frequent breastfeedings or pumping sessions, or if time constraints interfere with your ability to work on improving production. Partially breastfed babies still receive benefits from the nutrients and illness-fighting properties of your milk that are not found in any artificial baby milk/infant formula. Partial breastfeeding still allows you to enjoy the special closeness that comes with breastfeeding each baby. (See Chapter 18, "Full and Partial Breastfeeding.")

Flat or Inverted Nipple(s)

Flat or inverted nipples are fairly common structural variations of the breast. Often only one nipple is affected, or one may be flatter or more inverted than the other. Many women report that flat or inverted nipples improve during pregnancy. However, such improvement may appear to have been lost in the first several days after birth, especially if a mother received much intravenous fluid during labor and delivery. Stay calm. Improvement often reappears once any swelling subsides.

Many alert, full-term babies have no difficulty drawing out and latching on to an affected nipple, since babies actually latch on to the areola of the breast–not to the nipple. Some babies initially have difficulty grasping onto an inverted or flat nipple, but with a little time and patience they learn to latch on well.

- Mothers of multiples sometimes find that one baby has little or no trouble latching on to the same flat or inverted nipple that causes difficulty for another baby. If only one nipple is causing any baby difficulty, a baby more adept at latch-on could be assigned the affected breast until the other(s) becomes more proficient.
- Breast shells are hard, lightweight plastic domes that are worn inside the bra for short periods of time. They are often recommended for treating flat or inverted nipples, because the shell exerts a slight, steady pressure on the areola to help draw the nipple out. Some mothers begin to wear them during the last trimester of pregnancy, although the research support is not clear so the effectiveness of wearing shells is debatable. Be aware of the following concerns.

❑ Wearing breast shells during a multiple pregnancy may be considered an unnecessary risk for preterm labor. Do not wear breast shells during a multiple pregnancy unless your obstetric care provider approves their use.

❑ If you decide to try breast shells after giving birth, begin by wearing them for only 30 minutes before each breastfeeding. Some believe wearing breast shells may contribute to swelling in the area of the areola and nipple, making it more difficult for an infant to latch on.

Exposing the nipple to cold air or a cold cloth briefly, using RPS (see "Severe Engorgement" in this chapter) or applying a breast pump for a few minutes immediately before breastfeeding, often helps draw out a flat or inverted nipple. LLL Leaders and lactation consultants will be aware of other devices that some mothers have found helpful, such as a nipple shield or a suction device that draws out a flat or inverted nipple. Because inappropriate use of devices can hurt nipple tissue or affect milk production, it is best to get an LLL Leader's or lactation consultant's guidance before using any of them.

Plugged Ducts and Mastitis

A mother of multiples may be somewhat more susceptible to developing a plugged duct or mastitis than the mother of a single infant.

A *plugged (blocked) milk duct* feels like a lump or knot in the breast, and it usually is tender to the touch. When a plugged duct occurs at the nipple tip, it may be called a *plugged nipple pore* and usually appears as a white blister-like or skin-covered bleb on the nipple tip. When a milk duct becomes plugged/blocked, milk cannot move forward through that duct and "backs up" behind it.

Mastitis is associated with a red, swollen, tender area on the breast. It may follow a plugged duct, as backed up milk may lead to inflammation in the breast tissue surrounding the milk-making glands in that area. Mastitis differs from engorgement in that mastitis usually occurs in only one breast and any swelling tends to be in a particular area rather than the entire breast. The first sign of mastitis may be the flu-like symptoms associated with it. Mastitis occurring without a fever may be referred to as *inflammatory mastitis*. If a fever develops, it indicates the development of an *infectious mastitis*.

A mother of multiples may be somewhat more susceptible to developing a plugged duct or mastitis than the mother of a single infant. The factors that contribute to plugged milk ducts and mastitis are more common for mothers breastfeeding multiples, and they may have a greater effect on someone producing double, triple, or quadruple amounts of milk.

- When making so much milk, the body cannot adapt as quickly to a delayed, dropped, or missed feeding. Milk "build-up" may then contribute to a plugged duct or mastitis.
- Inadequate milk removal caused by poor breastfeeding technique or ineffective milk removal during breastfeeding or pumping is associated with plugged ducts and mastitis as well as for sore nipples, which was discussed earlier in this Chapter. Be more alert for the signs of a plugged duct or mastitis in a breast with a sore, red or cracked nipple.
- Some mothers of multiples find they are more prone to develop a plugged duct or mastitis if they become extremely fatigued or ill. Poor nutrition also appears to be a factor in some cases. All of these factors tend to lower a mother's resistance to illness.
- A number of mothers have developed a plugged duct or mastitis within days of preparing for and hosting a special event, such as hosting a party to celebrate a holiday or the multiples' christening. They almost always reported that such events were "stressful." Most of these mothers lost additional sleep in the days before the event, and a breastfeeding or two was delayed or missed while they were trying to get ready for or entertain guests. Trying to accomplish too much at home or at work are other sources of stress that appear to be associated with an occurrence of a plugged duct or mastitis. Both may be related to a mother's fatigue level and with inadvertent delays or missing breastfeedings/pumping sessions.
- Poorly fitting nursing bras and the constricting or "bunching" of a shirt under the armpit during feedings may contribute to a plugged duct. Either can put pressure on the breast's glandular (milk-making) tissue or milk ducts.

If you develop a plugged duct or inflammatory mastitis:
- Breastfeed babies frequently on the affected side to ensure that the affected breast remains as "empty" as possible.
- Rest and eat nutritious foods. Sure, "rest" and "multiples" sound like an incompatible combination! However, a plugged duct or inflammatory mastitis is your body's way of telling you to "Sit down and forget other chores, errands, and activities for a few days!"
- Use heat or cold on the area for comfort. Heat may be applied to the affected area in the form of warm compresses or a heating pad. Shower and let the warm water run over the area or immerse your breasts in a basin of warm water. Many women prefer to apply a cold compress or an ice pack to the affected area.
  - ❏ If part of or the entire breast feels hard or swollen, you may also be engorged. Applying cold may be a better idea.

❑ Consider taking an anti-inflammatory medication if an area of the breast is enlarged or swollen, as inflammation usually accompanies this. Talk to your health care provider for a medication recommendation.

• Massage the area while applying moist heat or after applying cold. Also, massage during breastfeeding. One form of massage is to move your hand above the plug and firmly massage over it and downward toward the areola and nipple. Another form is to firmly press in over the plugged duct with the heel of the palm of your hand for several minutes. Repeat either form several times.

• Try a breastfeeding position that takes advantage of gravity: Place one of the babies on her back on the floor (on a blanket or pad) or on a sofa. Then lean over, bending at the waist, to feed the baby. Use this position for several feedings a day until the plugged duct is no longer felt.

• Some mothers find it helpful to take extra vitamin C.

• If you develop a plugged nipple pore:
   ❑ Use a soft, clean cloth or gauze pad that has been soaked in hot water and apply as a compress just prior to breastfeeding or pumping on that breast.

   ❑ Remove the skin over the plugged pore after using the compress and before breastfeeding or pumping if prior breastfeeding/pumping has not opened it. You might rub over it with the compress cloth or use an extremely clean fingernail to "scrape" over the area. Contact your health care provider if this does not work.

   ❑ Keep the area clean and dry. Once a day wash the nipple tip with a non-antibacterial, non-perfumed soap and then rinse well.

• For repeated plugged ducts:
   ❑ Look at your breastfeeding or pumping routine. Many mothers continue to pump milk fairly frequently, even after babies can breastfeed effectively. It is one thing to have enough expressed milk to help with a feeding or two, but overdoing it may lead to problems, such as plugged ducts.

   ❑ Some mothers report they experienced fewer plugged ducts after they started taking supplementary lecithin. Contact an LLL Leader or lactation consultant for a reference regarding the usual recommended amount.

• Contact your obstetric care provider if there is no change in a plugged duct or if it has grown in size after several days of self-treatment.

If your *temperature is above 100.4°F (38°C),* call your obstetric care provider immediately as the elevated temperature indicates an infectious mastitis.

• In addition to following the suggestions for inflammatory mastitis, your health care provider is likely to prescribe an antibiotic for 10 to 14 days per current recommendations.

- Although almost all antibiotics are compatible with continued breastfeeding, ask your health care provider about the one being prescribed and ask for a different medication if there is a question about compatibility with breastfeeding.
- If you experience more than two bouts of infectious mastitis, it is likely that the antibiotic has not "killed" all the bacteria that caused the first bout. There are several reasons for and strategies to deal with this:
  - ❑ As they begin to feel better, busy mothers often forget to take the medication, or stop taking it as often as prescribed. It is important to take the full course of antibiotics if you want to decrease the chance of a recurrence.
  - ❑ Sometimes a care provider is not aware of the 10 to 14 day recommendation for antibiotic treatment with infectious mastitis.
  - ❑ If a less common bacteria is causing infectious mastitis, the medication may not be the right one for the job. Your health care provider may need to do more testing to discover which bacteria is causing the problem.

Overabundant Milk Production and Forceful Let-Down/Milk-Ejection Reflex

Mothers of multiples tend to worry that they will not produce enough milk, but many mothers find themselves coping with the opposite problem. Producing for multiple babies sometimes leads to "oversupply" or rapid "refilling" with milk. Generally, this is a good problem to have, but some babies quickly become over-full, which may cause them to spit up or develop stomachache symptoms. The combination of frequent spit-up and apparent intestinal discomfort may be signs of gastro-esophageal reflux disorder (GERD), which is more common for babies born preterm.

If babies frequently choke, sputter, or break away and cry within a minute or two after beginning a feeding, it may be due to a forceful let-down, or milk-ejection reflex (MER). Forceful let-down may occur alone, but it often occurs in conjunction with overabundant milk production. Most babies learn to handle a forceful let-down as they mature. In the meantime, the following ideas may help.

- Offer each baby only one breast at a feeding (if you have not already begun to do this). If overproduction continues to be an issue, assign each baby a specific breast for several days or weeks to see if production in each breast adapts to each multiple's nutritional needs. (You may want babies to switch sides for an evening feeding a few times a week so that each baby remains willing to feed from both breasts.)
- Do not limit feeding time on the one breast unless absolutely necessary. If you must limit feeding time to 10 to 20 minutes, you may find babies ask to breastfeed more frequently but for a shorter period.

- Offer the breast when you notice any baby's early feeding cues. This can help in two ways. The let-down is often more gentle and you may avoid overfull breasts.
- Breastfeed in an "uphill" position to slow both a forceful let-down and the rate of milk delivery. The let-down may be more manageable for babies, and they often can breastfeed comfortably for a longer period.
  - ❑ To breastfeed uphill, lean back in a semi-reclining position or lie down, and place one or two babies in the clutch, prone, or kneeling positions. (See "Simultaneous Feeding Positions" in Chapter 14.)
  - ❑ A double (or single) straddle in which each baby sits facing a breast while straddling one of mother's legs can slow the flow.
- Some find the side-lying position to be helpful when breastfeeding only one baby.
- Some babies are very good about knowing when to stop. These babies will refuse to take the breast again because their tummies are full, yet they still act interested in sucking after they have finished a feeding. Some mothers find that these babies are more content if offered a pacifier at these times.
  - ❑ Avoid offering a pacifier to any baby who does not breastfeed effectively or one who is not gaining weight appropriately. (See Chapter 15.)
  - ❑ Be aware of the potential for overuse of pacifiers, which is associated with early weaning. As much as possible hold and cuddle babies if offering a pacifier.
  - ❑ Encourage babies to "latch-on" to a pacifier similarly as to the breast by stimulating rooting and a wide-open mouth before inserting a pacifier in a baby's mouth.
  - ❑ Many multiples find a thumb or a finger more pleasant to suck.

- Overabundant production may put you at more risk for developing a plugged duct or mastitis. For some mothers overuse of a breast pump increases milk production well beyond the babies' need for milk, which may contribute to the problem.
- Contact an LLL Leader or a lactation consultant if overabundant production causes discomfort for you.

Milk Leakage

Milk leakage is not truly a breastfeeding problem, but it can seem a nuisance. It is more common during the early weeks or months of breastfeeding. Leakage usually diminishes as a mother's body gets used to babies breastfeeding, and it often stops altogether within several weeks or months. There are ways to minimize leaking in the meantime.

- Often you can halt leakage by immediately applying firm, direct pressure over the nipple with the heel of your hand. If at first that does not succeed, keep trying. To discreetly apply pressure to both breasts at once, lace your fingers together and spread your hands over your chest so that the heel of each palm is over a nipple. Then press inward firmly.

- Turn milk leakage to your advantage. When feeding only one baby, hold a clean cup under the other breast and collect the leaking milk. Pour it into a bottle or a milk-storage bag, and refrigerate or freeze it for later use. (See "Guidelines for Storing Human Milk" in the Appendix.)

- There are alternatives to the expensive nursing pads on the market. Large white handkerchiefs work, but washing all those hankies may be one thing you can live without when caring for multiples. White paper towels are another option. Fold one paper towel (or double it) in half lengthwise and then into thirds to make a disposable, inexpensive nursing pad. Many paper towels come in bulk packs, but choose a brand that is soft yet absorbent. Mothers also have cut disposable diapers (minus the outer plastic lining) or sanitary napkins for disposable nursing pads; however, some contain perfumes or deodorants that may be irritating to nipple or areola tissue.

Maternal Illness, Disability, or Health-Related Conditions

Mothers have breastfed multiples while coping with many different kinds of short- or long-term illnesses, physical disabilities, or other health-related conditions. Often their family, friends, or health care providers expressed concern that breastfeeding two or more babies might be "too much" for them, yet these mothers found breastfeeding actually simplified caring for more than one baby.

Physicians' greatest concern may be about the medications recommended to treat various illnesses and conditions. They may question whether a medication will get into a mother's milk and affect the babies. However, the risk or danger to babies of not receiving their mother's milk usually is much higher than the potential risk from a medication. If you or your doctor is unsure about the effect of any medication for the babies, contact an LLL Leader, a board-certified lactation consultant, or the babies' pediatric care provider. They often have scientific references about a medication's effects on human milk. A few medications are not compatible with breastfeeding, but in most cases there are alternative medications that may be prescribed instead.

Sometimes a mother's illness or health condition requires medical or surgical treatment in a hospital. (See Chapter 17 for more information.) Some mothers find that milk production decreases temporarily after a surgery or with an infectious illness. It may be related to the mother's recuperative needs or she may not have been

Mothers coping with illnesses, physical disabilities, or other health-related conditions often say that breastfeeding actually simplifies caring for more than one baby.

able to breastfeed or pump her breasts as often as necessary. However, a return to frequent breastfeeding or pumping sessions quickly reverses any reduction in milk production.

Breastfeeding multiple babies can be confusing enough without developing sore nipples, severe engorgement, or a plugged duct, or wondering whether it is possible to produce enough milk. Since most mother problems are related to a minor snag in breastfeeding management or one multiple's mechanics at the breast, the majority of these problems go away once the management or mechanical issue resolves. Get help immediately when a problem develops; do not let a problem persist without seeking help. No mother caring for multiple babies should have to devote extra time to handle these kinds of problems for any longer than necessary.

KEY POINTS

❑ If you ever develop sore/painful or damaged nipples/breasts, immediately contact a La Leche League Leader or a lactation consultant.

- Sore nipples are most often related to the "mechanics" of how the breast and each baby's mouth "fit" together.

- If a structure(s) in a baby's mouth is the cause, the structural issue may need "fixing."

- A fungal (yeast) infection, such as thrush, can cause nipple soreness/damage.

❑ The breasts may feel more full and heavy at about 2 to 6 days after birth when the milk is said to have "come in."

❑ A mother's breasts become hard, lumpy, and painful with severe engorgement, and the nipples/areola may be too tight for the babies to latch on easily.

- If treatment is begun quickly, severe engorgement usually resolves in 12 to 24 hours.

❑ The most common reason for insufficient milk production is a lack in milk removal. A suckling difficulty in one or more babies and trying to "schedule" breastfeeding are common causes.

❑ A few women have physical issues that interfere with producing enough milk.

- Galactogogues (herbal or medication) may improve milk production if used in addition to frequent milk removal.

- Partial breastfeeding is worthwhile if milk production is too low.

❑ Flat or inverted nipples may affect a baby's ability to latch on during early breastfeeding.

❑ Mothers of multiples may be more prone to a plugged/blocked milk duct. When a plugged duct leads to poor "emptying" in an area of one breast, it may result in mastitis.

- Increased milk removal and rest are the best way to treat a plugged duct or mastitis.

- Call your health care provider if you develop a fever of 100.4°F (38°C).

❑ Breastfeeding more than one baby may lead to overabundant milk production.

❑ Many mothers have breastfed multiples while also coping with a short-term or chronic illness, physical disability, or other health condition.

- Most medications are either compatible with breastfeeding or an alternative medication is available so that breastfeeding can continue.

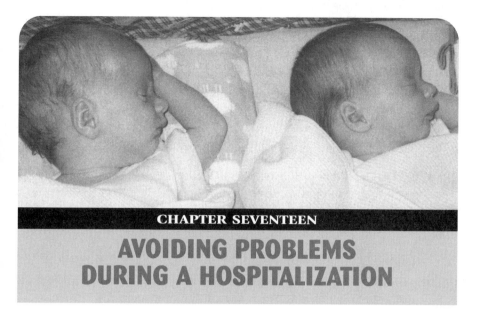

CHAPTER SEVENTEEN

AVOIDING PROBLEMS
DURING A HOSPITALIZATION

Occasionally, a mother or one of her multiples has a health problem that requires hospitalization. (Such situations occur more often with multiples than singletons due to preterm birth or other multiple-pregnancy issues.) Sometimes a close family member must be hospitalized, and the mother's presence is needed for that relative. No matter who is hospitalized, a mother of multiples often feels torn between the demands of the situation and each baby's needs.

If a mother faces hospitalization, she may feel concerned about separation from her babies and a possible drop in milk production in order to meet her health needs. Mothers often feel pulled when one baby must be hospitalized, and the needs of that baby must be weighed against those of the other(s) remaining at home. When a close family member is the patient, a mother may feel she belongs in two places at once–at home with the babies and at the hospital to support the family member.

No matter who is hospitalized, the ideal is for a mother and her breastfeeding multiples to stay together for the duration of a hospital stay. This ideal often is attainable, but it will be up to you, and possibly your husband or partner, to pursue it. As a parent, you not only have the right, you also have the responsibility to see that the needs of your babies are met in the best possible way.

Exploring Options

Some parents have changed physicians or hospitals to keep the breastfeeding family intact.

If you find that you, one of your babies, or someone close to you is facing a hospitalization, there usually are options to help you meet the needs of all involved.

- Explore alternatives to actual hospital admission with the physician. Often diagnostic tests, treatment interventions, and even surgery can be done on an outpatient basis.
- Ask whether elective procedures could be postponed safely for a period of time.

- If you ever feel uncomfortable with a physician's explanation of a health problem, the reason for a particular treatment, or the need for immediate intervention, continue to ask questions until you are completely satisfied. Ultimately, you are responsible for your health care and that of your family. Never feel inhibited about seeking adequate information. It is your right.

- When hospitalization is unavoidable, arrange to take the babies to the hospital, especially if the hospital is many miles from home. Some parents have changed physicians or hospitals to keep the breastfeeding family intact. It is reasonable to expect the hospital staff to help you find some way to accommodate your babies' need for close contact with you during the hospitalization. Taking both babies has worked well for many mothers of twins, although it gets more complicated when higher multiples are involved.

  ❏ It may be less complicated to rotate babies. Some mothers of higher-order multiples keep two babies with them; a helper picks up one or both babies and drops off another one or two every few hours.

  ❏ A "rotation" plan may also work better if you have twins and you or another family member is the patient. Most mothers recruit extra helping hands. Having someone with you to help with babies is crucial when you are the patient, but it is also very important if you must be available to a hospitalized baby or family member.

  ❏ The next-best arrangement is to have the babies brought to the hospital–together or one at a time–several times a day. In many areas babies may be brought directly to a patient's hospital room. When this is not possible, there is always some area on a hospital unit or on another floor where you and the babies can be together for a while. (Insist that the babies be brought to the unit/same floor as your room if you are the one hospitalized and babies are not allowed in patient rooms. If you continue to ask, a place to visit will usually be found.) When a baby or another family member is hospitalized in an intensive care unit, there is usually a family lounge or waiting area nearby.

- If one of the babies or a family member is the patient and you are not allowed to bring in all of the babies, another option is to leave the hospital a few times each day to go to the babies. However, it is easy to become exhausted if constantly running between hospital and home (or hotel), so develop an alternative plan in case this does not work for you.
- When a brief hospitalization is anticipated, express milk ahead of time for any baby who is to remain at home. For example, a surgical procedure requiring an overnight hospital stay was planned for one of twins. Rather than take the well twin back and forth to the hospital for breastfeeding, that baby stayed home with family members. The mother expressed enough milk to feed the "at home" baby for the 18 to 24 hours she would be at the hospital with his twin. (See the Appendix, "Storing Human Milk.")
- Whether the babies stay throughout a hospitalization or are brought in every few hours, certain items may help everyone feel more comfortable while at the hospital. Some items may be available at a hospital, but others must be brought from home. Items may include: a rocking chair (a folding lawn-chair type will do), a baby sling or carrier, a lightweight single or double stroller, and disposable diapers. If any baby enjoys playtime in an infant seat, be sure one is available. Take extra changes of clothing for babies, unless each can wear hospital-issued gowns.

Emergency Situations

Sometimes hospitalization is necessary for a sudden health need or an actual emergency. Immediacy may be unavoidable for some surgical or medical treatments. In these situations, there may be little, if any, time to explore alternatives for keeping the breastfeeding "team" together. Yet many mothers have continued to breastfeed multiples during or after such unanticipated events.

To maintain breastfeeding with an unanticipated hospitalization, begin by maintaining milk production. Express milk as soon as possible–soon after you get to the hospital or as soon as you think of it. Whichever comes first! You will also want to express milk at regular two to three hour intervals during the day and when you wake or are awakened at night. If you are the one who is ill or had surgery, you may need your husband/partner, a nurse, or a close relative or friend to help you use a breast pump for the first 12 to 24 hours. After 12 to 36 hours of treatment or after surgery, many mothers find they are ready to have babies brought to them in the hospital.

> Explain, and repeat as many times as necessary, that it is impossible to treat one member of your breastfeeding team without affecting every member of that team.

Be sure the hospital staff understands the consequences of delayed or missed breastfeedings when a mother is producing milk for multiples. Frequent breastfeeding or pumping helps prevent complications by decreasing the risk of severe engorgement or the development of a plugged duct or mastitis.

- If contact with the babies must be limited due to your situation, ask whether a breast pump is available on the hospital unit where you are staying. A breast pump should be available if the hospital has a birthing unit, but, if possible, call the hospital before admission and ask about breast pump availability.
  - ❏ If you already have a double collection kit, take it with you. It may be the same brand as the hospital pump, although a hospital able to provide a breast pump is usually able to also provide a collection kit.

- A high-level "personal use" breast pump—one designed for frequent daily pumping—may be adequate if milk production is well established and around-the-clock pumping is necessary for only a few days.
- Some mothers have found it necessary to rent a breast pump to take into the hospital.
  - ❏ If you take a rental pump, be sure it is compatible with any collection kit you already have or you will probably need to purchase a new kit.
  - ❏ To prevent theft, some mothers chain a rented breast pump to the frame of the hospital bed with the type of chain and lock used for securing a bicycle.

- It is not unusual to experience a temporary decrease in milk production during a hospitalization, so do not panic if this occurs. The physical and emotional stress, plus a decrease in the usual number of breastfeedings or pumping sessions, may contribute to reduced production,

> **Frequent breastfeeding or pumping helps prevent complications by decreasing the risk of engorgement or the development of a plugged duct.**

- To get milk production back on track, do what you would do any time milk production is not up to the babies' needs. Breastfeed each baby (or pump) more frequently, eat a balanced diet, drink adequate fluids, and minimize other activities so you get enough rest.
- If you and your babies have been separated, they may cling to you when you return. On the other hand some babies ignore their mother initially after being reunited, which may include resisting breastfeeding for several days. Increasing skin-to-skin contact with them usually helps in either case.
  - ❏ Consider taking a "babymoon"–a few days of round-the-clock breast-feeding in bed, with everyone's shirt off for skin-to-skin contact and "room service" for all meals. (Meals are brought in by family and friends.)

When Breastfeeding Is Contraindicated

Breastfeeding can continue, and should be encouraged, during most health-related situations. Weaning is *rarely* necessary for health care problems or because of medications a mother must take. A health care provider may know a great deal about a specialized area of health care yet know little about breastfeeding and lactation. If you are told to wean, ask for an explanation from the health care provider. Then call a La Leche League Leader or a lactation consultant for additional information. She can help you explore whether alternatives to weaning may be available in your situation. Most health care providers are happy to listen to or read available research evidence about breastfeeding for a special situation or to accommodate realistic options to weaning.

> **Weaning is rarely necessary for health care problems or because of medications a mother must take.**

When exploring options for keeping your breastfeeding team intact during a hospitalization, your physician or family members may be concerned that keeping your multiples with you when possible will be too taxing. There are several points you may want to make when arranging for your babies to be with you.

- Explain, and repeat as many times as necessary, that it is impossible to treat one member of your breastfeeding team without affecting every member of that team. Some health professionals or family members may not understand how it benefits you to keep milk moving or how it benefits babies to receive mother's milk without interruption. They may not grasp the intimacy of the breastfeeding relationship or that you and your babies work together to achieve a physical harmony.

- Only you can help others understand that the greater burden would be separation from your babies or that worrying about their welfare and feeling torn about whose needs are greatest would create an even more stressful situation.

Although others may not understand that breastfeeding is more than a way of getting food into babies or that it provides a sick baby with the perfect nourishment for healing, make your intentions clear, develop a plan, and let each person know how to help you carry it out.

The hospitalization of a family member is a source of stress no matter when it occurs or what the circumstances. That stress may be compounded if a mother must juggle the intense needs of multiple breastfed infants with the needs of the family member requiring hospitalization. If you have any questions or concerns about breastfeeding and meeting the needs of your babies during any family member's hospitalization, contact an LLL Leader or a lactation consultant for information and support.

KEY POINTS

❑ Sometimes a mother, one of her babies, or a family member is hospitalized during multiples' infancy–the period when each has an intense need for mother's presence and her milk.

❑ Outpatient testing or procedures may negate or delay a need for hospitalization.

❑ For an unavoidable hospitalization, it may be possible to bring babies for some/all of the time.

  • A helper is needed when all babies are at the hospital with their mother.

  • Sometimes only one baby may remain with mother, so multiples "take turns" with mother.

  • If not "taking turns," have someone bring babies to the hospital to breastfeed.

❑ To prevent breastfeeding problems, breastfeed or pump at least 8 times in 24 hours.

  • Hospitals often have a breast pump (and collection kit) available.

❑ Milk production may drop briefly with the stress of hospitalization, especially if not able to breastfeed or pump frequently.

  • Milk production will "bounce back" with extra breastfeeding or pumping and mother-babies skin contact.

❑ Weaning is rarely necessary for a mother's or any baby's health care situation.

❑ Remind health care providers, relatives, and friends that you and your babies are a breastfeeding team–all are affected when one is ill or needs medical treatment.

❑ An LLL Leader or a lactation consultant can give you support and options for continuing to breastfeed, which can be shared with health care providers.

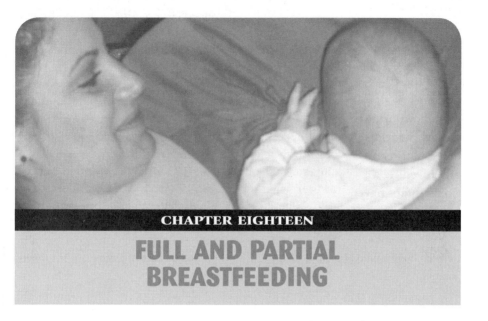

CHAPTER EIGHTEEN

FULL AND PARTIAL BREASTFEEDING

It makes sense that Nature would design human milk to be the perfect food for human babies. Most human infants grow and develop best when fully breastfed for their first six months. However, Nature also designed the typical human to give birth to only one baby at a time. Technology, not Nature, is mainly responsible for both an increase in the number of multiple births and the improved survival rate for these multiple-birth infants.

Although technology has not found a way to give a new mother more hours in a day or provide additional arms so she can care for multiple babies more easily, Nature apparently did anticipate a boom in multiple births when it created breast-feeding and human milk. Human milk and the process of breastfeeding can adapt to the number of babies that need to be fed. Most women are able to produce enough milk for several babies. In addition, human milk produced after a preterm birth is different and contains more of what preterm infants need than milk produced at full term. Even the later milk of a mother with preterm babies is different than full-term milk. A mother's milk is the only infant food that continually changes as babies grow and develop.

What does a mother do when Nature gives her the ability to breastfeed multiple babies, but she and her babies did not have ideal conditions for initiating breast-feeding? What does she do when it seems there are not enough hours in every day to cope with 8 to 12 feedings for each baby? What does she do if, in spite of good lactation management, milk production is not adequate for multiple babies?

The physical demands of a multiple pregnancy and birth and the round-the-clock care for two or more newborns creates situations that a mother breastfeeding a single infant never encounters.

What does she do? She does her best. For one mother this may mean fully breastfeeding each multiple for several weeks or months; whereas, another mother may have to offer the babies her milk or an infant formula by another method at times.

The physical demands of a multiple pregnancy and birth and the round-the-clock care for two or more newborns creates situations that a mother breastfeeding a single infant never encounters. To make breastfeeding decisions that are best for their multiple babies and for themselves, mothers must weigh the benefits of full and partial breastfeeding and then examine their particular family situation. It may also help to be aware of some of the pitfalls that can lead to unnecessary supplementation when breastfeeding multiples.

When partial breastfeeding is or becomes the goal, a realistic plan may make the difference between long-term breastfeeding and untimely weaning.

Breastfeeding Definitions

New mothers may be unfamiliar with some of the terms that lactation consultants and other health professionals and La Leche League Leaders use to refer to breastfeeding. Several of these terms refer to breastfeeding "quantity," and others refer to aspects of different types of feeding a baby may receive.

Multiples nourished only by breastfeeding are said to be *fully, exclusively, or completely breastfed.* Fully breastfed babies receive no other liquids or solids. When a baby *is almost fully breastfed,* the baby may receive vitamins and minerals or an occasional feeding of some other liquid.

A baby is *partially breastfed* when the baby is regularly fed by an alternative method, such as by syringe, feeding tube, infant feeding bottle, etc. Such feedings usually consist of some food other than the mother's milk, including infant formulas, water, juices, or any type of solid food.

When expressed human milk, infant formula, or any other infant food is regularly offered to a baby after a breastfeeding, it is considered a *complement* to breastfeeding. In some areas a complement feeding is called a *top-off* feed.

A *supplement* replaces all, or most, of a breastfeeding. Instead of breastfeeding first, a baby receives only expressed human milk or infant formula at a particular feeding.

The term *breast-milk-feeding,* or *human-milk-feeding,* may be used when a baby is fed expressed human milk by an alternative feeding method or by using a bottle. Some mothers fully human-milk-feed one or more multiples for days, weeks, and even several months. Other mothers breastfeed directly for some feedings, but one or more babies are human-milk-fed at other feedings.

Benefits of Full and Partial Breastfeeding

Nature intended for babies to receive full or almost full breastfeeding during their first several months, and Nature had very good reasons for designing human milk and the process of breastfeeding to nourish human babies as it did. Human milk creates a balance within the fully breastfed baby's body systems, so the human infant can easily absorb essential nutrients, eliminate waste, and minimize exposure to potentially allergenic or disease-causing substances. Introducing a foreign substance, such as infant formula, interferes with that balance. Still, multiples benefit when they receive any amount of their mother's milk.

Receiving almost any amount of human milk is associated with better health for babies.

Because of the antibody properties found only in human milk, fully, or almost fully, breastfed babies have the lowest rates for many common bacterial or viral illnesses. Partially breastfed babies still are less likely to contract many common infant illnesses than babies receiving only infant formula. Receiving almost any amount of human milk is associated with better health for babies.

The degree of difference for the rates of several common infant illnesses depends on the percentage of a partially breastfed baby's diet that comes from mother's milk and the percentage that comes from other sources. The more breastfeeding or human milk a baby receives, the healthier that baby is likely to be. The less babies breastfeed or receive human milk, the more the illness rate approximates that of babies on diets consisting only of artificial infant milk or other foods.

In addition to being the optimal way to deliver human milk, the process of *direct breastfeeding* ensures close contact with mother. A computer-age mother may not worry as much as her stone-age counterpart about keeping a baby physically safe from saber-toothed tigers and other environmental hazards, but each baby's need for the emotional and physical comfort provided by close contact with mother has not changed for tens of thousands of years.

Multiples must share mother from before birth. Once babies arrive, infant care can too easily become a series of tasks rather than an opportunity for building a relationship with each baby. No matter how much round-the-clock attention multiples require, each still is an individual with the same need for physical contact as any single baby. Any amount of direct breastfeeding provides an important means of close contact with mother.

Dealing with Temptation

What if your multiples have arrived and all are breastfeeding well? The babies' diaper counts are good and each is gaining weight. That still leaves you with at least eight and up to 12 or more daily feedings times two, three, or more. Even if two always breastfeed simultaneously, you are feeding babies for many hours of every day.

There are days, and nights, when most mothers feel willing to try anything if it might calm two or more crying babies. Yes, supplementing is mighty tempting when

No matter how much round-the-clock attention multiples require, each still is an individual with the same need for physical contact as any single baby.

multiples are howling, they have demanded extra feedings all day, and you are wondering if you have enough milk. Or it may be the prospect of an entire night's sleep a few times a week that makes supplementing sound so appealing.

Family, friends, and health professionals often pressure mothers of multiples to complement or supplement breastfeeding even when all babies are doing well. Some think it is not possible to produce enough milk for multiples. Many worry that breastfeeding multiples is too hard on a mother.

No matter what form temptation takes, you are not alone if you find yourself thinking at times that there has got to be an easier or better way than fully breastfeeding multiples. Many mothers ask themselves at least once a day, and usually well before that fifteenth feeding, "Why am I doing this?"

To get past these temptations, answer the question. Why are you doing this? You can remind yourself and others that you are doing this because you want all of your babies to get all of the physical and emotional benefits of breastfeeding and your milk.

Repeating "self-talk" statements may help. Some mothers post various one-liners in conspicuous spots.

"This is a short period of time in my life, but it is a crucial time in my babies' lives."

Feedings should meet babies' need to be held in mother's arms as much as they meet babies' need for nourishment. Breastfeeding ensures they receive both. The period of at least 8 to 12 or more daily feedings per baby lasts a relatively short time. In a few months all will be ready to add other foods to their diets, and they will begin to gradually drop breastfeedings. Before you know it, each will be weaned and off on adventures away from home.

"I know I'm making enough milk because each baby has enough wet and soiled diapers, and each is gaining a normal amount of weight."

Frequent breastfeeding increases milk production. Typically, each baby should breastfeed at least 8 and up to 12 (or more) times in 24 hours, but different babies have different breastfeeding needs. It can be confusing, but it is quite normal for one (or more) to need to breastfeed at least 10 to 12 times in 24 hours while another is satisfied and growing well with 8 to 10 breastfeeds in the same period. Having different breastfeeding patterns is especially common for dizygotic (fraternal) multiples.

Babies, like most adults, sometimes want to eat for reasons other than hunger. And like adults, some of their daily feedings may be more of a snack or to quench thirst than for a big meal.

"Look what I did! My babies have gained a total of ___ pounds!"
Post this self-talk statement with the babies' latest weight total. Do not forget to pat yourself on the back every time you read it. There may not be a better feeling in the world than watching multiple babies grow–all on mother's milk.

"It takes time to prepare bottles and clean feeding equipment. I am giving that time to my babies" or "In the time that it would take to warm a supplement, I could sit down and breastfeed and my babies would be happy."
When fully breastfeeding two or more babies, supplementing may sound like a way to make life easier. Other feeding methods are often presented as if the time and effort required for multiple feedings will *magically* disappear! No method can do this. It takes extra time–and extra effort–to feed two or more babies no matter how they are fed.

Supplementing multiples can further complicate a mother's hectic life. If help is rarely available at feeding times, alternative feedings offer no advantage and often add work. In surveys, mothers of bottle-fed multiples complained most about the amount of time required for preparation and clean-up of feeding equipment. Mothers who breastfeed multiples after artificially feeding a previous child often say they like the fact that breastfeeding is always "ready to go"–no making a baby wait and no cleaning up.

> Family, friends, and health professionals often pressure mothers of multiples to complement or supplement breastfeeding even when all babies are doing well.

Some mothers are encouraged to offer their young babies infant cereal at bedtime, as it was once thought that it would help babies to sleep longer. Several studies have shown that this practice does not affect babies' sleep patterns. If given before several months of age, babies cannot digest solid food well, so most of the nutrients are wasted and they miss a meal or take less of mother's highly digestible milk. More importantly, giving cereal or other foods too early may expose babies to possible allergens unnecessarily.

Confidence is what a mother needs if she is to avoid *unnecessary supplementation.* When tempted to offer supplements, keep answering the question of why you chose to fully breastfeed. Remember how you feel when the babies are weighed and you know that all those pounds are from your milk alone.

Recruit family, friends, and health professionals for their support, and ask them to avoid any discouraging words. Let them know how much it means to you and your babies to breastfeed. Remind them that multiples require more time and effort no matter how they are fed. Tell them when you are in need of someone to listen while you vent and when you could use some positive cheerleading due to doubting your ability to breastfeed.

Partial Breastfeeding

Multiples may be partially breastfed for many reasons. Many mothers planned to fully breastfeed, but partial breastfeeding was thrust upon them when babies were born prematurely or one or more was sick at birth. If one or more babies experience an ongoing breastfeeding difficulty, a mother of multiples does not always have the time to work through the problem as a mother with a single baby can. Recovery from multiple pregnancy and birth conditions or the side effects of related treatments, sometimes affect a mother's ability to fully breastfeed. Occasionally, a mother has a physical condition that affects her body's ability to produce enough milk for multiple infants. Other mothers find their family situations simply do not allow the time it would take to breastfeed each baby at least eight and often more times a day.

Some mothers decide during pregnancy to partially breastfeed once their multiples arrive. Knowing themselves and knowing their family situations, they know they will need help with some feedings. Mothers sometimes choose partial breastfeeding after several weeks of full breastfeeding so they can begin to have regular relief for some feedings. These mothers may find that it helps them cope if someone offers a baby a supplementary feeding when two or more babies "cluster" feedings at the same time of day. Some mothers choose partial breastfeeding so they can get a few hours of uninterrupted sleep. They delegate someone else to handle one of the night feedings on a regular basis. Other mothers initiate partial breastfeeding when they return to an employed position.

Full Breastfeeding as a Goal

Many mothers have moved gradually to full breastfeeding as babies' ability at the breast or a mother's physical condition improved.

The more babies in a multiple set, the more likely it is that some difficulty will affect a goal of full breastfeeding. Do not let that discourage you if full breastfeeding of your babies is your goal. It may be necessary to supplement with your milk or an infant formula initially, but many mothers have moved gradually to full breastfeeding as babies' ability at the breast or a mother's physical condition improved. (See Chapter 12, "Making Up for a Poor Start," and Chapter 15, "Breastfeeding Difficulties in Young Babies.") This may take weeks, and occasionally months, for any given multiple, especially if babies were extremely preterm, any was in severe distress, or time to work with a particular baby is limited.

There are times when fully breastfeeding multiples is never going to become a reality. For the mother who wanted to fully breastfeed her babies, this realization can bring feelings of terrible disappointment. Often a mother will grieve for what she and her babies will miss as she lets go of this goal. Sometimes it helps to shift the focus to the many benefits of partial breastfeeding and to partially breastfeed in a way that allows babies to breastfeed for as long as they would like.

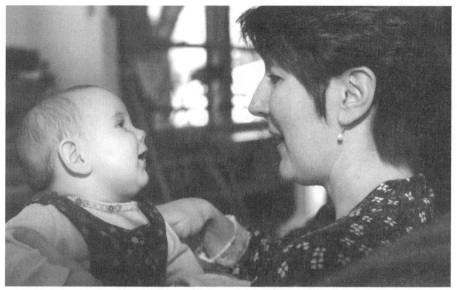

Breastfeeding helps a mother form individual attachments with each multiple.

Partial Breastfeeding as a Goal

Partial breastfeeding is a valid goal. Each mother knows her family situation best, and full breastfeeding may not be a realistic consideration for some mothers caring for multiples. If the choice is between partial breastfeeding or full bottle-feeding, obviously any amount of breastfeeding is the better choice for the babies. Partially breastfed multiples often continue to breastfeed into toddlerhood, and they can experience natural weaning the same as multiples that were fully breastfed during their first months.

Successful Partial Breastfeeding

The less "partial" the partial breastfeeding is, the more likely it will continue without unanticipated weaning. When possible, establish breastfeeding and adequate milk production by fully breastfeeding or pumping, or by using a combination of breastfeeding and pumping comparable to full breastfeeding, for the first week or two after birth. Once milk production and breastfeeding are well established and milk production is plentiful, partial breastfeeding can be initiated. When you plan to breastfeed the babies for several months or longer, bottle-feedings should be introduced on as limited a basis as possible.

> If the choice is between partial breastfeeding or full bottle-feeding, any amount of breastfeeding is the better choice for the babies.

- Complementary feedings given after breastfeeding first are more compatible with long-term, partial breastfeeding than supplementary feedings.

- Mothers choosing to offer a bottle usually do so in the evening, when babies tend to "cluster" feedings, or during the night. After breastfeeding first, dad might top off each baby's evening feeding, or a baby might be supplemented if he wants to eat again within an hour or two of the last breastfeeding. Another option is for dad to bottle-feed one (or more) during the evening or night while mother breastfeeds the other(s). Perhaps dad bottle-feeds all babies for one night feeding and mother breastfeeds all at the next one.
- Some mothers partially breastfeed, but their babies still receive only mother's milk. These mothers pump their milk once or twice every morning, and dad or someone else offers mother's expressed milk to the babies later in the day or during the night.

In order to reinforce breastfeeding oral (mouth) behaviors if bottle-feeding, you (or a feeding helper) should:

- Place baby in an almost upright (sitting to semi-sitting) position with one hand supporting baby's neck and shoulders. (When properly positioned, baby's chin will tilt slightly upward–not toward the chest, and baby will sit with legs "bent" outward from the hips–not bent at the waist. Baby should not look slumped over.)
- Gently touch the tip of baby's nose with the bottle teat/nipple before stroking down from baby's nose and over her upper lip to stimulate the rooting reflex, which encourages baby's mouth to open wide. When baby's mouth is open wide, let baby "latch" onto the bottle teat as you want baby to latch onto your breast.
- Baby is likely to pause after a few minutes of feeding. Take advantage of this natural pause to give baby a sense of the ebb and flow that occurs during breastfeeding by allowing the baby to stop occasionally. Resume the feeding when the baby signals readiness or after at least 20 to 30 seconds.
- A relaxed pace should guide bottle-feeds. If the average time a baby spends "emptying" the first breast during early breastfeeding is about 10 to 30 minutes and 5 to 15 minutes as baby grows, Nature must be trying to tell parents something. Take another look at bottle-teat flow rate when a young baby empties a 60 to 120 ml (2 to 4 oz) bottle in less time than 10 to 15 minutes or an older one finishes a feeding in less than 5 to 10 minutes.

Alternating Feeding Methods with Twins

Health professionals or concerned family members sometimes suggest that a mother of twins alternate breastfeeding and bottle-feeding. The mother is told to either breastfeed all babies for one feeding and bottle-feed all at the next, or she is told to breastfeed one and bottle-feed the other at every feeding–rotating which baby is breastfed and which is bottle-fed. Following this feeding plan often leads to early weaning from the breast.

Alternating feeding methods can interfere with long-term breastfeeding of twins for a number of reasons. Mothers with twins tend to have less regular household help than mothers with higher-order multiples. Unless a mother has someone else who prepares for and cleans up after all supplementary feedings, alternating feeding methods means a lot more work. This mother is investing twice the time because she has the equivalent of one fully breastfed baby and one fully bottle-fed baby.

In addition, when almost half of the babies' calories are coming from infant formula, milk production drops. Infant formula takes longer than human milk to digest, so babies will not "cue" to breastfeed often enough. This means less milk is removed from the breasts, which contributes to a decrease in milk production.

Once milk production decreases, the babies may not seem as content. Most mothers find it is difficult to cope with two full-time feeding methods and dwindling milk production. Before long something has to go. Rebuilding milk production can seem a daunting task. So before the mother knows it, her babies are weaned from the breast and both are artificially fed.

If you do breastfeed twins half-time, yet you want your babies to breastfeed for several months, the following suggestions may help.

- To maintain adequate milk production and avoid unanticipated weaning, you still want to breastfeed (or pump) often enough to equal at least 8, and up to 12 or more, feedings a day. For example, breastfeed (or pump for) each twin at least 4 to 6 times in 24 hours for a daily total of at least 100 and closer to 120 to 140 minutes of breastfeeding/pumping.

- If weight gain is an issue, monitor the diaper counts and weigh any baby as needed. Consider test-weighing, which is described in Chapter 12, "Making Up for a Poor Start." Then you can adjust the amount of expressed human milk or infant formula to suit the individual baby's circumstances.

Number of breastfeedings needed every 24 hours to maintain adequate milk production for long-term partial breastfeeding (for first 6 or more months):

	Fully Breastfed Singleton	Twin	Triplet	Quadruplet
Number of Breastfeedings in 24 hours	At least 8 and up to 12 to 16	At least 4 per baby-More as possible	At least 3 per baby-More as possible	At least 2 per baby-More as possible
Total number of Breastfeedings (or Pumping Sessions) in 24 hours	8 or more	8 or more	8 or more	8 or more
Typical number of minutes in 24 hours spent breastfeeding	100 to 150	50 to 75 per baby	35 to 50 per baby	25 to 40 per baby
	Breastfeed in response to infant feeding cues	Increase breastfeeding for one if other has a breastfeeding difficulty (or pump to make up difference) to reach total	Increase breastfeeding for others if one has a breastfeeding difficulty (or pump to make up difference) to reach total	Increase breastfeeding for others if any has a breastfeeding difficulty (or pump to make up difference) to reach total

- Limit the amount of any infant formula given in daily bottle-feedings, so babies will "ask" to breastfeed often enough. Although each baby might be willing to take 3 to 4 ounces (90 to 120 ml) from a bottle, each may be satisfied after drinking 1 1/2 to 3 ounces (45 to 90 ml).
- If babies' requests for breastfeeding drop or you notice signs of decreased milk production, begin to pump your breasts as often as needed to make up any difference in the number of feedings.
- As babies begin to eat solid foods, cut back on the number of bottle-feedings rather than the number of breastfeedings. (See Chapter 28, "Breastfeeding, Starting Solids, and Weaning.")

Alternating Feeding Methods with Higher-Order Multiples

Alternating breast and bottle often works better for mothers feeding higher-order multiples, especially when a household helper manages the bottle-feeding. A mother may breastfeed one (or two) of triplets for all feedings around the clock, rotating which one or two are put to breast. This routine can be flexible so that two babies breastfeed at some feedings, but only one may be breastfed at others if needed or desired.

Mothers of quadruplets sometimes breastfeed two simultaneously while the other two babies are bottle-fed by a helper. At the next feeding, babies are switched so the two bottle-fed at the previous feeding are breastfed for this one.

- To maintain adequate milk production with higher-order multiples, you still want to breastfeed (or pump) often enough to equal at least 8 and more like 10 to 12 feedings a day. Breastfeed (or pump for) each triplet at least 3 to 4 times, and each quadruplet at least 2 to 3 times in every 24-hour period. This should equal at least 100 but closer to 140 minutes of daily breastfeeding/pumping. (See the chart above.)

- When possible, limit the amount of formula the babies receive and pump as needed as per the bulleted items in the previous section for mothers of twins.

- Mothers of triplets and quadruplets sometimes alternate breast and bottle-feedings for part of the day or night, but they breastfeed all the babies for several consecutive feedings at other times. The time of day varies depending on the mother, the babies, and the family situation.

For instance, one mother fed her triplets on a three-hour schedule during the daytime. She developed a rotation plan, so each baby breastfed twice and bottle-fed once over three feedings. During the night all three babies breastfed based on their individual cues. With her husband's help, the mother simply rotated babies in and out of her bed during the night. (This mother had no household help, so for daytime feedings she would breastfeed two babies simultaneously using the double clutch position. The third baby was given a bottle while sitting in the crook formed by her leg when she rested her left foot on her right knee.)

Another mother of triplets chose to do the opposite. She fully breastfed all three babies during the day, but her husband bottle-fed one (or two) while she breastfed one (or two) for one or two evening feedings and all the night feedings.

- Some mothers find they are able to continue breastfeeding higher-order multiples only by alternating breast and bottle for all feedings. At least one baby and often two are breastfed at all (or most) feedings, and babies alternate so that all babies get this special time with mother a few times a day.

Human-Milk-Feeding

When babies are given a mother's expressed milk from a feeding bottle or other alternative feeding device rather than breastfeeding directly, it is often referred to as *breast-milk-feeding* or *human-milk-feeding*. Babies who regularly receive expressed human milk definitely receive the nutrition and antibody benefits available only from human milk, although expressed human milk is not precisely the same product as human milk obtained directly through breastfeeding. Collecting, storing,

There are no rules! Do what works for your situation while protecting your milk production.

refrigerating, freezing, and heating affect some of the nutrients or antibody activity in human milk. Most of the effects are minimal, and feeding expressed human milk is highly associated with better health for babies compared with infant formula.

The process of feeding human milk from a bottle also differs from direct breastfeeding. Having help with feedings is one of the reasons a mother may choose occasional human-milk-feeding. There can be times when everyone's needs might be better met if a helper holds and feeds a crying, hungry multiple. On the other hand, too much help with feedings may interfere with a baby's social development and the mother-baby attachment process. Mother should be the one holding and cuddling each baby for as many feedings as possible, no matter how they are fed.

Full Human-Milk-Feeding

Occasionally a mother opts to fully bottle-feed all multiples with expressed human milk. Usually this occurs when a mother has higher-order multiples and one or more experience an ongoing breastfeeding difficulty; however, twins present a similar situation if both continue to have difficulty breastfeeding. It may not be possible to continue working with two, three, or four babies until they improve their breastfeeding skills when also making sure they receive the complementary or supplementary feedings needed for weight gain *and* fitting in at least eight daily breast-pumping sessions to maintain adequate milk production. Even when one baby breastfeeds well, a mother may find it difficult to breastfeed that baby and still provide the care the others need.

No mother gets more than 24 hours in a day no matter how many babies she has, and a mother may feel physically and emotionally exhausted after days or weeks of trying to "do it all"–juggle breastfeeding, alternative feedings, and pumping sessions. So, some mothers human-milk-feed one or more of their multiples for long periods.

- Most of these mothers pump at least 8 and up to 12 times a day for 6 or more months to provide their milk for babies' full or partial human-milk-feedings.
- A full-size rental electric breast pump with a double collection kit is preferred by most mothers for long-term pumping. These pumps are associated with obtaining higher amounts of milk most quickly.

Physical Conditions that Affect Sucking

When a baby is born with a physical condition that affects breastfeeding ability, such as cleft lip/palate or Down syndrome, a mother may choose to fully human-milk-feed that baby. (A breastfeeding decision should not be made on the basis of a diagnosis alone. Many of these babies breastfeed well with little extra effort.) If breastfeeding ability has been affected, a mother may continue to work with that baby at the breast when possible but human-milk-feed to ensure the baby receives adequate nutrients. (See "Breastfeeding Only One" in the section that follows.)

Temporary Human-Milk-Feeding

When any multiple's temporary breastfeeding difficulty lasts longer than a few days, a mother may choose to fully human-milk-feed one or more of her multiples for several days. This "breather" may allow an overwhelmed mother to get some rest after she has been juggling "practice" breastfeeds, pumping sessions, and supplementary feedings for two or more babies. Since milk production can decrease when any baby is not breastfeeding effectively, a few days of only human-milk-feeding may let a mother focus on increasing milk production by giving her more time for pumping sessions. The mother still offers the baby her breast when possible, and she resumes more intense efforts when she feels ready, but the pressure of feeling that one has to "do it all" may be reduced.

Breastfeeding Multiples When Mother Is Employed

Breastfeeding provides additional benefits when a mother works outside the home, and many mothers have continued to breastfeed multiples after resuming full- or part-time employed positions. Because babies fed human milk are less likely to become ill, mothers generally miss fewer workdays caring for sick babies. This can be a particular advantage for employed mothers with multiples, since illness in one baby often leads to illness for the other(s). After being separated during work hours, breastfeeding is an easy yet wonderful way for a mother and each baby to reconnect. Mothers say they like the fact that breastfeeding is one thing a sitter cannot do for their babies, so their role as mother remains special.

The increased availability of effective portable breast pumps has made it easier for employed mothers to continue breastfeeding. Employed mothers of multiples usually recommend renting or purchasing an electric, self-cycling model to maintain optimal milk production. Most find they pump more milk in less time when a breast pump is used with a double collection kit.

Establishing a pumping routine is especially important for a mother maintaining milk production for multiple babies. Many mothers begin to pump once or twice each morning for two to three weeks before their return-to-work date. Then they pump every two to three hours when away from the babies, especially if babies are less than six to eight months old and not yet ready for any solid food. To maintain adequate milk production, a mother of multiples' routine may include an additional 10 to 15 minute pumping session compared to that of a mother of a single baby. It often takes a couple of workweeks to develop a daily pumping plan that fits a mother's workday while maintaining milk production.

Try to breastfeed before leaving the babies with a sitter, and breastfeed as soon as you and the babies are reunited. Some mothers breastfeed their babies before getting ready for work and then breastfeed again immediately before leaving for work. When leaving work, a call to the sitter can let her know you are on your way, so babies do not get fed too much when you will soon be available. Breastfeed frequently on any day you have off.

Frequent pumping should maintain milk production, but if you notice signs of decreased production, look at your routine. A feeding or pumping session may have been delayed or dropped inadvertently. Increasing the number of breastfeeds or pumping sessions for two or three days usually takes care of any problem. Contact a lactation consultant or LLL Leader if you have any ongoing issue with milk production.

Some employers may be concerned about employee productivity when a returning new mother needs to pump as frequently as every two to three hours. They may not be aware that providing human milk usually means less illness for babies, which means fewer sick days for an employee. Also, some studies have shown increased employee productivity when employers support women's efforts to breastfeed. Employers may be more understanding when they learn that you will not require as many pumping breaks once babies have begun to enjoy other foods.

See "Employment Issues" in Chapter 7, "Getting Ready: Preparing for Multiples," for additional ideas. For "Human Milk Storage Guidelines," see the Appendix.

Lower Milk Production

Mothers of multiples often cite low or insufficient milk production as a reason for partial breastfeeding. True and perceived milk insufficiency are discussed in more depth in Chapter 16 under "Insufficient Milk Production."

Adopted Multiples

Many women have induced lactation, or "brought in" milk, to breastfeed adopted children, including adopted multiples. Milk production varies greatly depending on the individual, but most adoptive mothers must depend on at least some supplementary feedings to meet their babies' nutritional needs. Whether supplementing a little or a lot, "successful" breastfeeding mothers of adopted multiples often rely on an at-breast feeding-tube system to provide supplementary liquid. (See "At-Breast Feeding-Tube Systems" in Resources.) An at-breast feeding-tube system is also an excellent alternative for supplements when babies latch on and suckle well but mother's milk production is not adequate for multiple infants' needs.

In addition to using an at-breast feeding-tube system during breastfeeding, strategies for inducing lactation are similar to those for the mother with lower milk production. They generally include frequent sessions using a full-size, hospital-grade electric breast pump to "tell" the breasts that milk production is desired. Galactogogues, herbal preparations or medications thought or known to have milk-increasing properties, are often recommended as well.

When ongoing supplementation is required because milk production cannot meet all of the babies' needs, many mothers have found it necessary to redefine "success" as it applies to breastfeeding. This is more difficult for some, especially when full breastfeeding had been the goal. As noted earlier in the section "Full Breastfeeding as a Goal," it may help to focus on the physical benefits of partial breastfeeding and especially on the emotional benefits. The closeness of the breast-feeding relationship—for each baby with mother and for mother with each of her multiples—has high long-term value, even when full breastfeeding is not possible.

A lactation consultant or La Leche League Leader can provide more in-depth information and the support you may need when inducing lactation, increasing milk production, learning to use an at-breast feeding-tube system, or revising breast-feeding goals.

Breastfeeding Only One

Breastfeeding means more than food to babies and to a mother. Breastfeeding is a gift of self that a mother gives to her babies, providing babies with close physical contact and the most perfect nutrition available, and it does this in a form that only a mother can deliver. For this reason fully breastfeeding one (or more) and fully bottle-feeding the other(s) should be avoided except in extreme circumstances, such as when one multiple has a physical condition that makes breastfeeding that baby impossible.

> **Babies' feedings are as much a social and emotional experience for them as they are a way of getting food–just as meals are for older children and adults.**

When any multiple is fully breastfed, it means that this multiple receives optimal nutrition and immunity factors against illnesses. Unless human-milk-fed, the other(s) is exposed to a potential allergen in a food that is less perfectly suited to human infants and one that contains no disease protection. Most important, fully bottle-feeding one while breastfeeding the other(s) may contribute to differences in a mother's feelings for her babies, even if the bottle-fed baby is receiving only mother's milk in those bottles.

When possible, a better option may be to breastfeed each baby as much as possible and supplement each as necessary. Not every multiple may require supplementation. Mothers have fully breastfed one (or more) and partially breastfed the other(s). With this plan, all babies are breastfed for at least some feedings.

In the rare instance when completely different feeding methods are necessary, a mother should be aware of the physical and emotional implications of fully bottle-feeding one baby. Look for opportunities, during and between feedings, to increase skin-to-skin contact with the bottle-fed baby. This *kangaroo care* is an excellent way to increase contact no matter what the baby's age or development. (See Chapter 10, "Multiples in the Newborn Intensive Care Unit.")

When one "loses interest." Occasionally, a mother will report that one of her multiples appears to have "lost interest" and has weaned abruptly or is weaning rapidly. However, few babies naturally wean from the breast before their first birthday. Since this is not a common behavior for a fully or almost fully breastfed baby, suspect some underlying issue. Often the baby's feeding pattern, the number of breastfeeds, and the related number of supplemental bottles are at the heart of the problem. If any baby stops "asking" to breastfeed or appears to be weaning prematurely, treat the situation as a *nursing strike* to get the baby back to the breast, and contact an LLL Leader or lactation consultant for additional information and support. (See "Nursing Strikes" in Chapter 28, "Breastfeeding, Starting Solids, and Weaning.")

Early Weaning

Sometimes a mother of multiples finds it necessary to discontinue breastfeeding altogether. If you are considering weaning your babies from the breast or from human-milk-feeding, but breastfeeding has been an important goal for you, first contact an LLL Leader or a lactation consultant to discuss whether there might be other options. The early weeks with newborn multiples can be very chaotic. You may wonder, and family or friends may tell you, that other feeding methods will make your life easier. During the first couple of months, mothers sometimes make decisions about weaning that they later regret. If you are thinking about weaning from the breast or discontinuing pumping, ask yourself if six months from now you are likely to still feel you made the best decision. Your answer will give you insight into which direction to turn.

Try to continue your efforts to breastfeed if the babies have been home less than four to eight weeks. (See the discussions above about partial breastfeeding and read Chapter 12, "Making Up for a Poor Start.") Babies change a lot from week to week during their first months. Their current breastfeeding abilities probably do not reflect what their abilities will be in a few weeks. Also, you probably will feel better about any feeding decision you make if you wait until you have recovered more fully from the pregnancy and birth. There is no easy way! Multiple babies require more time and effort to feed no matter what method is used. Although mothers say it takes time to breastfeed, they also say it is the easiest method once babies have learned to breastfeed well.

If you decide weaning is best in your situation, you can feel good about the length of time you were able to breastfeed or human-milk-feed. No matter how brief it may have been, studies indicate that any amount of breastfeeding, or human milk, has a positive impact on babies' health. Any breastfeeding is better than no breastfeeding or no human milk at all. It may not have been easy in your situation, but you provided your babies with the best possible start.

To decrease milk production. If milk production has not been an issue, it is more comfortable and easier for babies if you can avoid abrupt weaning. There is no button one can push to suddenly turn milk production to "off." It takes time for breasts to get the message to stop production completely. Unless your babies are already getting numerous formula supplements, you are producing a lot more milk than the "average" new mother. If you abruptly stop, you could develop severe engorgement or mastitis.

> You can feel good that you provided your babies with the best possible start.

Gradually decrease milk production by slowly decreasing the number of breastfeedings or pumping sessions, and gradually lengthen the time between breastfeedings or pumpings. You might begin by breastfeeding one less baby at each feeding, or try to shorten pumping sessions by a few minutes for several days. When your body adapts, delete a feeding or pumping session every few days while increasing the amount in their supplementary bottles by 1/2 to 2 ounces (15 to 60 ml).

Certain medications or herbs are associated with decreasing milk production. A lactation consultant or La Leche League Leader should have information on the use of anti-galactogogues. Certain types may require a consultation with your health care provider.

If you become engorged or develop a plugged duct or mastitis, maintain the current number of breastfeedings or pumping sessions. Do not attempt to decrease breastfeeding or pumping further. (See Chapter 16, "When Mother Has a Breastfeeding Difficulty," for suggestions for coping with a specific problem.) Depending on the severity of the problem, you may need to increase milk removal by increasing the number of breastfeedings for some of the babies. You could add brief pumping sessions instead, such as pumping just to the point that relieves fullness. You can resume the weaning process, but perhaps more slowly, once the problem resolves.

You still can contact a La Leche League Leader or lactation consultant for help if you do decide to wean. She may have additional ideas to make the process more comfortable.

Babies' needs after weaning. Discontinuing breastfeeding does not change your babies' need for your presence and your touch. Holding them skin to skin, as in kangaroo care, taking turns so each spends time in a sling or carrier, rocking one or more in your arms, bathing with one or another–all are ways to increase contact. Of course, one of the best ways to provide physical contact is to continue to be the one who holds each baby for their bottle-feedings most of the time.

To develop a sense of trust and feelings of security, babies need a primary, which means "one," caretaker. Babies' feedings are as much a social and emotional experience for them as they are a way of getting food–just as meals are for older children and adults. Babies learn to trust and feel most secure when the same person generally is the one who replaces their hunger pains with a pleasurable feeling of fullness. Your babies still need you to hold and cuddle them for most of their feedings–no matter what method you use to feed them.

A mother of multiples is in need of the best possible breastfeeding start, yet she is the least likely new mother to get it. When circumstances interfere, breastfeeding does not have to be "all or nothing." There are many ways to continue to include breastfeeding while also coping with the additional demands of multiple infants.

KEY POINTS

- ❑ Although many mothers have fully breastfed twins or triplets for several months, full breastfeeding is not always possible with multiples.
- ❑ Partial breastfeeding is a good option if full breastfeeding is not possible. Some breastfeeding is a lot better than no breastfeeding at all!
  - Partial breastfeeding still provides nutritional and immunological benefits.
  - Physical issues for a mother or her babies may lead to partial breastfeeding or partial breastfeeding may be chosen due to a family situation.
  - Some mothers fully breastfed multiples at first and then moved to partial breastfeeding; others began with partial breastfeeding and then moved to full breastfeeding.
- ❑ Giving mother's expressed/pumped milk is called breast-milk-feeding (EBM-feeding) or human-milk-feeding.
- ❑ For adequate milk production, be sure to "empty" the breasts by direct breastfeeding or milk expression/pumping **at least** 8 times in 24 hours.
- ❑ If thinking about weaning multiples:
  - Try to wait until at least 4 to 8 weeks after giving birth. It may be difficult to make a good decision during the confusing first several weeks.
  - Consider "weaning" to partial breastfeeding or human-milk-feeding.
  - If you do wean completely, continue to provide lots of cuddling and skin-to-skin contact. Be the one who still usually feeds each baby.
- ❑ Call a lactation consultant or a La Leche League Leader for ideas and help to develop a plan that will work for you and your babies.

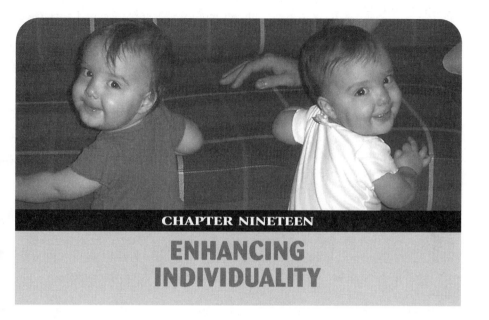

CHAPTER NINETEEN

ENHANCING INDIVIDUALITY

Most parents want each of their multiples to grow into a self-confident, unique individual. At the same time they want their children to enjoy the special relationship that only multiples can share. This often leaves parents feeling as if they are walking a tightrope over an alligator pit! However, it is possible for multiples to have both. When each is treated as an individual, each is free to savor the special bond found only among multiples.

Breastfeeding is a wonderful way to begin to appreciate each multiple as an individual because it removes the temptations that could compromise close contact. For two persons to get to know one another as individuals, they must spend a lot of time together. The close contact and interaction inherent with frequent breastfeeding helps a mother slowly form individual attachments with each multiple–whether or not she is aware of it at the time. When breastfeeding is based on each multiple's feeding cues, a mother quickly appreciates that her babies have individual needs and approaches to life that are present from birth.

Attachment to Each Baby

The formation of an attachment for a mother (or father) with each baby provides a multiple with the foundation to be an individual while also enjoying being part of a set. This process may be influenced by multiples' type (monozygotic/identical or dizygotic/fraternal) and by the effect their births had on a mother's early interaction with each.

The close contact and interaction inherent with frequent breast-feeding helps a mother slowly form individual attachments with each multiple.

Forming attachments seems to be a very different process for a mother with her multiples. Nature designed humans to form close bonds with one person at a time. A mother often feels an intimate closeness with her single newborn within hours, days, or at least within several weeks. It takes more time to get to know two or more babies with that same degree of closeness. It is more difficult to fall in love with two persons at the same time. In addition, the attachment process with multiples is often complicated by factors beyond parents' control. Attachment formation with multiples seems to fall into three categories: 1. unit attachment, 2. preferential attachment, or 3. flip-flop attachment.

Unit attachment. When healthy newborn multiples are in a mother's care from birth, she may find she feels very close to, and protective of, the unit of babies first. Once attached to the unit, or set, a mother (and father) can become acquainted with each unique personality within it. This may take months or even well into the babies' second year.

This may explain the sensation some mothers describe during their babies' early months. They say that although they know they have two (or more) babies and they certainly can see each one, it seems as if they are caring for only one baby who keeps them busy around the clock. (Only other mothers of multiples seem able to understand this phenomenon.)

Unit attachment may be one reason some parents feel compelled to dress multiples alike. When dressed in look-alike clothing, the babies almost take on a single image.

Preferential attachment. Certain situations that commonly occur with multiple births are more likely to lead to the formation of a stronger attachment, or a preferential attachment, with one baby. A long-term preference for one particular multiple can have profound consequences for the entire set, including the one receiving preferential treatment.

It is fairly common for one (or more) of preterm multiples to require a stay of several hours to several days in a NICU while the mother cares for the other multiple(s) in her room and at home. When separated from only one for even a brief period, mothers often report they quickly feel closer to any baby who was in their care and not separated from them. It seems logical that a mother would bond initially with a baby who was able to respond to her constant care and was with her without interruption before she develops this closeness with a multiple that must always share her with the other(s).

Sick newborns often behave as many older children and adults do when acutely ill. They tend to withdraw from those around them, because interacting with others requires too much of the energy they need to get well. Just as the ill child or

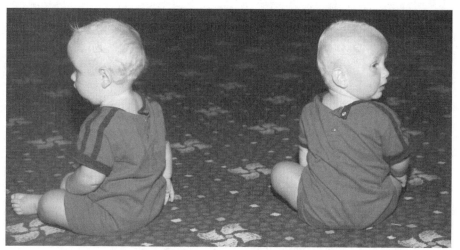

Each multiple needs to grow into a unique individual.

adult regains an interest in her surroundings as her condition improves, the same is true for a sick newborn. The newborn begins to respond more as his condition improves. When multiples are preterm or sick at birth, they usually do not make progress at exactly the same rate. Therefore, one may be ready to respond and interact before the other(s). It is natural for a parent to feel drawn to, and form an attachment first with, any multiple able to respond to her.

Few have "surprise" twins or triplets now that ultrasound and other diagnostic tests have become commonplace, but occasionally a woman still gives birth to a second baby whose presence is not detected until the first baby's arrival. Many mothers of undiagnosed twins say they initially felt more of an attachment for the baby born first. Because the bond between a mother and child begins to form before birth, it is not surprising that a mother may think of the firstborn twin as "her baby."

One baby simply may be easier to fall in love with! Most persons find they instantly connect with certain new acquaintances while others must first "grow" on a person. Some studies have found that without intervention, a preference for one multiple often continues, which can result in poorer treatment for the other(s). Because of its detrimental effects, it is important to recognize a preference for one and then act to improve the bond with each baby. Ideas for coping with preferential attachment follow later in this chapter.

Flip-flop attachment. If a parent finds her attention ping-pongs from one multiple to another–and back again, it may be referred to as flip-flop attachment. In this instance, a parent may spend a few days or weeks getting to know one multiple and then switch to pay more attention to another.

Many parents begin to flip-flop attention after first attaching to their multiples as a unit. Flip-flop attachment differs from a preferential attachment since the parent focuses on each baby in turn rather than always focusing on a particular one.

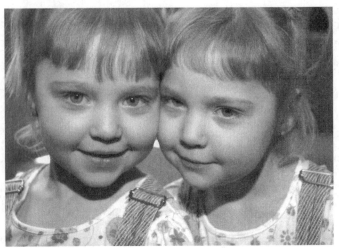

No matter how similar multiples' traits may seem to be,
they still vary in how each expresses those traits.

Other Factors

Differentiation

The process of comparing and contrasting multiples' appearances and behavioral traits may be called *differentiation*. Differentiation helps parents move past the unit/set and get to know the individuals. Generally, the more different multiples are, the sooner parents see beyond the set to the individual persons that comprise it.

- Dizygotic (fraternal), different-gender (opposite-sex) twins tend to be the most different in appearance and behavior, which may be the reason they tend to be regarded as individuals sooner than same-gender twins. Their differences can lead to unnecessary concern when parents compare babies with different, yet both normal, developmental timetables.

- The physical appearance, temperaments, growth, and development of same-gender dizygotic multiples may be very similar or quite different. These multiples may be very close or vary widely in their approaches to breastfeeding and to life in general.

- Because monozygotic (identical) multiples have all their genetic material in common, they are always the same gender. They not only look more alike, but they often behave more alike and operate from built-in body clocks set for the same or a similar "schedule." When their clocks are in sync, a mother will usually find she is feeding and handling two at once. This lack of one-on-one time may contribute more to unit bonding than their similar appearances, and it may influence how long it takes to form an attachment to each.

- The more multiples in a set, the more complicated the attachment process becomes. Not only are there more individuals to form an attachment with, but the twin types comprising the set affect getting to know the different babies. In the majority of higher-order sets, all multiples are dizygotic due to the use of fertility-enhancement methods for conception. However, any given set may include all multiples of the same gender, or one, two, or several babies may be the opposite. Also, monozygotic triplet, quadruplet, and quintuplet sets occasionally do occur. A combination of twin types, such as a set of monozygotic twins and a dizygotic triplet, is fairly common among spontaneously occurring sets, but combinations also occur in sets resulting from fertility-enhancement techniques.

> **It is more difficult to fall in love with two persons at the same time.**

No matter how similar multiples' temperament traits may seem, especially those of monozygotic multiples, they still vary in the degree to which each expresses those traits. For instance, all may be calm, easygoing babies or all may be high-need babies, but one is likely to be calmer or more high need than the other(s). Do not be surprised, however, if the moment you begin to figure out the difference(s) in degree, the babies add interest to the attachment process by flip-flopping traits, or taking turns, as to which is calmest or which is higher need. Flip-flopping traits seems to be more common with monozygotic multiples. Also, it occurs more often during multiples' first one or two years, although they may occasionally flip-flop traits for years–even into adulthood for many sets.

Unit Thinking

Watch out for unit thinking–a desire to always treat multiples equally. It strikes most parents of multiples at an early date. Although this desire is a normal response to having two or more at once, if unrecognized or unchecked, unit thinking can interfere with individual attachment formation.

Multiples do not deserve to be treated exactly the same. Each is a different person, including monozygotic (identical) multiples. Each has different needs, and their individual needs will vary and flip-flop as they grow. For instance, today's high need baby really needs your extra time and attention. Another multiple may not need the same amount of time now, or she may need more of you later. Responding to the individual multiples' "demands" helps a parent focus on developing a relationship with each baby rather than simply accomplishing baby care tasks for the unit.

When you find yourself worrying about spending equal time and attention with each, stop and ask yourself whether you would be so concerned about treating two babies exactly the same if they had been born a year apart. Most likely you would simply have responded to their individual needs.

Helping the Attachment Process Along

The more multiples in a set, the more complicated the attachment process becomes.

There are many actions a parent can take to enhance attachment with each multiple. Although the different categories of attachment are noted, many of the suggestions could apply to any set of multiples.

Unit Bonding. If you feel closer to the unit, or the set of multiples, several activities may help you get to know the individuals.

- Consciously **look for differences**. There are always physical and behavioral differences, no matter how alike the babies may seem. Frequently one of identical twins has a fuller face or a different look about the eyes. Look for a distinguishing mark, such as a freckle or a birthmark.
- Most mothers of monozygotic or similar-looking dizygotic multiples can quickly **tell them apart**. (Fathers often take longer.) However, if you cannot yet tell one from another when they are ready to leave the hospital, take home an extra set of identification bracelets; continue to bracelet one until you are certain you know each. Paint a fingernail or toenail of one baby. (Mothers of monozygotic triplets or quadruplets may need to use different colors of fingernail polish for each.) Use different-colored wristbands or bracelets for each. Iron the first letter of each one's name on t-shirts. (This won't work if multiples are given alliterated names.)
- Go out of your way to **call each baby by name**. Every day you have numerous opportunities to make eye contact and call each by name during feedings, diaper changes, and cuddling. Encourage others to do the same. It may be unrealistic to think the lady up the street or the grocery clerk will remember one from the other(s), but it is reasonable to expect relatives, friends, and close neighbors to call each by name.
  - ❏ Discourage references to them as "the twins" (or "the triplets," "the quads," etc.), "twin" or "twinnie"–especially in their presence, to avoid reinforcing the "set" rather than the individuals.
  - ❏ Never admit to anyone if you ever have trouble telling them apart, especially when one or more of your multiples is within hearing distance. Can you imagine how you would have felt as a child if your parents were not sure who you were?
- **Photograph each baby alone,** as well as with the rest of the set. Unless each baby has a very distinct look, label photos after processing. This helps others learn to identify each baby. If photos are not labeled, you may be surprised years later when you have trouble identifying who is who in some photos.
- Do not feel too concerned if you find yourself **dressing infant multiples alike.** This may be one aspect of unit bonding–a way that the babies "take

on" a single image. However, if you find yourself changing every baby when only one soils an outfit, you may want to consider your actions more closely.

❑ Many parents say they dress multiples alike for fear that others may think they like one baby better if one baby is perceived as wearing a cuter outfit than another.

❑ You can revisit the issue of look-alike outfits as multiples become toddlers. By 18 to 24 months, they can help choose their clothing if given some simple options. Three- to six-year-olds often develop definite, and individual, senses of style that should be respected–within reason.

❑ A solution that combines the urge to dress multiples alike with a desire to treat them as individuals is to color-code their clothing. The babies wear the same outfit, but each dresses in a different color. For instance, one of male twins may be assigned to always wear the color blue and the other always wears another color. (For same-gender triplets there would need to be at least two assigned colors, same-gender quads would need at least three assigned colors, and so on.)

Color coding same-gender twins helps others identify one from another. When one of a set is always in a particular color, others soon learn to call him by name based on the color he wears. The one wearing a different color is identified by process of elimination. It is helpful when a neighbor can call an escaping toddler by name before he runs into the street. However, if someone comes to depend on the color of multiples' clothing, it may interfere with learning to distinguish the children by other means.

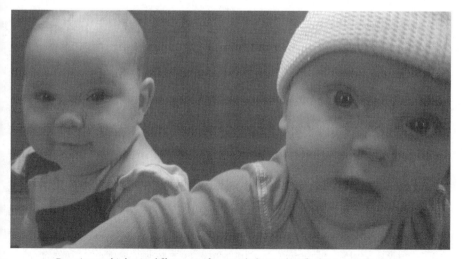

Dressing multiples in different outfits may help to identify them as individuals.

Preferential Attachment. The attachments you form with your multiples influence your interactions with each. This in turn may affect each one's sense of identity and social development. Because of the long-term implications of a preferential attachment, it is crucial for a parent to recognize when feelings of attachment are stronger for one (or more) than for the other(s).

If you do feel closer to one, remember it is a fairly common feeling, especially if you were able to care for one before the other(s). Do not waste energy by feeling guilty about a situation that began beyond your control. Instead, invest that energy positively by taking action to rectify the situation. It often takes a conscious effort to become as attached to the one(s) with whom you feel less close.

- Go out of your way to listen for and ***respond immediately*** to the cues and cries of any multiple with whom you feel less close.
- Make ***eye contact*** with that baby and talk to him often.
- Increase close contact with this baby by placing him in a ***baby carrier or sling*** more often than the other(s).
- Use ***kangaroo care*** with this baby. Hold or breastfeed him skin-to-skin. Massage him; take him in the bath with you.
- You will still want to meet the needs of the multiple(s) you already feel close to, but most mothers do not find this to be a problem. They usually continue to respond quickly to their "preferred" baby, too.

> **Multiples do not deserve to be treated exactly the same; each is a different person.**

Differentiation and Making Comparisons. Parents of multiples are often told they should not compare their babies. No matter how well meaning, this advice is absurd! Most parents of a singleton compare their baby with other babies. It is a way of trying to figure out if a baby is growing and developing at about the same rate as peers. However, most parents do not have a built-in peer comparison.

Comparisons are a way of examining each individual's behaviors. Comparison may be part of the attachment process with multiples, because it helps parents sort out their babies' different traits and approaches to life. This sorting out is part of ***differentiation***. It allows parents to look at their babies' similarities and differences and note both changing and ongoing behaviors. Still, there are pitfalls to avoid when comparing multiples:

- Do not label multiples (or let anyone else do so). Labels can stick. Saying, "Baby A is outgoing, but Baby B is unsociable," or "Baby A is the dominant twin; he can make his passive brother do anything," unfairly categorizes both babies. A child can carry a label long after a behavior has disappeared or taken a new direction.
- There are normal variations for most behaviors associated with infant growth and development. Multiples may accomplish new tasks on very similar or very different timetables, yet all may be within the range of

normal. Invest in a reliable reference about normal infant growth and development, and refer to it when you feel concerned about multiples' different developmental timetables. (See Resources.) Share any concerns with their pediatric care provider. You do not want comparisons to cause you to worry unnecessarily, but identification of and early intervention for developmental delays can make a big difference in eventual outcomes.

- When babies are preterm, they may not "act their age" for several months to more than a year of age. Ask their pediatric care provider how much to adjust developmental timetables to accommodate their original full-term due date rather than their actual birth date(s).

Celebrity Status. By giving birth to more than one baby, parents of multiples gain a sort of celebrity status by default. You may as well enjoy it–sometimes praise from an adoring public can help a mother get through a long day. However, do not let instant celebrity tempt you to reinforce the unit of multiples at the expense of the individuals. It is normal for the ego to inflate a bit with recognition as a celebrity. There is no reason to feel guilty about it, unless you lose perspective and become a victim of the celebrity syndrome.

> **Always announcing a child's status as part of a multiple set could cause him to wonder which you value more–his uniqueness or his place as part of a unit.**

You might be taking celebrity too seriously if you find you must always mention the existence of the other(s) even when out with only one multiple. You may be taking advantage of your celebrity if, by their third birthday, you often find yourself calling them "the twins" ("the triplets," "the quads," etc.) instead of calling each by name or if you are still compelled to dress them alike when you all venture out.

Each of your multiples, and others, are watching and listening. Always announcing a child's status as part of a multiple set could cause him to wonder which you value more–his uniqueness or his place as part of a unit. Relatives and friends take their cues from you. When your emphasis is on the individuals, they will learn to look at each child that way, too. If you express unit thinking or label your multiples, they will do likewise. When your multiples and everyone else know each is recognized as a unique person, there will be no difficulty with the concept of individuality for your multiples or their enjoyment of the special bond multiples share.

KEY POINTS

❑ Developing a close attachment with each of multiples is different than with a single baby. It often takes longer to "fall in love" with two or more separate little persons.

❑ Breastfeeding is a good first step due to the close contact and the need to learn how each baby indicates hunger.

❑ Babies learn that each is special when parents respond to each baby's cues and do not try to treat all exactly the same.

❑ A parent often begins to bond with multiples in three ways:
  • Unit attachment–a parent first feels closer to the entire set of multiples.

  • Preferential attachment–a parent feels close to or prefers one particular baby in the set, and this feeling continues as babies grow, unless the parent works to change it.

  • Flip-flop attachment–a parent pays more attention to one particular baby for a few days or weeks, and then the parent's attention moves to a different baby in the set.

❑ Most parents compare their multiples, which may be called differentiation.
  • Compare but do not "label" babies by saying, for example, "This is the good twin; the other one is bossy." Babies change, but labels can stick.

  • Do not immediately worry if multiples do not grow or develop at the same rate. Do check with their pediatric care provider and read a book on infant growth and development.

❑ Unit thinking comes from a desire to treat multiples equally. Unchecked unit thinking may interfere with attaching to the individuals in the set.

❑ Some people treat parents of multiples as celebrities. Enjoy it, but do not let being a celebrity get in the way of treating each multiple as an individual.

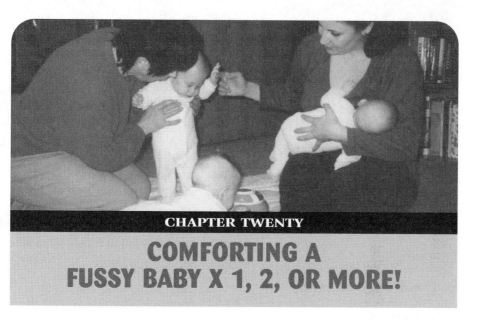

CHAPTER TWENTY

COMFORTING A
FUSSY BABY X 1, 2, OR MORE!

There should be a contract that promises parents of multiples that because they are caring for two or more babies, none of the babies will be a fussy or high need baby. There *should* be a contract like that but, of course, there is not.

Many babies have fussy periods, especially during the first few months. As with singletons, one or more multiples may have prolonged fussy or crying periods. One or more may be a "high need" baby who needs almost constant contact and attention. If babies fuss at different times during the day, a mother may feel as though each day is one big fussy time. (And she's more than half right!) On the other hand, it can be extremely difficult when two or more babies share fussy periods.

Any mother who has felt the helplessness and frustration of caring for one uncomfortable or high need baby can only imagine contending with another at the same time. When only one is affected, it still requires extra energy to meet the needs of that multiple plus the needs of the other(s). It can be more than doubly or triply frustrating.

This may be the point when a mother feels ready to throw in the towel, put the babies in cribs or automatic swings, walk away, and let the babies cry it out. However, the only thing the babies learn if left to cry it out is that no one is there for them when they most need comfort. Put yourself in each baby's place and imagine life from his or her perspective.

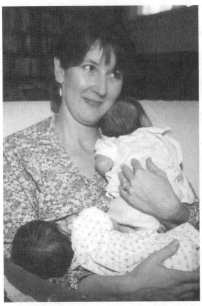

A baby cannot yet speak. Crying is one of the few ways babies have to communicate. A baby's cries are supposed to bother parents; they are designed to gain *needed* attention. And it is normal for a mother to want to respond and soothe her crying baby; it is supposed to be difficult to ignore a baby's cries.

No matter how frustrated and overwhelmed a mother may feel, the babies feel even more so. No baby "chooses" to have a high need or more irritable temperament; no baby "chooses" to have a physical issue that results in colic; no infant "chooses" to be fussy. Imagine how terrible it would be to feel physically or emotionally uncomfortable and not understand why or know how to communicate the nature of the discomfort.

Mothers soon learn how to comfort one fussy baby while feeding another.

> The only thing the babies learn if left to cry it out is that no one is there for them when they most need comfort.

General Causes

Unrealistic Expectations. Many first-time parents have had little experience with newborns, which may result in unrealistic expectations of babies' abilities, their need for human contact, and their sleep needs. Television and other media lead one to believe that most infants do nothing more than sleep or sit in an infant seat staring happily at a mobile. No wonder new parents are surprised when a newborn requires so much time and attention. This surprise only intensifies when multiples arrive.

From birth, babies are "wired" to seek interaction with other humans, and some are more wired than others. Being held and carried from place to place stimulates brain development, affecting babies' motor function, cognitive development, and socialization. Babies are not supposed to sleep their days away; they are not supposed to spend hours staring at a mobile. They are supposed to be in arms, learning how to live in their new environment. The need of each multiple for this stimulation does not change because he or she arrived as part of a set.

Temperament and High-Need Babies. Temperament refers to each multiple's behavioral style or behavioral approach to all the various stimuli in both their internal and external environments. Because about 50 percent of temperament has a genetic basis, it is not surprising that monozygotic (MZ/identical) multiples generally have more similar behavioral styles than dizygotic (DZ/fraternal) ones.

Temperament is not something parents can change, especially during infancy. Temperament does evolve, however, as each infant grows and develops.

Physician-researchers Alexander Thomas and Stella Chess identified nine temperament traits with each trait varying along a continuum from one person to another. These traits are:

- activity (level),
- (ability for self-) regularity,
- initial approach/avoidance (related to new persons/situations),
- adaptability (to major/minor change in activity, situation, etc.),
- intensity,
- mood,
- persistence/attention span,
- distractibility, and
- sensory threshold.

The overall result can be seen in the range of babies who are considered "easy" or calm to those viewed as more challenging or "high need."

Any multiple whose temperament is higher on the activity, irritability, intensity, or distractibility scales and/or lower on the regularity, adaptability, persistence/ attention span, mood, or sensory threshold scales may be more sensitive to internal physical sensations and external stimuli and more difficult to soothe. Greater difficulty developing a daily wake-sleep pattern is common. These babies often require more physical contact–day and night–and environmental stimuli are more likely to interfere with current activity, including sleep.

From birth babies are "wired" to seek interaction with other humans, and some are more wired than others.

Physical issues that cause or contribute to infant fussiness are likely to have greater impact on babies with a more sensitive temperament. Therefore, it is important to rule out possible physical causes that may be exaggerating temperament traits.

Physical Causes
Colic

The word colic refers to the colon (large intestine) and intestinal-related discomfort. Although colic has become a catch-all word for bouts of infant fussiness and crying that begin within a few weeks of birth, it generally refers to daily, or almost daily, several-hour periods during which babies seem to experience spasms or waves of pain. Babies respond to apparent spasms with shrieking cries and the drawing up of their legs. A baby is difficult to console until a spasm resolves. An individual baby's colic period often occurs at about the same time of the day, and it frequently disappears between three to four months for babies born at full term.

Food sensitivity or allergy

A sensitivity or allergy to the protein in cow's milk and other dairy products is a common cause of colic symptoms.

Although allergy to a mother's own milk is virtually unheard of, certain proteins passing through mothers' milk may affect some babies. This is more likely if there is a strong history of allergy on either side of a family. Most foods eaten by mothers do not create problems for babies. Babies thrive on the milk produced by women from all cultures and their mothers eat all sorts of different diets.

If you suspect one or more babies is sensitive to something in your diet, eliminating the offending food from your diet is likely to result in a happier baby. Although it often takes two to three weeks for the offending food to be out of the system completely, some relief from symptoms is often seen during the first week.

A sensitivity or allergy to the protein in cow's milk and other dairy products is a common cause of colic symptoms. (Mothers who must eliminate dairy products often ingest goat milk/cheeses and soy milk without a reaction from their babies.)

The protein in cow-milk-based artificial formulas, even when given in small amounts, causes a reaction in some babies. Other food proteins more highly associated with food sensitivity and colic symptoms include: soy, wheat, corn, peanuts, egg white, and shellfish.

In addition to protein sensitivity, other substances a mother ingests may contribute to fussiness:

- Caffeinated beverages seem to affect some babies, especially when a mother consumes several cups of coffee, tea, or soft drinks daily. (Most coffee mugs hold at least two cups.)
- A few medications mothers take may contribute to discomfort resulting in fussiness. If you have any question about medication side effects, contact your babies' health care provider, an LLL Leader, or a lactation consultant for information.
- Tobacco product use is associated with infant fussiness and lowered milk production, especially for those who smoke (or use the equivalent of) a half pack or more daily. Cigarette smoke irritates babies and nicotine and other chemicals are excreted in human milk. Furthermore, babies exposed to secondhand smoke are much more likely to suffer upper respiratory infections, bronchitis, and asthma. Parental smoking is also associated with a higher incidence of Sudden Infant Death Syndrome (SIDS).
  ❏ If you cannot quit smoking completely, cut down as much as possible and always smoke outdoors so babies are not exposed to the smoke. (Smoke absorbed into clothing and hair also exposes babies to secondhand smoke.) In addition to limiting one's smoking, do it immediately after–not before–a breastfeeding.

Hormonal contraceptive pills and devices, especially those containing estrogen, can decrease milk production and result in fussy behavior.

Progesterone/progestin-only pills or injections do not appear to affect milk production, especially if introduced after a mother's milk supply is well-established. However, some women do report a decrease in milk production after progestin-only contraception is initiated. Therefore, a form taken by mouth may be a better choice, as it is easier to stop and reverse the effect if decreased milk production occurs.

Consider whether inhalation of or skin contact with something in the environment may be contributing to fussy or colicky behavior.

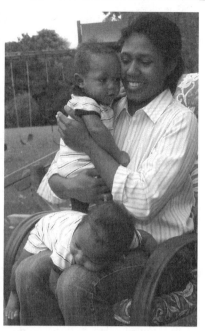

It takes time to discover what works best to comfort each baby.

- Some babies appear to react to something in infant supplemental vitamin or mineral drops, infant medications, etc. Food dyes or added flavorings are common culprits.
- Some babies react after inhaling particles from sprays or powders.
- Some babies are sensitive to substances, such as perfumes or other chemicals, added to soaps or detergents. They react to skin contact with certain soaps or when clothing, bedding, and so on were washed in an offending detergent.

Lactose overload

True lactose intolerance is *extremely rare* during infancy and through a child's first three to four years. Lactose is the sugar found in the milk of all mammals, including humans. Because our species' survival has depended on its ability to digest lactose during infancy and early childhood, full-term infants and young children produce the enzyme lactase to break lactose into two smaller sugars—glucose and galactose—for absorption by the body.

A temporary lactase insufficiency may occur during infancy under certain circumstances. Many preterm infants do not yet produce enough lactase and full-term newborns may not produce enough to deal with particularly large amounts of lactose. Also, diarrhea-causing illnesses or medications such as antibiotics can cause changes in the intestinal tract and damage the lactase-producing cells, resulting temporarily in low lactase production. When the amount of lactose is more than available lactase can handle, lactose overload occurs and bacteria in the large intestine (colon) ferments the extra lactose, releasing gases and causing symptoms similar to lactose intolerance.

The baby affected by lactose overload often experiences uncomfortable gassiness, resulting in irritability and fussiness. His stools may be watery–looser than normal human milk stools–and often are greenish in color and/or look bubbly or frothy. To avoid or minimize lactose-related digestive issues:

- Allow each multiple to decide when a breastfeeding ends rather than set some arbitrary time at the first breast, such as 10 or 15 minutes. (Babies self-detach on their own when finished breastfeeding.) The amount of fat in a mother's milk increases as feeding progresses; some call this higher-fat milk *hindmilk*. In addition to providing important calories for growth, the fat in mother's milk slows the emptying time of the stomach, allowing lactase more time to digest lactose. Only each baby knows when he has ingested enough milk fat.

- If a twin has an ongoing issue with symptoms associated with a lactase insufficiency, assign each baby a particular breast for at least a week and continue if this seems helpful. Always using the same breast allows each to self-regulate milk production in one breast, which may decrease lactose overload.

  Obviously, it is more difficult to assign a breast when triplets or more breastfeed. Still, a mother may assign a particular breast to an affected multiple while continuing to alternate the others to see if symptoms decrease for an affected multiple.

- Do *not* discontinue breastfeeding if an illness or medication affects an infant's intestinal tract. Mother's milk includes immunological substances that help heal the intestinal tract, leading to earlier replenishing of lactase-producing cells.

Infant Gastroesophageal Reflux Disease (GERD)

Multiples are more at risk for infant GERD because they are more likely to be affected by conditions associated with its development.

All persons, including babies, experience reflux–the reverse movement of stomach contents back into the esophagus. Although certain physical conditions can cause reflux, infant stomach anatomy and digestion physiology makes babies more prone to reflux. Reflux decreases as babies mature. Regurgitation or vomiting is an obvious sign of reflux, but reflux also may be silent. During silent reflux a baby may appear to gulp, choke, or cough when not actively feeding.

With most babies, reflux is mainly a laundry problem due to the excessive spitting-up/vomiting. However, some babies develop painful *gastroesophageal reflux disease (GERD)* when inflammation develops in the esophagus from exposure to acid in the regurgitated stomach contents. Ongoing re-exposure to stomach acid perpetuates the condition until the baby's anatomy and physiology mature. Multiples are more at risk for infant GERD because they are more likely to be affected by conditions associated with its development, such as preterm birth, low birth weight or small for gestational age (SGA), and other stressors associated with multiple pregnancy and birth.

Human milk and direct breastfeeding are associated with a lower incidence of GERD and less severe symptoms when it does occur.

Whether a baby has obvious spitting up/vomiting or signs of silent GERD, the discomfort caused by inflamed esophagus tissue may cause back arching or neck turning while a baby feeds. An affected baby is likely to become fussy and cry if placed flat on his back for a diaper change or to sleep soon after feeding. Respiratory symptoms and infections occur more often. These babies may begin to "resist" feedings if GERD pain becomes associated with feeding. Extremes in weight gain, both inadequate gain and too rapid weight gain, are more common for babies with GERD.

Human milk and direct breastfeeding are associated with a lower incidence of GERD and less severe symptoms when it does occur. Not only did nature design human milk for the human infant's immature digestive system, but it also contains properties that soothe and heal baby's esophagus. Also, babies control the amount of milk ingested during direct breastfeeding, so uncomfortable over-filling is less likely. Still, breastfed multiples can develop GERD, especially if physical or social circumstances create a need for regular supplementary feedings. To decrease the chance of GERD or to minimize symptoms in an affected multiple:

- Increase direct breastfeeding and limit any supplementary feedings as much as possible when an affected baby can breastfeed effectively. If direct breastfeeding is not an option, increase human-milk-feedings for this baby. Sometimes a mother chooses to readjust the amount of her milk that each multiple receives, offering more to any affected by GERD, if there is not enough for every baby for all feedings.
- Sensitivity/allergy to foreign proteins, including any that "sneak" in via a mother's own milk, may contribute to GERD. Another possible contributing factor may be lactose overload. To rule out either as a possible cause or to decrease symptoms related to either, read the sections above on "Colic: Food Sensitivity or Allergy" and "Lactose Overload" and try the related suggestions.
- Babies with GERD usually seem more comfortable with smaller, briefer, more frequent meals that put less pressure on the esophageal sphincter and do not overfill their stomachs, which direct breastfeeding is more likely to offer. Do not encourage an affected baby to breastfeed longer or take more of a feeding when this baby indicates he or she is finished.

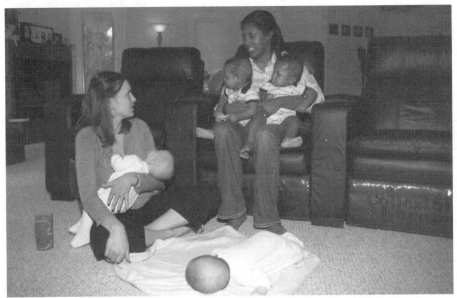

It can be very reassuring to be in contact with other mothers of multiple babies.

A few babies with GERD respond better to larger feedings that allow them to feed less often. It may take time and effort to find which feeding routine works best for a given baby. When two or more multiples have GERD, a feeding strategy that works for one may not be the one that works best for another.

- Offer a baby the same breast for several hours; many mothers of multiples already alternate breasts and babies no more than every 24 hours.
  ❑ If symptoms persist, assign each of twin multiples a particular breast as the ability to regulate production in one breast has helped multiples with GERD. (See "Lactose Overload" above.)

- Positioning baby in a more upright position during and after feedings allows gravity to help stomach contents stay in the stomach. An affected baby usually has less reflux when the spine remains straight, without slouching, and baby's head is upright at least 30° to 45°. In addition to being held more upright, these babies tend to be more comfortable in the left side-lying or prone/tummy position. Adapt breastfeeding positions as needed, using pillows, a foam wedge, etc., to help hold this baby in position.
  ❑ The straddle-saddle position in which a baby straddles a mother's leg as if it was a saddle and sits facing the breast keeps the affected baby in an upright position, and a second baby can feed simultaneously by sitting on her other leg facing the other breast. (See illustrations of simultaneous positions in Chapter 14.)

❑ To place this baby in the left side-lying position, position him in a modified cradle or side-lying position at the right breast and a modified clutch/football position at the left breast.

• The prone/tummy position is also more comfortable for many babies with GERD. To position one or two babies to breastfeed in a prone position, a mother lays back in a recliner chair or against pillows to create a similar angle in bed or on a sofa. The affected baby would lie with his tummy on mother's tummy and head at breast with the rest of the body directed down toward mother's legs. With mother in a similar position, some modify this position by cradling this baby in the crook of the right arm with baby's torso and legs down alongside mother's body. A second baby could be held and breastfed on the other side of her body.

Since the supine position used for necessary post-feeding diaper changes can trigger reflux and related pain, use a foam wedge or similar prop to change this baby in a more upright position. Avoid holding baby's legs up and over his head while cleaning baby's bottom, which can put pressure on the baby's stomach and trigger reflux.

If an affected baby is awake after feeding, it may be the perfect time for supervised tummy-time. Because the prone/tummy position is less safe when a baby sleeps, a sleeping baby should be laid down on her back. However, many parents place this baby in a more upright position by using a firm, foam infant sleep wedge. (See Resources, "Other Products: Infant Sleep/Relaxation Aids.") Make certain that the baby is placed securely on the wedge and cannot roll or slip into a less safe position.

If GERD does not respond adequately to other measures, medication may be prescribed. The medication that works best for one baby may not be the medication that works best for another. Also, babies grow quickly, so the dosage that works well today may be inadequate next week. Contact the baby's pediatric care provider if a medication either does not help or ceases to help control symptoms.

Overactive Milk Ejection/Let-Down Reflex or Lactation Overproduction

When a mother has a particularly forceful milk-ejection reflex (MER)/let-down or a multiple has difficulty handling mother's MER, some call this an *overactive let-down* (OALD). A few women have a physical condition that may cause *lactation overproduction,* but overzealous milk removal may also result in overproduction. Often OALD and overproduction occur together. The baby affected by OALD or overproduction may also show signs of lactose overload or reflux. (See "Lactose Overload" and "Infant Gastroesophageal Reflux Disease (GERD)" sections above.)

Because mothers with multiples are breastfeeding and/or expressing milk for two or more babies, they may be more at risk for either situation. Also, preterm infants may have more difficulty initially handling the sudden volume or flow rate of milk that occurs with MER. An affected multiple may cough, gag, push or turn his head away, etc., when MER occurs within the first few minutes of beginning to breastfeed. Symptoms of lactose overload or reflux or GERD also may occur for one or more multiples when OALD or overproduction occurs. Babies usually grow into and adapt to their mother's milk ejection pattern, and overproduction generally settles, unless a mother is overdoing or adding unnecessary breast expression sessions.

- Halt a breastfeeding if a baby shows signs of difficulty handling the let-down. The baby can go back to the breast when milk flow slows.
  - ❏ When it is difficult to stop and start the feeding because mother is feeding another multiple simultaneously, some mothers express/pump their breasts just to the point of MER and stop, wait and collect the milk flow in collection bottles, and then latch one or both babies back on once milk flow slows. The key to this strategy is to stop when MER occurs; overdoing it may result in overproduction.

- If a mother expresses/pumps her breasts on a regular basis, review the routine to see if overzealous milk expression may be contributing to OALD or overproduction.

- For an affected baby who is gaining well or has rapid weight gain, try comfort measures other than breastfeeding first when a baby fusses within an hour or two of the last feeding. Do not withhold breastfeeding if baby signals that other measures are not enough.

- Many of the strategies that help the baby affected by lactose overload or reflux/GERD also help the baby affected by OALD or overproduction.
  - ❏ Do not alternate breasts arbitrarily within a particular feeding.
  - ❏ Use the same breast for one baby for at least 24 hours or assign each baby a particular breast for a week to see if it proves helpful. Allowing each baby to regulate milk production in a particular breast often "calms" the MER and related milk flow for the affected baby.
  - ❏ Breastfeed using a more upright feeding position, which helps this baby control and slow the rapid flow with MER.

Central Nervous System Issues: Sensory Processing Disorders (SPD)/Sensory Integration Disorders (DSI)

Sensory processing refers to the way and the degree that an individual brain handles information from the environment that is constantly arriving via the senses. This includes touch, movement, and body awareness; sight; hearing; taste and smell. The brains of most children and adults organize, interpret, and respond to–or integrate–the incessant sensory information in a cohesive way and without effort. Sensory processing disorders (SPD), which may also be referred to as sensory integration disorders/dysfunction (DSI), manifest in the affected person's behavioral patterns.

SPD/DSI may be associated with over-responsiveness or under-responsiveness to sensory input. The over-responsive baby may arch his back and pull away or seem uncomfortable with cuddling or other kinds of touch; the under-responsive baby may seem unusually active or seem to need constant contact. These babies may lag behind in or exhibit poor fine and gross motor skills. Toddlers with SPD/DSI may be either overly cautious or risk-seeking daredevils. As these children grow, they may gain reputations as being defensive, aggressive, manipulative, or controlling. About 70 percent are eventually diagnosed with some type, of learning disability.

> **Multiples are more prone to SPD/DSI because they more often are exposed to environmental stimuli before their neurological systems are ready.**

Multiples are more prone to SPD/DSI because they are more likely to have been born preterm, low birth weight or SGA, or affected by intra-uterine stressors; they often are exposed to environmental stimuli before their neurological systems are ready. Also, it may be difficult to distinguish behaviors that are related to a more challenging temperament from those of SPD/DSI.

A mother who is concerned that the behavior or motor skills of one or more of multiples may be a result of a SPD/DSI should bring those behavioral symptoms to the attention of the baby's pediatric care provider and request an in-depth evaluation, as early intervention can make a difference in behavior. Usually evaluation for SPD/DSI is performed by an occupational therapist (OT) or physical therapist (PT) who specializes in these pediatric conditions and develops interventions that address the needs of the individual baby/child.

Respect this baby's cues for more or less direct touch or skin contact, which is simply an extension of responding to each multiple as an individual.

- Learn the behavioral cues that indicate a baby is over-stimulated, such increasing agitation or crying, arching the back, etc. It may take time to find the degree of increased or decreased contact a particular baby needs.
- Modify breastfeeding positions if the over-responsive baby needs a less hands-on approach to feeding. However, the under-responsive baby may be less happy if a position does not provide enough of a hands-on feel.
- Many of these babies respond better to gentle but firm touch. Light touch or light stroking may result in a more fussy or irritable baby.
- *Do not take it personally* when a baby indicates a need for less direct touch, as this is not a behavior the baby chose.
- Center a baby's body through a snug swaddle or by bringing baby's arms and hands to the middle of his body while gently but firmly holding the arms/hands in place to help this baby "organize." But stop if a baby becomes more agitated.
- Monitor environmental stimuli to avoid over-bright lighting, loud sounds, and movements more likely to cause startling.

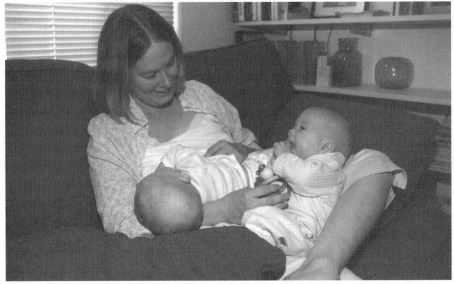

Mothers of multiples find themselves spending lots of time holding, cuddling, and feeding babies.

Parents may have to experiment to discover the cause of baby's distress. Also, each multiple is an individual. One may be affected by some physical cause when the other(s) are not.

Survival Tips

No matter what the reason for fussy or high need behavior, a mother still must find ways to cope. The following ideas, shared by mothers of multiples, may help you and your babies survive the fussy times.

- Hold and cuddle your babies. *Skin contact* often calms a fussy baby. Try kangaroo care with each fussy baby; take off your shirt and the babies' shirts, and put one or two of them directly against your chest. A shirt or a sheet can then be placed to cover mother and babies. Although cuddling may not always relieve the babies' discomfort, these actions let them know someone is there for them and cares.

   ❑ Kangaroo Care is not just for mothers; it is an activity that fathers can also enjoy with each of their babies–separately or two at once.

- Offer the breast. *Breastfeeding* is more than just food; it is also a way to comfort a baby. If you suspect overproduction, OALD, or GERD, refer to those sections in this chapter.

- *Dance* with the affected baby. Think waltz rather than rock. Soft classical or "new age" music tends to be more soothing. A smooth, rhythmic swinging or swaying motion is soothing for many babies.

- Place a fussing multiple in a *baby sling or carrier*. It is usually easier to carry a young baby at the front of the body when meeting only that baby's needs. When using most front carriers, a mother still has a free arm for a second multiple. If wearing one baby on the back, a mother usually can cuddle or breastfeed a second multiple at the same time.

  ❑ A baby may not settle the first few times she is placed in a carrier or sling. Movement, such as walking or swaying, may be needed to settle a baby new to a sling or carrier. A sling worn to the side of one hip allows a mother to carry one baby in the sling and hold or feed another on the opposite side of her body.

  ❑ Some mothers have carriers (and bodies) that allow them to carry one baby in front and one in back, both babies in front, or crisscross slings to carry a baby on each hip.

- When two or more multiples fuss at once, head for a *rocking chair.* Keep a rocking chair on every level of the house; store a folding lawn rocker in the car. Rhythmic rocking generally calms a distressed mother as well as her distressed babies.

> **Although cuddling may not always relieve the babies' discomfort, these actions let them know someone is there for them and cares.**

- Being wrapped in a *snug swaddle* position calms many babies. When snugly swaddled, a baby lays on a small blanket and her arms are held down along the side of her body as the corners of the blanket are folded over and tucked in. This swaddling is snug but *not* too tight; it should not interfere with a baby's ability to expand her chest during breathing. Swaddling blankets with Velcro® tabs are available. (See Resources.)

  ❑ Snug swaddling has been shown to help babies settle when they are placed on their backs for sleep. This strategy should be used only after making certain that the multiple is not hungry and cueing to feed.

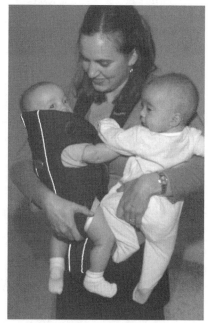

A baby carrier can make it easier to comfort two fussy babies.

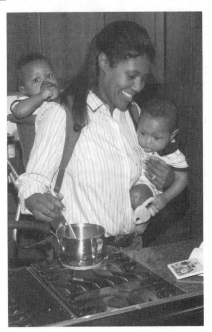

A backpack carrier can help a mother manage simple tasks.

• Take the babies for a walk. Wear a fussy baby or two in one or more carriers or slings while outside. Dress everyone appropriately and enjoy the fresh air whenever possible; walk the halls in an enclosed mall during inclement weather. (If multiples were born preterm and winter cold/flu season is an issue, ask the pediatric care provider about winter-related illnesses if the plan is brisk walking without stopping, which should minimize contact with others.)

• Go for a drive with babies. Keep a book, paperwork, sewing, etc., in the car. The movement of the car often "rocks" babies to sleep during a drive. When weather allows, many mothers let babies snooze while they read or work in the car, taking advantage of the peace and quiet. Some mothers take their multiples for a drive every day because their babies nap better. (For ideas about getting out of the house with multiples, see Chapter 23, "Getting Out and About.")

• Perform colic massage on any high need multiple during diaper changes. Massage tends to be more effective in decreasing overall fussiness when performed during the baby's calmer periods rather than during a crying bout. Massage takes about five minutes, but enjoy this close contact with one baby for longer periods if another is not "calling." (For more information about infant massage, see Resources.)

• Few, if any, child care experts would suggest picking up and holding two babies at the same time, unless one is secured in a carrier. However, it is unlikely that these experts ever had to listen to the symphonic sound of crying multiples. Carrying two is dangerous because a mother has no way to break a fall, so she or her babies could easily be injured if she slips or trips. Carrying two while walking up or down stairs is particularly hazardous. Avoid such situations as much as possible. However, if you must ever carry two babies:

❏ Walk slowly.

❏ Be constantly alert. Watch for objects on the floor or for irregular spots in carpet or flooring that could cause you to trip.

❏ Sit or put a baby down as soon as possible.

❏ Never let others hold two babies at once. You are adapting constantly to small changes in their weights and each baby's ability to balance her body. Unless another person, such as their other parent, holds and cares for the babies every day, it is extremely dangerous to allow anyone else to carry two babies at once.

- Bathe in the tub with one baby at a time. The warm water usually relaxes baby and mother.
  - ❑ Do not step in or out of a tub with a baby in your arms because of the potential for slipping. Instead, have someone hand a baby to you once you are seated. If no one is available to help, place a baby on a towel on the floor or in an infant seat next to the tub and reach for him after you sit down.
  - ❑ Sharing a warm bath can be a nice way for a father to get extra skin contact with each of his babies, too.
- Although cuddling comforts most tired babies and helps them drift to sleep, some babies become fussier and cry harder if not put down when tired. Continued handling results in over-stimulation for these babies. This baby's crying literally "winds down" once she is put down.
  - ❑ If a baby is laid in a crib/cot and crying persists without noticeable winding down within several minutes, laying baby down is probably not the answer for decreasing fussiness. More likely the baby is telling you that she is in need of your arms again.

Equipment

High touch beats high tech every time. However, since mothers of multiples are not given extra arms, there may be times when you must depend on equipment to "console" a baby or two while you care for the other(s).

Breastfeeding one (or two) while coping with another crying, hungry multiple is not relaxing for mother or babies. Still, many mothers of multiples find themselves dealing with this situation during their babies' early months. It may help to lay the crying baby close to you as you feed the other(s).

- Try swaddling her snugly first, or place your hand gently but firmly over and along her arm to hold it toward the center of her body as she lay next to you.
- Another idea is to place the crying baby in a cradle, buggy, stroller, or rocking infant seat, and use your feet to rock it. Some mothers find the baby in a seat calms if she "wraps" her bare feet around that baby's body.
- Many mothers of multiples swear by a bouncer seat, since a baby's own movement causes the seat to move up and down. Others find an automatic swing to be a godsend at these times.

Certain sounds tend to have a calming effect on babies. The same soft classical or "new age" music that you and a baby waltz to is also the best choice for soothing background music.

- Many parents recommend a recording of the sounds a baby heard when in the womb.
- Rhythmic white noise, such as the sound of a vacuum cleaner or the static heard when a radio is set between stations calms some babies. There are also white noise recordings on the market.
- To create white noise make a long, slow "ch" or "sh" sound, repeating it until baby calms. This often works more quickly when done while swaying or rocking babies.

The High Need Multiple and Maternal Guilt

Many mothers have been surprised to find they feel closer to a high need baby sooner than to a calmer one.

Many mothers have been surprised to find they feel closer to a high need baby sooner than to a calmer one. This is probably due to the extra contact the high need multiple requires. Mothers also say they then feel guilty that they are not paying as much attention to their more patient babies. Actually, they are treating each baby as an individual by responding to each one's cues for time and attention.

If this occurs, spend any extra time with the calmer baby but do not feel guilty when there is no extra time. Several daily breastfeedings provide even the most patient baby and her mother with opportunities for time together. Also, the calmer, more patient multiple eventually flip-flops with the fussier one(s), "demanding" her turn for more time and attention when she needs it. (See Chapter 19, "Enhancing Individuality.")

Colic generally disappears by the time babies are a few months old; GERD or food sensitivity may take longer to resolve. When temperament contributes toward high need behavior, a child is more likely to remain high need; however, this child will change and express sensitivity in different ways. With appropriate intervention a child can learn to manage behaviors associated with SPD/DSI. For more information on high need babies/children, see Resources, Related Parenting Books: Fussy or High Need Baby/Children.

KEY POINTS

❑ Sometimes one or more of multiples is considered high need because parents did not know how much time and attention young babies require.

❑ Temperament traits, which form a baby's behavioral "style," have a genetic basis so a baby cannot change these traits.

❑ There are a number of physical causes of fussiness.

- Colic appears to be related to spasms, or waves, of pain in a baby's intestinal tract. Sensitivity to a food or something else in a baby's environment may lead to colic symptoms.

- An uncomfortable form of reflux (regurgitation/vomiting) is called gastroesophageal reflux disease (GERD).

- Overactive let-down (OALD) of milk or lactation overproduction bothers some babies and may be associated with lactose overload or reflux and GERD symptoms.

- Sensory processing disorders occur when a baby has difficulty interpreting the information that is sent to the brain from sight, sound, smell, taste, and touch.

❑ Many of the same strategies work for several physical causes of fussiness.

- Breastfeed or give expressed mother's milk as close to fully as possible.

- Eliminate dairy products from baby's diet by eliminating dairy products in the diet of the breastfeeding mother and avoiding or minimizing exposure to cow's milk-based infant formula.

- When two multiples breastfeed effectively, alternate breasts and babies no more than every 24 hours or assign each baby a breast.

- Use positions that allow an affected baby to remain in a more upright position while breastfeeding.

- High need babies tend to be high contact babies. Strategies that are high-touch, low-tech usually make these babies happiest.

❑ Many babies become calmer when their shirts are removed and they are placed skin-to-skin on a mother's or a father's bare chest.

❑ Slings or other on-body carriers allow a parent to carry the fussy baby while caring for another or completing some household task.

❑ Massage, including colic massage, often helps these babies if performed during calm–not fussy–periods.

❑ Since babies cannot tell night from day, high need babies are likely to need more contact during the night.

❑ Mothers often find they soon feel closer to a high-need multiple. This may be due to the amount of contact these babies need.

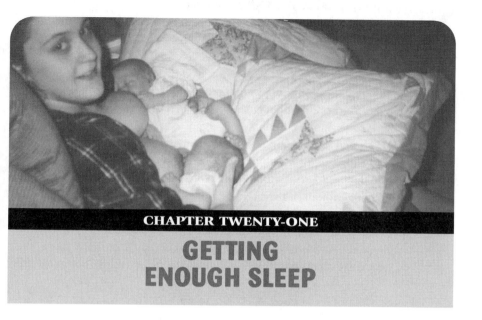

CHAPTER TWENTY-ONE

GETTING ENOUGH SLEEP

Most mothers say they can cope with any number of multiples *if* they get enough sleep. In addition to needing rest to keep up with multiples during the day, sleep also contributes to recuperation from a multiple pregnancy and birth. However, with two or more babies waking for night feedings, getting enough sleep is no simple quest.

A few babies sleep through the night–a four- to six-hour stretch–within a few weeks of birth, but most babies *cannot* do this. They are not physically ready or able. They need to eat every few hours; they also rouse more easily to wake from lighter sleep than older babies/children. Babies are not born telling time; they do not associate daytime with activity or sleep with night. They will get the idea eventually, but it may be months before one or more can be counted on to sleep for a several hour stretch without waking. Most mothers of multiples learn to get adequate rest on a "catch as catch can" basis!

Babies' cries need a quick response no matter what the hour. They are learning to trust the person who answers their calls and realizing that they are worthy of response. Babies who continue to wake at night do not interrupt their parents' sleep on purpose, yet their nighttime needs do not negate a mother's (or father's) need for adequate sleep.

Sleep Deprivation

Sleep deprivation is a real problem for many mothers of multiples. It especially affects mothers during the early weeks postpartum when they are recuperating from pregnancy and birth. And it is physically and mentally draining if weeks or months pass without a several hour stretch of uninterrupted sleep a few times a week. Some mothers report they begin to feel numb after operating for several days with very little sleep. Many find that small annoyances are magnified and they feel "on edge" or irritable. Occasionally mothers say they became so exhausted that they felt unable to respond to a waking baby; they literally felt paralyzed and could not make their bodies move.

Dad must be ready to help when a mother becomes too exhausted to care for babies, and suggestions for how dad can help are included below. If your partner cannot be relied on to awaken, you may need to ask a relative or friend to stay over when you recognize the signs that you are reaching a critical point of sleep deprivation.

Although exhaustion is understandable when a mother is recuperating from multiple pregnancy and birth, the babies still need someone who can respond when they cry. Parents must find sleep solutions that meet the babies' needs as well as fulfilling the mother's need for sleep.

Encouraging Sleep

The following ideas have helped many mothers "make it through the night."

- *Wake each baby more often during the day,* to see if it lengthens the time they sleep at night. This strategy does not mean cutting out daytime naps, as many babies also sleep better at night when they have had needed naps during the day. It may mean shortening one or two nap periods.
  - ❑ *Babies wake more easily from light sleep,* so watch for signs that a baby is in a lighter sleep state, such as stretching arms and legs, grimacing of the mouth, blinking or movement behind the eyelids, and grunting or making other noises. As with coordinating feedings, some babies are better able to go along with attempts to change their body clocks than others.

- *If babies were preterm and have been awakened every few hours on doctor's orders,* ask if it is all right to begin letting each set her night feeding routine on an individual basis once any demonstrates appropriate wetting and stooling patterns and is gaining adequate weight.
- *Some parents find their babies sleep longer when they massage each baby every evening as part of a bedtime routine.* Infant massage techniques are simple to learn. There are several books that illustrate the movements that babies find relaxing. (See Resources.)

- *Play the same soft classical music each evening when any baby looks sleepy.* The babies may learn to associate the music with falling asleep. Do not expect this to work immediately; it may be weeks or months before they make this association.

> Babies' cries need a quick response no matter what the hour.

- *Try snug swaddling each baby immediately before bedtime to help them settle and sleep for a longer period.* In snug swaddling, each baby's arms are held alongside the body folding a corner of the blanket over one arm, tucking it in, and then doing the same with the opposite corner over the other arm. Swaddling blankets with self-adhesive tabs are also available.

- *Younger babies may settle more easily if they hear the rhythmic static of white noise, such as a vacuum cleaner, a radio set between stations, etc., in the background.* Recordings of such noises are available. Also, some babies respond to recordings of womb sounds–the soft, rhythmic sounds of a mother's heartbeat and blood rushing through an umbilical cord–or sounds of the surf or rainfall.

- *By two to three months babies generally soil diapers less often,* and it may be possible to double–or triple–diaper babies, or get by with a nighttime disposable, to avoid the stimulation of nighttime changes. Heavier diaper liners may also help extend diapers during the night.

- *Unless you find night feedings the perfect time to interact with one baby*–and some mothers do–keep night feedings as businesslike as possible if you want babies to learn that nighttime is sleep time. Cuddle and give kisses but:
  ❑ Dim the lighting
  ❑ Leave the TV, radio, or CD player off
  ❑ Keep conversation to a minimum.

Sleep Arrangements

Nearness to adults is associated with safe infant sleep. The safest sleep arrangement for babies is one that places them in the same room close to their parents. A separate nursery, no matter how beautifully decorated, how high-tech the baby monitor, or how many babies share it, has been found to be the least safe place for babies to sleep. In addition to babies' safety, keeping babies close to parents has other advantages.

- Night feedings, diaper changes, and comforting one or more are more easily and efficiently accomplished when babies are within an arm's reach. All usually return to sleep more quickly.

- Young babies regulate their breathing patterns and heart rates better when they sleep near parents.

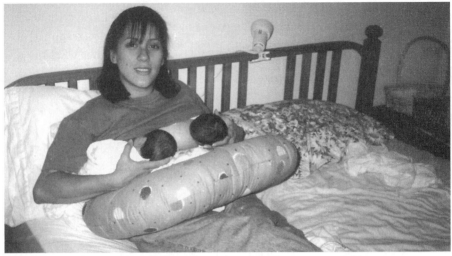

Some mothers find it easier to sit up in bed to nurse two babies.

Having babies nearby rarely affects physical intimacy for new parents of multiples. Most couples are creative enough to figure an alternative "approach" when they wish to be intimate and babies are in their bedroom. (And most parents of infant multiples usually are thinking of sleep rather than sexual relations when they propose going to bed!)

> The safest sleep arrangement for babies is one that places them in the same room close to their parents.

Co-Bedding

When two or more multiples share a single crib/cot, it is called co-bedding. Multiples spent months together in cramped quarters during pregnancy, so they tend to sleep for longer stretches or find comfort from the nearness of the other when they share a crib/cot. Also, multiples' sleep cycles become more similar when co-bedded–something most parents prefer. Co-bedding provides one way to keep all babies in the safety of their parents' room for a longer period.

Preterm multiples are often co-bedded in a NICU or special care nursery. However, round-the-clock monitoring was available and in place.

To lower potential risks with co-bedding:
- Always lay infants on their backs in bed/crib/cot.
- Place multiples next to each other with both/all heads toward the head of the crib and all feet toward the foot of the crib to avoid entanglement of head or extremities between slats along the side of a crib.
- Do not separate babies in the crib by placing a pillow, rolled blanket, etc., between them.
- Do not use loose bedcovers. (If covering babies, use a light cover and tuck the ends under the mattress.)

- Do not place toys, stuffed animals, bumper pads, etc., in a crib/cot that a baby may pull over his face.
- Avoid overheating the babies. Do not use too many or heavy coverings, especially when warm night clothing is used–and do not overdo night clothing.
- Co-bedding is not associated with an increase in multiples' body temperatures, but the close contact should reduce a need for anything more than light covers.
- Room temperature should feel "just right" to a lightly clothed adult.
- Only a light blanket is needed to swaddle a baby snugly. Also, proper snug swaddling technique involves a baby's body from the shoulders down, so the blanket should never

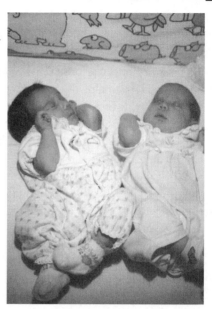

Babies often sleep better when placed together in one crib.

be high enough to cover any baby's nose or mouth to interfere with breathing. With good swaddling technique, no blanket corner can become loose and possibly cover the nose or mouth of another multiple during sleep.

Many parents of twins use only one crib for their babies' first three to six months. Young babies rarely disturb one another even when one stretches on top of another. There is no arbitrary date when multiples should be separated in bed. Usually, their sleep behaviors loudly and clearly "tell" parents when it is time.

Cosleeping/Bedsharing

Cosleeping refers to having babies sleep in the same room, close to their mothers. Bedsharing means bringing one or more babies into bed with one or more parents. Whether to bring a baby (or two or three) into the parents' bed has become a matter of debate for parents in Western culture. However, human mothers sleep with their babies in almost all cultures worldwide. There is nothing new about parents and children sharing a bed. For tens of thousands of years mothers have appreciated that everyone in the family copes better during the day when they have gotten enough sleep the night before.

In addition to more sleep for parents, bedsharing offers the benefit of close human contact for babies with mother. Research has shown that babies are breast-fed for longer durations when a mother brings a baby into bed with her for breastfeeding. Even when a mother does not plan to fall asleep, breastfeeding hormones may encourage her to drift off while feeding one or more babies in her bed. Fortunately, studies also have found that a sober, unimpaired mother tends to fall asleep in a protective position–facing baby with an arm placed in a way that prevents a baby from moving up or down in the bed. Breastfed babies rouse from sleep more readily, which is a protective mechanism. Also, the sleep of breastfeeding mothers and their babies are more in tune with one another.

Recently, some pediatric care providers have attributed bedsharing as a contributing factor in some cases of Sudden Infant Death Syndrome (SIDS). Parents also may worry that they might hurt or even suffocate a baby by rolling on her. However, no research has found an increased risk to a baby cosleeping on a safe surface with a sober (unimpaired by medication or substances), non-smoking, breastfeeding mother. It is impossible to eliminate all risk no matter where babies sleep, and multiples born preterm or affected by intrauterine growth restrictions are at somewhat higher risk for SIDS; still, such happenings are rare and safe sleeping measures reduce potential risk factors.

- When a baby sleeps in the crook of mother's arm (or there is a multiple in the crook of each arm), it is nearly impossible to roll on a baby.
- Many mothers sleep on one side facing a baby with one arm encircling the area above the baby's head. This may be more difficult to accomplish with two babies, whether mother is turned toward both (on one side of her) or one is on either side of her.

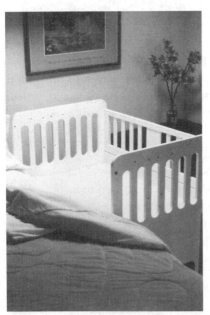

Portable cribs that attach to the side of parents' bed can provide extra room for multiple babies.

Parents of multiples have discovered many ingenious ways to get more sleep by bringing babies in bed for at least part of the night. Safe cosleeping when there are two or more babies to care for at night is a little more complicated, but with a little imagination it can be done.

- Many parents remove one side-rail from a standard crib/cot. It is fastened securely against their bed with the crib mattress adjusted to the level of their mattress. Most suggest placing one baby between the mother and her partner while another sleeps in the crib. Mother then rolls from side-to-side to meet babies' breastfeeding needs during the night.
- Portable cribs that attach directly to the parents' bed have been developed to give everyone more space when cosleeping or bedsharing.

Safer Cosleeping/Bedsharing for Parents and Multiples

LOW Risk IF

Any cosleeping/bedsharing baby is:
- In supine (on back) position during sleep
- With mother/parents who are:
  - Non-smokers
  - Unimpaired by alcohol, medications/ drugs, excessive fatigue, or illness
- Breastfed
- With mother who assumes (typical) protective position with her body and arm around baby
- On firm, flat mattress that fits tightly in frame or against wall(s)
  - With sheets that fit mattress snugly
- Unlikely to become overheated, due to:
  - Light bed clothing
  - Light bed covering(s)
  - Room temperature below 70°F/20°C
- Unlikely to have nose or mouth covered by:
  - Fluffy covers/duvet
  - Soft mattress pads
  - Loose sheets/covers and pillows
  - Loose objects in bed
- NEVER left alone when in/on an adult bed.

Risk Effect Is UNKNOWN IF

Any cosleeping/bedsharing baby is:
- Born "borderline" preterm (less than 38 weeks gestation but healthy)
- Small for gestational age (SGA) even if full term (less than 5lb 8 oz/2500 gm) and healthy
- Put to sleep with a pacifier
- In parents' bed with another multiple:
  - More difficult for mother to assume a typical, protective position with two/more babies
  - No data regarding two/more on either side of mother vs. sharing space on same side

Increased Risk IF

Any cosleeping/bedsharing baby is:
- Asleep on stomach (prone) or lying on side
- Affected by a health issue, anomaly, or preterm (especially if less than 36-37 weeks gestation)
- With mother/parent who is:
  - Smoker (even if adult does not smoke in bed/home)
  - Impaired by alcohol, medications/drugs, excessive fatigue, or illness
- With a sleeping adult on:
  - Sofa, armchair
  - Waterbed
  - Sagging or "fluffy" mattress
  - Mattress with spaces between frame and wall(s)
- In bed with
  - Someone other than mother/parent
  - Older child/sibling (reduced risk if a parent sleeps between baby and older child)
- Exposed to objects that could cover nose or mouth:
  - Fluffy, loose coverings
  - Pillows (near baby)
  - Ill-fitting/loose sheets
  - Impaired adult
  - Older child or pet
- Overheated due to
  - Too much clothing/covering
  - Room temperature greater than 70°F/20°C
- Alone in or on
  - Room separate from adults
  - Adult bed
- Formula-fed
- Bottle-fed (even mother's milk) while cosleeping/bedsharing

- When a mother remains awake after feeding a baby, she can place the just-fed baby back in the adjacent crib/cot with a co-multiple.
- Some parents refuse to be limited by standard bed sizes. When even a king-size bed seems too small with two or more babies sharing it, the width of a bed can be extended by placing another mattress (or two/more) side by side. Be certain that mattresses fit tightly against one another so that no gaps or cracks are created which a baby could slip into. It may be safest to place the mattresses (and box springs) directly on the floor.
- Another option many use is to set up a crib/cot in the parents' bedroom near but not attached to their bed. Babies rotate in and out of bed with mother as they wake to eat during the night.
- Often babies begin nighttime sleep in the crib. When Baby A wakes, mother breastfeeds and possibly falls asleep with that baby until Baby B wakes to feed. Baby A is resettled in the nearby crib and mother breastfeeds and possibly falls asleep again with Baby B.
- Some parents place a mattress on the floor of the babies' room and mother sleeps there and feeds one or more babies.
- An option used by many parents during the early weeks or months at home is for parents to sleep in separate rooms—each responsible for one or more babies for the night. Dad brings the baby to mother for breastfeeding if he is unable to comfort him or her in other ways.

Simultaneously breastfeeding two multiples while lying in bed works for some mothers and not for others. Usually, it becomes easier as babies get older, although a few mothers achieve this from the start.

- Many mothers use a modified double-cradle position when in bed. Mother lays back—flat or propped in a semi-sitting position—and holds a baby in the crook of each arm. Babies' bodies extend down, along the sides of her body. This allows babies to remain on their back for sleep or be rolled slightly toward her body to breastfeed.
- By sitting up and leaning back against a bed-rest pillow, other mothers are able to breastfeed two babies at once while in bed. The safety of this position depends on the mother's ability to keep babies' in a position that does not allow babies to slide down and possibly entrap or cover a baby's nose and mouth should mother drift to sleep while sitting up.
- Although it may be more comfortable to breastfeed young babies simultaneously when sitting in a supportive recliner chair in the bedroom, recliners are not a safe sleep surface and are not recommended for a mother who tends to drift to sleep while breastfeeding because of the potential for infant head/face entrapment or falls.

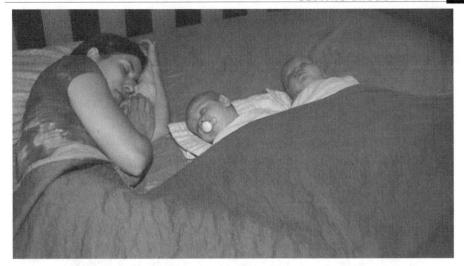

These babies are sleeping comfortably on their backs with no pillows or loose bed covers that could interfere with their breathing.

Mother's Sleep Style

How a mother chooses to cope with night waking and feedings, and getting enough rest, often depends on her sleep style. There seems to be two basic styles: 1) the mother who easily falls back to sleep after waking for feedings, and 2) the mother who has difficulty falling asleep again if she awakens too much or for too long for feedings.

> **Parents must find sleep solutions that meet the babies' needs as well as fulfilling mother's need for sleep.**

Mother #1 will want to coordinate babies' night feedings by waking two to feed at once or waking one immediately after the other. She figures this is the best way to get several hours of uninterrupted sleep. Mother #2 is more likely to bring whichever baby wakes into bed with her, help him latch on, and then drift back to sleep. If two babies wake at once, she will find a way to feed them simultaneously, allowing her to fall asleep again.

Mother #1 may not understand how Mother #2 copes with being interrupted so often at night, and Mother #2 cannot figure how Mother #1 gets any rest by waking for so long several times a night.

Mothers also have different napping styles. Mother A falls asleep at the drop of a hat when the babies (and older children) sleep; she wakes feeling refreshed and ready to take on the rest of the day. Mother B cannot fall asleep no matter how tired. On the rare occasion she eventually does drift off, she wakes from her nap feeling more tired than before and feels sluggish the rest of the day.

Mother A probably will want to take advantage of opportunities to sleep when all babies sleep–whether a daily or a rare occurrence. Mother B may feel more rested if she relaxes in some other way when babies sleep.

Ultimately, the idea is to meet the babies' needs and get needed rest–no matter which method(s) best suits a mother's sleep style.

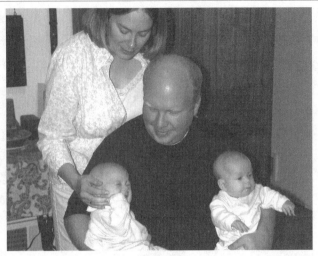

Caring for twins around the clock can be a challenge for both parents.

Dad's Involvement

It is amazing how much more sleep a mother obtains if dad gets up to bring babies to her or helps with the logistics of night feedings. He also can change a baby's diaper as necessary or soothe a baby waiting to be fed.

If a partner's schedule interferes with his ability to help at night, you and he may need to discuss ways for everyone to get enough rest. Dad's need for sleep is also important if he is to be alert on the job the next day. He may be unavailable many nights due to work travel or an "on call" schedule. Unfortunately, respect for his workload does not help you get needed rest. Perhaps he can agree to help more on the nights before his days off or during his off days.

- Consider napping during the day or evening or go to bed several hours early sometimes, leaving dad with expressed milk if babies must eat while you sleep.
- Some mothers regularly express milk to have available for one night feeding so dad can get up and feed one (or more). Depending on dad's availability or mother's level of exhaustion, dad (or someone else) may help with night feedings a few times a month to every night.

  ❏ In some families mother feeds one baby (or more) while dad feeds another, so all are able to return to sleep sooner.

  ❏ In other families dad is responsible for feeding all the babies for one feeding so that mother gets several hours of uninterrupted sleep one night. (Use caution if dad is responsible for more than one consecutive feeding due to double, triple, or greater milk production leading to an increase risk for plugged ducts, mastitis, lower milk production, etc.)

Night waking times two, three, or more can challenge even the hardiest of parents. Yet young babies cannot be expected to sleep long periods without waking. It takes time for babies to sleep several hours without interruption, but eventually a nighttime routine develops. However, even prolonged night waking has its silver lining. Never will a night of uninterrupted sleep be taken for granted–for the rest of a mother of multiples' life!

KEY POINTS

- ❑ Sleep deprivation is an important issue for many mothers of multiples; however, babies are not born understanding that nighttime is for sleep.
- ❑ Strategies for encouraging sleep must take each baby's needs into account while moving toward a nap and nighttime routine that every member of the family can live with.
- ❑ Safe co-bedding of multiples in a single baby crib/cot seems to comfort and prolong sleep for many multiples.
- ❑ Safe cosleeping of one (or more) multiples on a safe bed surface with his sober, non-smoking breastfeeding mother increases sleep for many mothers.
  - Simultaneous breastfeeding of two babies in bed with mother can be difficult but many mothers eventually find a position that works for all involved.
- ❑ Because mothers also have different sleep styles, ideas that work for one mother may not work well for another.
- ❑ Bringing babies to mother, comforting a baby waiting to breastfeed, or handling some night feedings are ways a father may be able to help with night feedings.
- ❑ Eventually, a nighttime routine develops and parents obtain several hours of uninterrupted sleep.

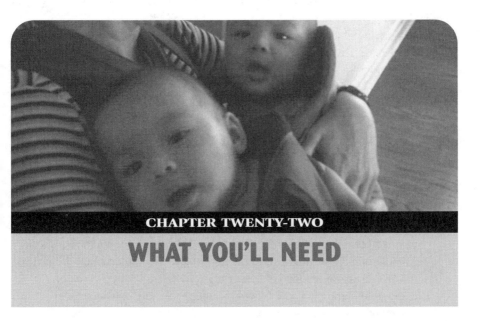

WHAT YOU'LL NEED

Infant gadgets and equipment often make life easier for a mother of multiples. Fortunately, few items are needed in double or triple quantities, and most can be purchased once you have begun to care for the babies at home and developed a better sense of what would be useful. When an item is needed for each baby or toddler, any offer from relatives and friends to lend clothing and equipment can be a budget saver. Consignment shops and neighborhood or mothers of multiples club sales may be other sources of used clothing and equipment in good condition. (Uses for various types of equipment are discussed in relevant chapters. Information for obtaining certain products is included in Resources.)

Anticipating the kinds and amounts of clothing and equipment you will need to have on hand for multiple newborns can be difficult, but newborns do not need much in the way of material goods. Beyond diapers and several changes of clothing for each, there are few items one "must" have on hand when the babies are discharged home.

Diapers

Each newborn will require about 8 to 12 diaper changes a day. (Older babies usually require at least 4 to 6 daily changes.) Standard cloth diapers, or nappies, usually must be changed more often than highly absorbent brands of cloth or disposable diapers. You will probably want to weigh the advantages and disadvantages of diapering options with potential cost. Since time is at a premium with multiple babies, do not cut convenience simply for the sake of low cost or you may find you pay in other ways.

- Laundering cloth diapers may seem the least expensive diapering option. Purchasing a week's worth of diapers is unnecessary, but unless you want to spend a lot of time in the laundry room, you will probably want at least 1 1/2 to 2 days of diapers (36 to 48) on hand. Prefolded diapers are more convenient than unfolded ones, but they cost more since different sizes are needed as babies grow. Flushable diaper liners are available, which may simplify diaper changes and laundry. Include the diaper hamper, laundry detergent, hot water, and wear and tear on appliances when figuring the total cost of cloth diapers.

- Disposable diapers are convenient to use, but the cost of 8 to 12 daily diapers times two, three, four, or more quickly adds up! However, you can easily change diaper sizes as babies grow. If you are interested in using disposables, ask other parents which brands they prefer and why. Check into discount department store brands, which often incorporate the favorite features of name brands yet cost considerably less. Many brands of disposable diapers are not biodegradable, and many consumers have voiced concern about their long-term effect on the environment.

- In areas where a diaper service is available, many parents have found it to be the most economical and convenient option for multiples. Since the delivery charge is part of the overall fee, multiplying the number of diapers for two or more babies often adds little to the total cost. Most services include the "dirty" diaper hamper(s). Hampers are returned later with service cancellation.

- Many parents combine diapering options. They use purchased or diaper service cloth diapers at home, but take disposable diapers for outings or travel.

Clothing or Layette

Newborns do not need much in the way of material goods.

Most newborns require a change of clothing two to three times a day due to diaper overflow, spit-ups, and so on. About five t-shirts or one-piece shirt/diaper covers (onesies) per baby and an equal number of stretch sleepers or gowns for each should be enough to get by for two or three days. Depending on the climate, each newborn may need a sweater and cap/hat or heavier outerwear. Have at least two smaller receiving blankets and, perhaps, one larger crib blanket available for each multiple. Some parents color-code blankets so they know which blanket belongs to which multiple.

Babies quickly grow through several sizes of clothing, so parents of multiples often look for durable used clothing at garage sales, flea markets, and consignment shops. Some parents of multiples groups sponsor clothing sales. Parents who can connect with another family having slightly older multiples of the same number and gender(s) may continue to purchase their gently used clothing for several years.

- Whether new or used, wash all clothing before the babies wear it. Using a special detergent for babies' laundry is rarely needed; simply throw their clothing in with the rest of the family wash.
- Few parents have to purchase fancy clothing for multiples. Friends and relatives tend to give dressy matching outfits as gifts.

> **"Lucky" parents connect with another family having slightly older multiples of the same number and gender(s) and purchase their gently used clothing.**

Breast Pumps

Few women need to purchase a breast pump prior to giving birth. If you must express your milk for babies, many hospitals provide the use of a self-cycling breast pump during the hospital stay as well as a double collection kit. After discharge, it will be necessary to rent a breast pump, however, the collection kit can be taken home by the mother and used with the rental pump. La Leche League Leaders and lactation consultants in your area should be aware of local rental stations if:

1. The hospital does not stock these items for use during your hospital stay
2. You must continue to pump after hospital discharge
3. A need for pumping does not occur until after discharge.

Whether rented or purchased, an effective self-cycling, electric pump saves time when expressing milk two or more times a day for daily supplements or when returning to outside employment while multiples still rely mostly on mother's milk for food. Usually a mother has plenty of time to rent or purchase a pump for these uses after babies are born and breastfeeding is well established. (Currently, only full-size, hospital-grade breast pumps were designed for use in establishing milk production.)

If expressing milk for occasional complementary feedings, a reliable manual (hand) or mini-electric pump probably will do. Some mothers purchase two one-handed manual pumps; mini-electric options with double collection kits are available.

Many mothers find the use of any breast pump is unnecessary when they fully breastfeed without complements or supplements and they learn the proper technique for hand-expression of milk. (This technique is simple for most mothers to learn and do.)

To discuss the advantages and disadvantages of breast pump options or manual expression, contact a La Leche League Leader or a lactation consultant. (Milk expression in different situations is discussed in relevant chapters. See Resources for breast pump company contact numbers.)

Car Seats

Infant car seats are required by law in many areas. Proof of availability and proper installation of a car seat for each baby may be required before the babies are discharged from the hospital. Some car seats adapt for newborn through toddler or preschool ages or weights. Other types are designed for a specific age or stage, but many can be used outside of the car as infant seats that fit in strollers, infant swings, and so on. Still other brands are for use only in the car and for a specific age level, which means parents must purchase separate sets of car seats for newborn and older multiples.

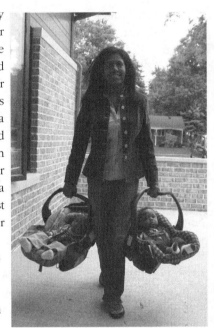

Infant car seats are required by law in many areas.

- Your multiples will use their car seats for several years. Age-related car seats may seem less expensive initially, but adaptable car seats often save money in the long run.
- Before purchasing car seats, measure the space(s) in your car where car seats will be placed and then match these with car seat measurements. Do not forget to measure for how car seats will fit before purchasing or using another car.
- Be certain that the car seats you buy can be anchored safely in your car, according to manufacturer directions.

Bedding

Sleepy newborns can drift off in any safe spot. The latest design in nursery furniture is not a requirement for safe, sound sleep. Since it is not always as safe or convenient to let multiple babies sleep with parents, most parents have some type of infant crib(s)/cot(s) available. (See Chapter 21, "Getting Enough Sleep" for a discussion of safe sleeping.)

Multiples may sleep better when placed with another baby, so a single crib for two babies may meet their needs for several weeks or months. The babies will let you know–loudly and clearly–that they want more space! Doubling up may not work in bassinets or small portable cribs, although those designed as an extension of the parents' bed often accommodate two younger babies.

- Whether you buy or borrow a baby crib(s), be certain that each meets all recommended safety guidelines. Babies have strangled after getting their heads caught between side-rail slats that were too wide and from constricting clothing that became caught on some attachment projecting from a crib. Also, suffocation has occurred when babies' heads become trapped between the frame and mattress. A mattress should fit snugly within the crib frame.

- A bed extender, which is similar to a portable crib, attaches to the side of the parents' bed, which makes it easier to keep babies close during the night. One to two multiples should safely fit in it depending on the length and width of a particular brand and the babies' sizes.

Multiple Stroller

A stroller that safely seats two (or more) babies or children is considered a must by most parents of multiples. They often rely on their double, triple, or quadruple-seat strollers until multiples are through the toddler or preschool years.

- A multiple-seat stroller must be durable enough to last several years, as it often is not practical or safe to chase after two, three, or more same-age toddlers and preschoolers running in different directions.

- High-quality strollers for multiples can be expensive, but most parents say a well-constructed stroller that adapts as their multiples grow pays for itself many times over.

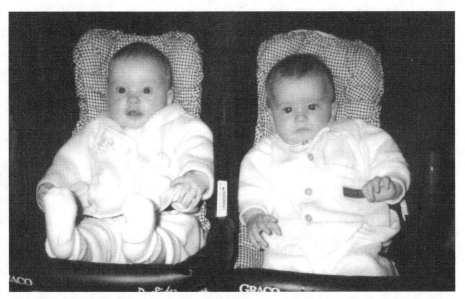

A multiple seat stroller needs to be sturdy enough to last for several years.

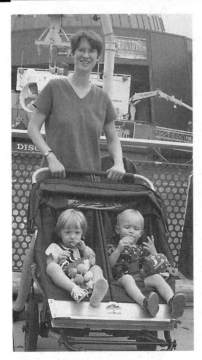

A sturdy stroller makes outings easier with toddler multiples.

❏ Many parents who have initially purchased inexpensive, less durable strollers report they ultimately spent more after that stroller fell apart from use and had to be replaced, or older babies or toddler multiples outgrew less adaptable models. A high-quality stroller also has resale value when your multiples no longer need it.

Compare features and costs before investing in a multiple-seat stroller.

Many parents delay investing in a stroller until after the babies' births. Since their babies are not going anywhere immediately after discharge, they want to gain a sense of which stroller, or stroller-baby carrier/sling combination, might best meet their needs. Parents today have more stroller options than ever before. Side-by-side models are becoming more compact. Strollers the width of a single seat come with all seats facing forward, one seat facing another, or with one or more seats that may be adjusted to face backward or forward. There are now stroller frames that allow for the addition of a variable number of seats. Double and triple jogging strollers are also available.

Before shopping for a multiple stroller:

- Ask other parents of same-number multiples which strollers they prefer and which type or brand they wish they had bought (and why).
- Consider how you are likely to use the stroller in order to compare features and cost and find one that best suits everyone's needs.
  ❏ The suburban family that is in and out of the car a lot may prefer a lightweight stroller that folds compactly for storage in their car's trunk or cargo area. On the other hand, the urban family that spends more time cruising uneven concrete sidewalks and curbs may look for a stroller with a shock-resistant frame and wheels. Both families will want a stroller that easily passes through typical 36-inch (1 meter) wide doorways and store aisles.
  ❏ Weight and portability are issues for a family living on the third-floor in an apartment building with no elevator or for a family that frequently travels on public transportation.

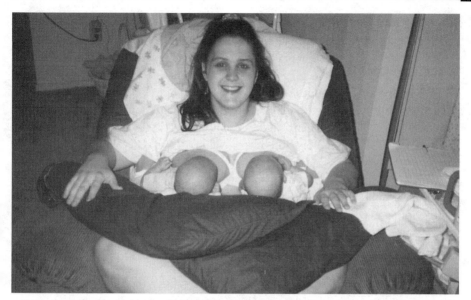

A comfortable recliner chair has helped many mothers learn to breastfeed two babies at once.

- Think about both immediate and long-term use. A stroller or carriage that is perfect for newborns may not offer enough room for toddlers to stretch their legs. Be sure the back of every stroller seat is completely adjustable from flat to sitting.
- Tandem strollers were developed for families having closely spaced children–those born 10 to 30 months apart rather than 10 to 30 minutes, and the flat position may not be available for every seat on some models. Although this type of stroller may not be the best option with two newborns, many parents begin using a tandem stroller once one baby can maintain a sitting position.
- If you have an older toddler or preschooler in addition to newborn twins or triplets, a stroller offering a variable number of seats may be the best option.
- Linking two umbrella-type strollers with a special stroller connector creates a compact and portable double stroller, yet allows for the convenience of a single stroller when desired.
  - ❑ Use a connector with two swivel-wheeled, umbrella-type strollers of the same brand. Measure the combined width of the two strollers and the connector, since the stroller combination must be narrow enough to pass through typical doorways when joined.

Rocking and Recliner Chair(s)

A rocking chair is so indispensable it should be tax-deductible for parents of multiples.

No parents should bring multiples home without installing a comfortable rocking chair on every level of the house! A rocking chair is so indispensable it should be tax-deductible for parents of multiples. Rocking not only soothes babies, the rhythm is also soothing for a frantic mother or older sibling. A well-designed wooden or upholstered rocker will hold you and your multiples for years.

- Place the most comfortable rocker where you spend the most time. This usually is not the nursery.
- Folding lawn chair rockers are an inexpensive option to place in other areas of the house. Keep one in the car to take for travel or visits away from home.
- Upholstered recliner chairs have been instrumental in helping many mothers learn to feed two babies simultaneously. The semi-reclining position and the upholstery combine to support babies' bodies, so a mother's hands are free to help the babies latch on.
- Many parents find they literally live in a rocker or a recliner for the first six months, and they recommend having at least one upholstered rocker-recliner combination.

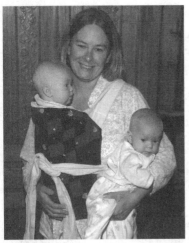

Mothers use all types of slings and carriers to meet their babies' needs.

Baby Carriers

Using a cloth infant sling or infant carrier that straps onto your body often makes life easier when caring for young multiples. A sling or front carrier allows a mother to carry and provide close contact with one baby while still having two free hands. The sling may be more practical with multiples because a baby can be carried at a mother's side in it, leaving a breast accessible for another baby.

Eventually parents may choose to obtain an extra one or two slings or carriers, so each parent can "wear" one or two babies. Some parents have carried two multiples at once in one roomy sling or by crisscrossing two slings on their upper bodies; others have worn two infant carriers with one baby on their chests and one against their backs.

Twin or triplet carriers exist, although the selection is limited. The most practical models have pieces that join to form one multiple-baby carrier or come apart for two single carriers.

A sling or front carrier allows a mother to carry and provide close contact with one baby while still having two free hands.

Many slings come in different sizes, and proper fit may affect comfort. Also, a brand that is a good fit for one mother's body may not be the best fit for another mother. When carrying two in different slings, some mothers use two slings of the same size and other mothers find a combination of one smaller and one in a larger size works better.

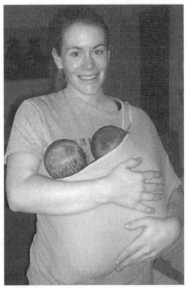

Some mothers find a way to carry two babies in one sling!

Other Equipment

The market is flooded with infant products that sound wonderful but are not crucial to comfort for either babies or parents. Budget and available space in a home for nonessential equipment are considerations before buying or borrowing such items.

- A changing table may be nice, but a waterproof pad placed on a carpet, sofa, or bed will work just as well and allows for assembly-line changing of two or more newborns. Changing babies on the floor eliminates the danger of a baby falling if another baby distracts a parent during diaper and clothing changes.
- An infant bathtub is fine for bathing each baby, but laying a newborn on a towel next to a sink for a sponge bath is just as effective for getting a young baby clean. Some infant seats can be used to prop babies for bathing in an adult tub. A parent can bathe with a baby by laying the baby across her/his chest or legs to bathe it, which is one way fathers can get more skin contact with their babies.
- Unless one baby has highly sensitive skin, special baby towels, soaps, or detergents are unnecessary. The towels and mild soap used by the rest of the family will do for most.
- Breastfed babies have such a nice scent of their own, why spoil it with artificial baby lotions or oils?
- A play yard or playpen may protect one or more infant multiples from an older sibling, and many parents find it works great as a large toy chest or laundry basket. However, young infants usually do not find a play yard or playpen a very interesting place to play.
- An automatic infant swing can be a great help when feeding one newborn

and another needs attention or it can rock one while you meet an older child's needs or prepare supper. However, a self-rocking infant seat or bouncer seat, some of which include a battery-operated mechanism that causes the seat to gently vibrate, may work as well or better. One swing or bouncer seat on the main floor of the house usually is enough when babies first arrive home. Depending on the individual babies' responses, you may want to buy or borrow additional swings or bouncing/rocking seats.

A word of caution. In one study of infants and equipment use, researchers found that babies less than two months old spent an average of six hours–and up to 12 hours–a day in some type of infant seat, such as infant or car seats, swings, etc. Because of their lack of muscle control, the babies' necks bent forward within 20 minutes of being placed in an infant seat. This positioning caused babies to regurgitate (reflux) more, and it partially blocked the airway, which researchers think may be related to an increase of upper respiratory infections. The researchers concluded that babies belong more in arms–not in devices.

Placing babies on their backs for sleep has significantly decreased the incidence of Sudden Infant Death Syndrome, but this position has resulted in an increased number of babies developing a flattened area at the back of their heads. This condition, which is more cosmetic than harmful, is called positional plagiocephaly. When young babies spend a lot of awake time in seats of various types, additional pressure is put on the back of their heads. Lots of time spent in arms plus some tummy time reduces the pressure on the back of their heads.

After 3 to 4 months, infant seats may pose a different problem. In some play seats a baby is virtually suspended in the sitting position. When this occurs, it is difficult or impossible for the baby to keep his feet flat on the floor. This may place unnecessary stress on the physical structures in a baby's pelvic area. Watch for this if babies are in walkers, saucer seats, or jumping seats suspended from a doorway or metal frame. If your babies enjoy any of these seats, limit their use and take a baby out of the seat after 20 to 30 consecutive minutes.

Equipment Use vs. Overuse

> It is too easy to overuse, or even abuse, equipment that gives a harried parent a break.

Infant equipment is beneficial, and some may be essential, when parents must meet the needs of multiple babies or toddlers in addition to other family members. However, it is too easy to overuse, or even abuse, equipment that gives a harried parent a break. Ultimately, the babies suffer.

A parent of multiples may need frequent self-reminders about the purpose of equipment. Regardless of multiples' current age and stage, equipment is meant to briefly help you–not replace you. A rocking chair or baby carrier will always be better equipment options because they include you. Automatic swings, infant seats, play yards, and so on can never replace your arms. Your babies, no matter how many of them came together, always need your touch. The wise use of equipment allows you to stretch yourself a little further without compromising babies' developmental needs.

KEY POINTS

❏ Extra diapers and clothing are need for multiples–but not 2, 3, or more times as many.

- Parents often buy "gently" used baby clothing and equipment at "parents of multiples" club sales, consignment shops, flea markets, etc.

- Be sure such items meet safety standards and are washed before using.

❏ Equipment considered "must haves" by most parents of multiples include:

- Individual car seats–all must actually fit in your car.

- Comfortable rocking chair for breastfeeding two at once.

- Multiple-seat stroller–one that can be used for 2 to 4 years.

- One or more infant slings and/or "on the body" infant carriers.

- One or more infant cribs/cots.

❏ Equipment that some parents of multiples consider important:

- Breast pump–type of breast pump depends on babies' age, how often a pump is used, how much milk a mother wishes to remove, and how quickly she wants to remove it. For occasional relief feedings manual (hand) expression works well and costs nothing.

- A changing table–although using a waterproof pad or sheeting on a bed or the floor allows for "assembly-line" changes.

- Infant washtub–using a sink is a less expensive option.

❏ Unless a baby has extremely sensitive skin, the family towels, mild soaps, and laundry detergent should do.

❏ Use caution when placing babies in bouncer chairs, infant swings, and other kinds of infant seats. These items can help when caring for two or more babies, but each multiple also needs lots of time in parents' arms to develop physically and emotionally.

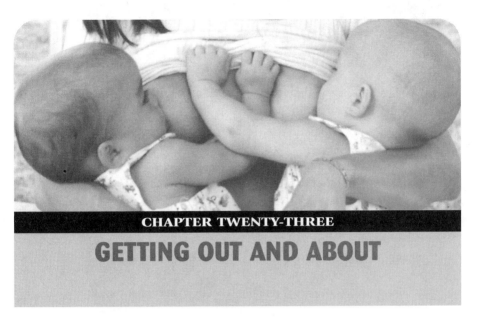

CHAPTER TWENTY-THREE

GETTING OUT AND ABOUT

It is important for a mother and her babies to get up and out of the house.* However, outings may be more complicated to organize with multiples. By the time everyone is ready for an excursion, a mother often feels too tired to leave home. Some mothers say they actually feel scared to go out when no other adult helper is available or if all the babies wailed in chorus during their last outing. Yet staying home because of fears, real or imagined, isolates both mother and babies.

The entire family benefits from the stimulation of fresh air, new sights and sounds, and meeting other people. Taking a stroll outdoors or in an enclosed shopping mall provides exercise that may help a mother relax and regain perspective when caring for multiple babies becomes overwhelming. The positive comments total strangers make about babies' adorable looks and actions or mother's obvious good care of them can be a real boost on days when doubt has set in.

Be Prepared for Going Out

To make outings more fun for everyone, try some of these mother-of-multiples-tested ideas.

- Find a large diaper bag that comfortably accommodates extra outfits and two diaper changes for each baby, a changing pad, diaper wipes, and several plastic bags for soiled items. Some mothers say a stick-type stain

* If multiples were preterm, ask their pediatric care provider if there are any health concerns or restrictions you should be aware of before including them on outings.

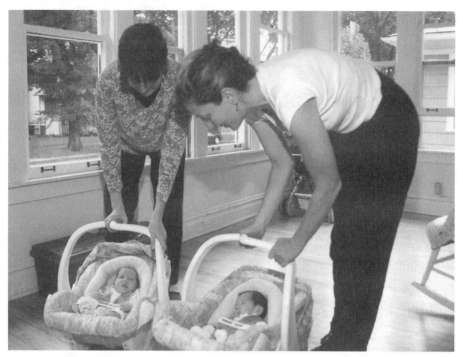

An extra pair of hands can be a big help to a mother of multiple babies.

remover is an indispensable diaper bag item. Also keep several small toys in the bag.

❑ Restock the diaper bag on a daily basis, so there is one less thing to remember and nothing is forgotten when ready to run out the door.

❑ Consider keeping a separate stocked bag in the car.

❑ Most mothers do not want a bag that can slide down the arm, leaving them to juggle babies and a bag. An expandable backpack with lots of pockets is often an ideal diaper bag. There are also diaper bags designed to fit on strollers.

❑ Valuables may be at risk when mother is preoccupied with babies' needs. Wallet, keys, credit cards, and so on should be kept in a hard-to-reach pocket of the diaper bag or in a separate purse. A small wallet or bag with a long shoulder strap can be worn across the chest. A waist pack for these valuables may be a better solution.

• A multiple-seat stroller may be the most valuable piece of child care equipment parents of multiples ever own. (For buying a stroller, see Chapter 22, "What You'll Need.") A good stroller can be used indoors or out in a variety of ways.

• Two or more babies in a stroller attract a crowd. There definitely are days when a mother can use some attention, but other days she may have errands and wants to keep moving. To minimize interruptions during outings with twins, place one baby in a baby carrier or sling and let the other ride in the stroller. A single stroller may do, but a double stroller provides an extra seat for storage. When mother is "wearing" one baby, many people will not notice the second.

> **Staying home because of fears, real or imagined, isolates both mother and babies.**

❏ Parents of higher-order multiples still have at least two in a stroller, so this strategy does not work as well. However, show-stopping attention may be minimized if each parent wears a baby. One or both can push another baby in a single stroller. If attention is unavoidable, at least the babies will enjoy some close contact while in the sling or carrier.

❏ Alternate which baby gets close contact in a baby carrier or sling. When one is fussy or high need, that multiple is likely to be "worn" more often for outings.

❏ The babies' pediatric care provider may feel more comfortable about early outings if a carrier or sling helps minimize contact with outsiders for one or two multiples more at risk for infection.

• Many families have a toddler or preschooler in addition to infant multiples. It is easier to keep an eye on everyone if a parent wears one multiple in a baby sling or carrier and lets the older child ride in one of the multiple stroller seats.

• Attaching a sign to the stroller that answers common questions about multiples may limit the number of times strangers interrupt an outing. A sign might include: 1) Yes, they're twins (triplets, quads, etc.), 2) They're __ weeks (months, years) old, 3) They are fraternal (identical)–two girls (two boys, girl/boy), 4) No, they're not small (large) for twins (triplets, quads, etc.).

❏ People often ask questions that are not worthy of a response, including personal questions about how the multiples were conceived, whether one is the favorite, and so on. Some parents develop snappy comeback lines, but do not hesitate to simply say, "I prefer not to answer personal questions," or "That really is not any of your business."

• Shopping carts at grocery stores and discount centers often have an attached infant seat or child seat facing the parent. A double seating area is attached to some of the newer carts for older babies and toddlers. ***Warning.*** Never leave any baby or child alone in a shopping cart for even a moment.

❏ Wearing one baby in a carrier or sling and seat-belting the other in an attached infant seat may be the easiest way to maneuver a shopping cart with infant twins.

❏ It may be necessary to place an infant seat in the body of a cart if: There is no attached seat, a baby cannot be placed in a carrier or sling for some reason, or a mother/parent is out with triplets.

> **Getting out and about with multiples takes more planning, but it is worth the effort.**

• It can be dangerous to pile groceries or other items around a baby in the body of a shopping cart. Instead, pull a second cart for these items. Those with quadruplets or more may also have to place a baby in an infant seat in the body of a second cart. If so, do not plan on buying many items when babies are in infant seats in the body of the cart or be sure to take another adult so it is possible to push an extra cart just for items.

❏ As the babies grow, one could be carried in a sling or backpack carrier while the other one or two are harnessed or seat-belted in the cart seat(s). (See Chapter 29. "Older Babies and Toddlers: Childproofing and Helpful Equipment.")

• An outing with young infant triplets or quadruplets may be feasible only if taking along a mother's helper.

• Arriving on time for appointments can be a challenge for anyone with multiples. If someone ever needed an excuse for being late, a mother of multiples really has one now. Besides having the diaper bag ready to go at all times (or keeping a second stocked bag in the car), there are ways to make appointment-keeping more realistic.

❏ To avoid having to keep two or more babies entertained for long periods when at the pediatric care provider, a baby photographer, etc., schedule appointments for times that require minimum periods in a waiting room. Usually this will be the first appointment in the morning or after a lunch break.

❏ Bring someone to help with the babies when taking two or more multiples for pediatric appointments. This is especially important when an office building cannot accommodate a multiple stroller. Even if you can take the stroller, you still may need extra arms to help in the waiting room and if it is necessary to attend to each baby individually during physical exams.

❏ For an appointment the first thing in the morning, dress the babies in "traveling" clothes the night before. An alternative is to leave them in sleep clothing and change nothing but their diapers–or not even diapers if babies are asleep when ready to place them in the car—until arriving at one's destination.

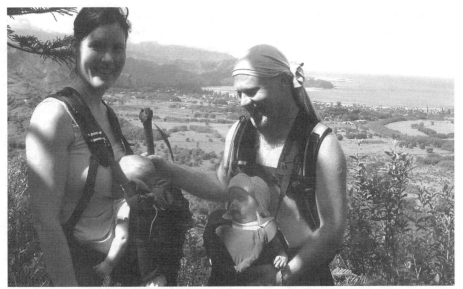

Mom, Dad, and babies enjoy fresh air and new sights.

- Most people understand a late arrival and are willing to accommodate a certain appointment time once the reason has been explained to them. This is a good thing considering Murphy's Multiples Law— No matter how well prepared, count on at least one baby to spit up or need an immediate diaper change the moment the last multiple has been fastened into the car seat or stroller.

The entire family benefits from the stimulation of fresh air, new sights and sounds, and meeting other people.

Additional Safety Precautions

1. **Develop a fire evacuation plan** for your home today. It should include a way to carry all babies out of the house at once. Keep a baby carrier, sling (or two), or backpack where the babies sleep, so both you and an adult partner could carry at least two babies in case of a fire. When babies sleep in a first floor bedroom and no stairs or steps are used to gets to the outside, an option is to wheel a multiple-seat stroller into the bedroom each night for possible emergencies.

2. Never drive with the babies unless a baby carrier, sling, or the multiple-seat stroller is in the car. These items may prove to be a lifesaver if a car breaks down or runs out of gas.

Getting out and about with multiples takes more planning, but it is worth the effort. You and the babies will enjoy the outside stimulation. Everyone will feel better–and often sleep better–when outings are part of the routine.

KEY POINTS

❑ Learn to take babies out of the house–whether for short or longer outings–so you do not feel "cut off" from others.

❑ A diaper bag, backpack, or stroller bag is always "ready to go" if items are replaced at the end of each outing or every evening.

❑ Although a multiple-seat stroller helps, experiment with stroller and infant sling/ front or back infant carrier combinations.

- A fussier baby is often happier when riding in a sling/carrier.

- Strangers are less likely to stop when one baby rides in a sling/carrier, because they do not recognize there is a set of multiples.

- Wearing one in a sling or carrier may also simplify shopping where grocery-type shopping carts are used.

❑ If an infant seat with one multiple is in the body of a grocery cart, it is not safe to pile groceries or other items around the seat. Wearing one in a sling/carrier instead of placing a seat in the cart or pulling another cart for shopping items are safer strategies.

❑ A parent of triplets or quadruplets will probably need to have another adult along to help on outings during early infancy.

❑ Being on time for appointments or scheduled events is more challenging when getting two or more babies ready to go.

- Requesting the first appointment of the day or immediately after a lunch break often means less time spent in a waiting room.

- Ask another adult to go with you if possible to help manage babies when going to the pediatric care provider's office.

- Explain why you may arrive a few minutes late when making an appointment or agreeing to a scheduled event.

❑ In case of emergency:

- Always keep a multiple-seat stroller and/or an infant sling/carrier in the car.

- Develop a *home evacuation plan* that includes a way of carrying two or more infants from the home at once.

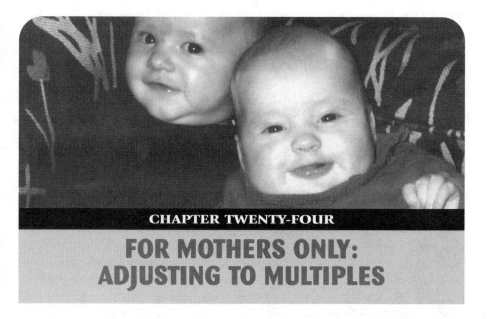

CHAPTER TWENTY-FOUR

FOR MOTHERS ONLY: ADJUSTING TO MULTIPLES

One dictionary defines the word ***intense*** as:

1) Occurring or existing in a high degree, very strong;
2) Strained to the utmost, earnest;
3) Having or showing strong emotion, great seriousness;
4) Characterized by much action or emotion.

With its positive and negative connotations, ***intense*** is a perfect word to describe life with young multiples. Nurturing multiples can be extremely intense during their first years.

A sentiment often expressed by women during the last months of a multiple pregnancy is the desire to "get back to normal." Expectant mothers tend to idealize babies during pregnant daydreams. Daydream babies seldom fuss, spit up, or have leaky diapers. Pregnant parents acknowledge that caring for multiple babies will keep them constantly busy, but imagining "constantly busy" and living "constantly busy" are seldom the same.

It can be a shock to discover that the postpartum year is even less "normal" than 30 to 40 weeks of a multiple pregnancy. Who could anticipate all of the ***sudden*** physical and emotional changes that giving birth brings about? Change is always disruptive for routine-loving humans, but change, and the accompanying disruption in household routine, lasts longer when a new addition turns out to be two or more new additions.

The new mother of multiples must begin to cope with two or more unique, yet immature and totally dependent, new human beings in her life, a task that can make the strongest woman feel vulnerable. And she must care for these new, very little persons while recovering from a more demanding pregnancy and birth that may leave her wondering if she is inhabiting a stranger's body. Although the new mother may be the one most personally involved, the entire family is affected by change.

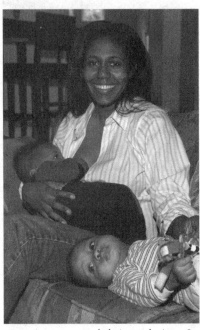

Learning to meet a baby's needs times 2, 3, or more can be challenging.

A New Role
Oldest but Not Only

When multiples are a couple's first children, a woman usually needs time to adjust to her new role and the title "Mother." Ambivalent feelings about learning this role with two or more different babies are not unusual, Learning to meet baby needs times two, three, or more while shifting career gears is a tremendous change. Still, some first-time mothers think it is easier to have multiples first since they know nothing else!

Babies do not realize if their mother has never had one baby before–much less two. They do not care that you may be feeling inept at first–babies know only that someone cares. They come to know this when you are the one who quickly answers most of their calls, relieves hunger in such a pleasant, high-contact way, and speaks with each in a soft voice after making eye contact. Any awkwardness is forgiven.

Recurring Role

The mother who has an older child usually feels relaxed about handling babies and more confident about mothering. Having multiples is a very different experience, however. In many ways a mother starts all over again–unless she has given birth to her second set of multiples.

The thought of nurturing two or more newborns at once may seem almost frightening at times to the experienced mother. She already knows how much time it takes to meet the needs of one baby and has some idea of what the care of multiple infants will entail. Physically managing multiple newborns may require a completely different set of caretaking strategies from the ones used for a single infant.

Having felt a special attachment with a previous baby, the elusiveness of a similar intimacy with the individuals within the set of multiples may be frustrating. The experienced mother understands the luxury of having a moment to look into a baby's face; she know the feeling of closeness that developed when she was able to devote hours a day to one baby.

Concern for an older child, especially if that child is a toddler who still needs a lot of mother's time and attention, adds another dimension for this mother. Ideas for coping with multiple newborns while helping other children adjust are in Chapter 26, "Older Siblings of Multiples."

Attachment

The process of maternal-infant attachment is very different when a mother must get to know more than one baby. The intimate closeness that develops within hours, days, or at least within several weeks, may take months or even well into the second year with each multiple. It simply is more difficult to fall in love with more than one person at a time. (For more on the attachment process, see Chapter 19, "Enhancing Individuality.")

Fortunately, as a breastfeeding mother of multiples, you are in close contact with each baby. The increased contact provides opportunities that maximize the attachment process. With time at a premium or because it often takes longer to form individual attachments, a mother may feel that she is missing out on the emotional benefits she had anticipated with breastfeeding, which can be disappointing.

The need to develop a special relationship with each baby is as important as each baby's need for your special brand of mothering, but accept that breastfeeding may be different with multiples and the emotional benefits of breastfeeding may be postponed for you as their mother. However, your babies enjoy all the advantages that breastfeeding offers from the beginning. Be patient. Allow breastfeeding and bonding the luxury of time. Let the bond between you and each baby grow in its own time. Then you will discover that breastfeeding multiples has its own emotional rewards–different but as special as those felt when breastfeeding a singleton.

Developing a Routine

After the birth of a single infant, a new routine usually begins to emerge after the first four to eight weeks. Most mothers begin to feel really in tune with the baby at about the same time. A mother of a singleton adapts to slight day-to-day changes in her baby's breastfeeding style and overall development without even being aware of the change because these changes are so subtle.

It generally takes longer–sometimes months longer–for a routine to develop after the births of multiples. Change is constant and usually there is nothing subtle about it. The developing routine will (and should) shift based on current circumstances. A change in breastfeeding style, the achievement of a developmental milestone, or a minor illness for even one multiple often has a noticeable effect on the delicate balance in the household. A mother simply cannot adapt as effortlessly as she would with a single infant. In addition, as a household routine emerges, the busy new mother of multiples may not have time to recognize it.

Learning to cope with the physical and emotional changes created when multiples are introduced to a household can be a lesson in flexibility for control-oriented adults. Do not fight to hold onto some old idea of your "normal" routine. Let go of expectations. Caring for two, three, four, or more babies can never be like caring for a single baby. Let go and give a brand new "normal" routine the time it needs to evolve.

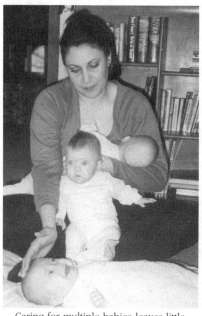

Caring for multiple babies leaves little time for anything else!

The Myth of the SuperMOM

There is a cultural myth that implies that everything, including infant-feeding routines, family sleep patterns, and a mother's body should quickly fall into place after giving birth. Help? There must be something wrong with a woman who needs help. New mothers are supposed to zip up their pre-pregnant jeans, nurture any number of newborns, and energetically resume all prior responsibilities within several weeks of giving birth. Right?

Wrong! Few mothers of a single-born infant can meet the unrealistic expectations of this Supermom mythology. Yet mothers of multiples (MOM) or their family members often impose the same unhealthy myth on themselves and their special situation. At times it may be difficult to remember, or for husband, relatives, and friends to understand, that a MOM continues to need extra help.

When hearing that another new mother seems to have settled into a routine with her baby, you may wonder if you are doing something wrong. You are doing nothing wrong. You simply have two, three, four, or more times as many newborns as the average new mother!

When you find yourself saying, "I should be doing...," ask yourself, "What am I trying to prove and to whom am I trying to prove it?" Give yourself a break. Do not feel that you need to give in to a stressful mythology that places unrealistic expectations on you. Let go of all you think you "should" be doing, and do only what really must be done.

- The Supermom cultural myth makes it difficult for a new mother to ask for help. To get the help you need and deserve, you must get over the idea that you cannot ask for help. Relatives, friends, and acquaintances may never completely understand the intensity of mothering multiples, but you owe it to yourself and your family to learn to ask for their help when you feel pressured or overwhelmed. Others may watch and think you are juggling babies and a hectic household with the greatest of ease. No one can read your mind. You have only yourself to blame if you fail to ask for help when you need it.

> **Few mothers of a single-born infant can meet the unrealistic expectations of this Supermom mythology.**

- *Never* deprive someone of an opportunity to do a good deed. Take whatever aid concerned family and friends offer. Some time in the future you will have the chance to pay back all the good deeds. Someday others will need your help, and you will have the time and energy to give it. For now, *it is your turn.*

- Ask helpers to assume tasks that give you more time to care for your babies. Extra hands may be needed at times to meet the needs of two or more babies and you may appreciate others' help as you learn to mother multiple babies, but an overdependence on helpers could interfere with gaining confidence in your ability to mother your babies.

- Cut *extra*curricular activities to the bone until multiples are older. These *extra* tasks add unnecessary *extra* pressure and take *extra* energy. The earth will keep turning and the task will be completed if you are not the one to bake the cookies, collect the donations, or work the auction booth at an organization or school event.

  Leaving your babies for meetings or activities means they will have less of you than they already do just by being part of a set. It may seem hard to believe now, but your multiples will be babies for a very brief time. All those extra activities will still be available when you are under less pressure and your constant presence is a little less important.

Riding the Emotional Merry-Go-Round

With the lack of time and routine during multiples' early weeks or months, a mother may feel as if she has jumped on a merry-go-round that cannot be slowed, much less stopped. Like the painted ponies going up-and-down on a carousel, emotions may cycle only from high to low without a period of feeling on an even keel for months after the babies' births. Mothers often say they feel as if they have lost any control of the environment. Ambivalent feelings about being the "lucky" one who had multiples are common.

> **You owe it to yourself and your family to learn to ask for their help when you feel pressured or overwhelmed.**

Highs and lows can occur in cycles of days or weeks–and sometimes within minutes. When everything is going smoothly or a mother has actually gotten several hours of uninterrupted sleep, she may feel fantastic–proud of the way she is handling the situation and meeting the babies' needs so well. However, after babies take turns crying all day, an older child seeks attention by constantly getting into mischief, the laundry is piling up again when there has not yet been time to fold the loads washed days ago, the last frozen casserole was baked the night before and the cupboards are bare, and she has not had more than 1 1/2 hours of uninterrupted sleep in a week, a mother may reach a deep dip on that merry-go-round.

When feeling low, feelings of guilt usually are not far behind. After all, here you are with these beautiful babies. How can anyone so lucky claim the right to complain? All right, so you are lucky. You know it. Still, feeling lucky cannot lessen the intensity of the situation. Knowing you are lucky does not give you more time or more sleep.

When multiples are the result of fertility-enhancement treatment, mothers sometimes heap on extra servings of guilt. Those lucky enough to hit the multiples jackpot are not "allowed" to feel ambivalent, tired, blue, and so on. Nope, no negative feelings are allowed for you. You asked for this. Isn't that right? Never mind that multiple babies mean multiple feedings, changes, cuddling, and round-the-clock care no matter how they were conceived.

If Things Go Wrong

How are you supposed to feel if you are not so lucky? Perhaps one or more of your multiples requires extra care for a short-term or a chronic health condition, or maybe one was born with a congenital anomaly. This multiple needs you in a special way, but the other babies need you, too. Plus, you still must form a close attachment with each.

Mothers Are Not All the Same

Every mother of multiples is different. Their responses are different, too. Your personality, the number of multiples and their conditions, the babies' temperaments, the number and ages of other children, the amount of help you receive, your family situation, and many other variables all influence your adjustment to multiple newborns.

Do not be surprised, however, if your mood fluctuates between *high* and *low* without hitting a plateau for awhile. There is no advice that will eliminate the dramatic ups and downs reported by many new mothers of multiples, but there are coping ideas that may help.

Acknowledge and accept your feelings, whatever they are today. Multiples are both a blessing and a burden. It is possible to feel glad you gave birth to multiples yet also envy women who have only one baby to care for. You can feel thankful but overwhelmed, excited yet isolated and alone–all at the same time. You may feel

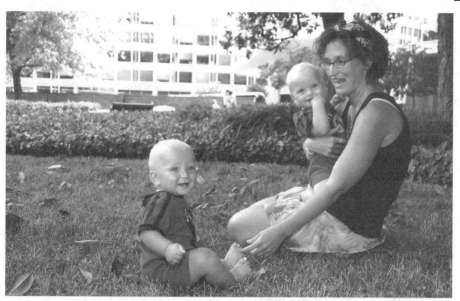

Take time to enjoy the special moments.

grateful for the help of relatives and friends, yet also resent being unable to manage alone. It is okay to want your children and your house to yourself.

Positive and negative feelings often coexist. But to paraphrase two old sayings, actions speak louder than feelings. You cannot help your feelings; however, *you do control your responses to them.* And your response is what really matters.

Remind yourself several times every day that you are doing your best, and *no one, not even you, can expect more of you than your best.* Say it aloud and listen to yourself, "I am doing my best today to cope with this situation."

Accept that "best" is a relative term. Your best will differ from day to day. Do the best you are capable of today. If occasionally your best seems rather low, get help so that the babies' and other family members' needs are taken care of.

Guilt is born along with babies. Mothers feel guilty that they cannot give each multiple the same time and attention they could give one baby. They feel guilty that they no longer have enough time to spend with an older child. They feel guilty that they are neglecting their husbands, their friends, their jobs. They feel guilty when they have ambivalent feelings. *Stop wallowing in guilt!* It is an unproductive use of needed energy.

Make guilt your friend instead of an enemy. It may be trying to tell you that something is out of balance in your life, or you may be falling victim to what you think you should be doing. When you feel guilt, examine it. What is it really about? Is it something you can, or should, do anything about? If the answer is "no," let it go and stop wasting precious time on it. If you truly believe the answer is "yes," than ask yourself what you can do to change the situation. Then do it. If you cannot do anything about it currently, accept that there is nothing you can do at this time but "revisit" the situation in the future. In any case, deal with guilt–then let go of it.

Enjoy the highs when you feel so capable of dealing with everyone and everything. When experiencing a low, remind yourself that it soon will be followed by a high.

Live one day at a time. This may enable you to enjoy the highs more and cope better when you feel low. During periods when even one day seems an eternity, try living from meal to meal instead. "I made it through the babies' night-wakings to breakfast, I can make it to lunch; I made it to lunch, so I can make it to supper; I made it to supper, I'm sure I can make it through colicky time to bedtime."

Do not look too far ahead. Look behind to gain some perspective of how far you have come. You may not appreciate how much progress you and the babies have made, especially if you are having a temporary setback.

Take Care of Yourself

When caring for the needs of multiples and other family members, keep in mind that *you have important needs, too.* You owe it to yourself, and your family, to regularly recharge your giving batteries. The earth will keep turning and your house still will be standing if you do something for you instead of accomplishing some household chore when a few minutes of peace and quiet come your way. A little clutter never caused a house to collapse. Your home will fall apart in a much more crucial way if you fail to take care of yourself.

> **Make time for you every day....Your home will fall apart in a much more crucial way if you fail to take care of yourself.**

Make time for yourself every day. With multiples and other responsibilities, no one is going to give you time. You must take it. You may be able to grab only 15 to 30 minutes daily when babies are small, but they add up. Savor moments alone, but accept that these time treasures may be brief.

Do something you really enjoy if a few minutes of uninterrupted calm unexpectedly come your way. Forget tonight's supper, the dirty laundry, or the dustballs under the chair. Of course, if you find it relaxing to clean and cook, go to it! Just do not feel guilty if you would rather take those minutes to read, exercise, nap, work on a hobby, etc.

Find a socially acceptable physical outlet when you feel tension building. Make bread dough, and when the recipe calls for you to "punch it down," really let that dough have it! (This is a very productive tension reliever, since you will also have something for dinner.) Don boxing gloves and attack a punching bag. Hit tennis balls against a backboard or a solid wall. You can jump rope, pedal a bike, jog, or take a walk. (With the proper equipment you can engage in the same activities indoors.) All of these activities easily fit into any few minutes you can find–or make.

Physical exercise increases rather than depletes energy stores, but take it easy at first. Even if your spirit is raring to go, your body may be weaker after a multiple pregnancy and birth. If you were on prolonged bed rest during pregnancy, you may want to consult with a physical therapist or fitness trainer to develop an appropriate reconditioning exercise program. (Even short-term bed rest diminishes muscular strength and endurance, and results in cardiac deconditioning.)

Physical exercise also results in improved mental health. In addition to toning muscles and cardiac conditioning, feelings of depression are less common for those who get regular exercise, such as a 20 to 30 minute brisk walk several times a week.

> Laughing is good for you. A sense of humor can help you keep babies' needs and breastfeeding marathon days in proper perspective.

Laugh. A lot! Face it–adapting to the addition of two or more babies leads to lots of laughable moments! Laughing is good for you. A sense of humor can help you keep babies' needs and breastfeeding marathon days in proper perspective. People who laugh are physically and mentally healthier.

- You say you have just changed the twelfth soiled diaper between babies' alternating nonstop feedings, and the day simply is not funny anymore? Tape your favorite comedy series or rent a silly movie to watch, or listen to a comedy CD or audiotape while feeding the babies. With the amount of time you spend each day breastfeeding, you should have plenty of time to meet your daily laugh allowance!

- Have you ever been describing a ridiculously laughable moment and your laughter suddenly turned to tears? Give in and let go if tears threaten at times. There is nothing like an occasional good cry for releasing bottled-up tension. Trying to hold it in only gives one a headache, a stuffy nose, burning eyes. Do not think you have to be alone to give in to tears.

A good cry can be more effective when others are present. They finally may get the message that you are feeling a little overwhelmed and a lot sleep-deprived. You will be treated with respect and tenderness for at least a couple of hours.

> There is nothing like an occasional good cry for releasing bottled-up tension.

If tears threaten many times a day rather than occasionally, consider whether you may be affected by postpartum depression. (See "Postpartum Depression" later in this chapter.)

Eating Well

Nutritional needs when breastfeeding twins or more will be as great, or greater, than during multiple pregnancy. Producing milk for two or more babies is big business; you burn a lot of calories when making so much milk. Breastfeeding mothers of multiples usually have a tremendous thirst and appetite. Most mothers place this need for extra calories high on the list of personal advantages of breastfeeding multiples.

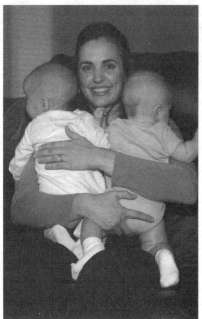

A mother needs a healthy diet in order to feel her best as she breastfeeds and cares for multiple babies.

Of course, you probably have no time to prepare all that food—much less sit down and enjoy it. When busy with multiple infants, the key to eating well is to select easily prepared finger foods. Eat while breastfeeding a baby or two, and always have a beverage available.

1. Create a breastfeeding station next to the chair or sofa you use most for feedings. Stock a small table with nutritious snacks within arm's reach, so you still can grab a few bites even on the most hectic days.

2. Store quantities of sliced or diced fresh fruits and vegetables in individual plastic bags to grab on the run. If you have no time for slicing and dicing, delegate by asking someone else to do it. Many supermarkets now sell bite-size pieces of fruits and vegetables by the bag or at a salad bar. Take advantage of this convenience. If these nutritious ready-to-eat items cost a bit more, remind yourself how much you are saving by breastfeeding.

3. Cheese cubes or slices and shelled nuts are good sources of protein that can be eaten on the run. Both are available in finger-food form at many markets.

4. Eggs are another excellent source of protein, plus a number of vitamins and minerals. Hard boil them to eat as is or to make an egg salad, which can be spread on a slice of whole grain bread. One mother of twins always kept her egg skillet ready to go on the stove. (She said she washed that nonstick skillet once a week whether it needed it or not!) She quickly scrambled or fried an egg, which she then "threw" onto pieces of toast. Voila! As her babies breastfed, she enjoyed a nourishing sandwich.

5. Whip up a pitcher of nutritious milkshakes in the blender every morning. Combine milk, yogurt, ice cream, or ice milk, with fruit, wheat germ, etc. (If you or any baby is sensitive to dairy products, puree fruit with crushed ice and leave out the milk.) Grab a glassful from the refrigerated pitcher throughout the day.

Drink to thirst. Sometimes breastfeeding mothers are told to drink X amount of liquid a day; however, there is no evidence that drinking large amounts of liquid translate into higher amounts of milk. Actually, one can overdo it. Rather than measuring the liquid you are putting in, check the color of what is coming out. As long as urine is pale yellow, you probably are getting enough fluid. If urine becomes dark yellow, drink a bit more.

- Invest in a large sports mug that holds at least 16 to 24 oz (about 450 to 700 ml) of liquid. Sports mugs usually come with a fitted lid that has a large straw in the middle. This is perfect for keeping at your breastfeeding station; this type of mug will not require constant refilling and is less likely to spill if bumped.
- Squeeze fresh lemon or lime into water for a more refreshing drink when keeping up with increased thirst. These citrus fruits are also good sources of vitamin C.

Speak to your health care provider before taking additional vitamin/mineral supplements while breastfeeding. Many mothers say they have more energy when taking supplements at higher levels. The vitamin and mineral content of human milk is generally stable, but high levels of certain vitamins and minerals may be harmful for you.

When a mother has *little appetite* or experiences *a rapid weight loss* while breastfeeding multiples, it may be a sign of a physical disorder, such as a thyroid dysfunction–occurring more commonly after the physical disruption of pregnancy and birth, or a postpartum mood disorder, such as postpartum depression. See a doctor if experiencing either of these symptoms.

Anemia and Menstruation

Postpartum anemia is more common after a multiple birth, because postpartum hemorrhage is a more common complication. Even the usual bleeding tends to be heavier and last longer. Anemia, or "low blood," can contribute to fatigue, decreased energy level, and lower resistance to some diseases. Diet plays an important role in rebuilding red blood cells and replenishing iron stores.

Exclusive, or almost exclusive, breastfeeding has an important role in resolving anemia, as it generally delays the return of menstruation. This gives a mother's body time to renew itself without losing additional blood through the monthly flow. Although having two or three times as many babies does not guarantee two or three times the delay in resumption of the menstrual cycle, mothers who have breastfed a previous infant often report a later return of menses by several months when breastfeeding multiples.

Menstruation does not occur during the months of exclusive breastfeeding because the hormones that regulate copious milk production inhibit the hormones that regulate ovulation and subsequent menstruation. The suppression of ovulation and menstruation by breastfeeding is called lactational amenorrhea. In many parts of the world, the lactational amenorrhea method (LAM) is the chief form of contraception. LAM is extremely effective when a couple understands how it works.

Exclusive breastfeeding for several months, frequent feedings–including some night feedings, and delayed initiation of solid foods all influence the length of lactational amenorrhea for any given woman. Whether complementary or supplementary feedings for multiples affect lactational amenorrhea when the daily total number of breastfeedings still computes to the exclusive breastfeeding of at least one baby is uncertain. For more information about lactational amenorrhea, see "Resources."

Self-Esteem Issues
Body-Image

During a multiple pregnancy, it is not uncommon to hear a woman exclaim, "I can't wait to get my body back!" It can be a shock when she discovers that the body she gets back seems to belong to someone else. Plus, there usually is little time for personal grooming when caring for multiple infants and other family members. Some days there may not be time for basic personal hygiene.

> **When you take a little time for your appearance, you will probably feel better about everything.**

It can be demoralizing to realize that it is already 4:30 PM and you have not had time to change out of your robe. Not to mention the flaps of your nursing bra have been down all day–including the time you opened the front door for a delivery man, one of the babies spit up down the front of that infamous robe at noon, and another waited until 1:30 PM to have an explosive bowel movement while on your lap. Now the flour that spilled down the front of you while you tried to throw supper together is clinging to the dried spit-up. And today you had planned to have everything organized when your husband walked in the front door, which should occur in about 45 minutes.

It does not take a psychic to figure out that you probably are not feeling your most attractive at this moment. Unlike situations portrayed in movies or on television, there is no time for a relaxing bubble bath. There is no live-in housekeeper who can watch the babies while you bathe, curl your hair, apply make-up, or get a manicure. Still, when you take a little time for your appearance, you will probably feel better about everything. The following ideas were used by other mothers of multiples to maintain "neat and clean" even if they do not quite measure up to gorgeous.

- Get a good "wash and wear" haircut a month or two before the babies are due, since multiples have been known to arrive early. Once you've gotten the basic cut, it should take little time to maintain it. With a good haircut, the style falls into place as hair dries.
- Schedule a shower or a quick wash and wipe bath every day at about the same time. It may be easiest to bathe during a naptime. Any baby still awake can be placed in an infant seat or automatic swing in the bathroom

or just outside the door. If you sing in the tub or shower, baby probably will enjoy your bath time as much as you do. A bright mobile hung over a crib or play yard may keep a baby or two occupied for the time it takes you to shower. As babies get older, putting one or two in a large play yard placed just beyond the bathroom door usually provides a safe environment during the brief time you need to bathe.

- Don't panic–at least not yet–if you find it difficult to drop those last few pounds of pregnancy weight gain. Many mothers find it takes months for those last pounds to melt away just as it took months to gain that important weight during pregnancy. It is unrealistic to think it will all magically disappear the moment the babies are born. If you ate a balanced diet during pregnancy and you continue to eat a balanced diet afterward, you will lose the weight.

- If you find your body has been rearranged even after most of the extra weight is gone, give yourself at least a year to shift back into the shape you remember. Your body needs time to recover from this more physically demanding pregnancy. However, a multiple pregnancy can have lasting effects on abdominal skin and muscles. It's simply impossible to be certain in the first year whether an effect of pregnancy is short term or will have lasting consequences.

- Whether you have a few or many pounds still to lose or you are wondering if your abdomen will be accordion-pleated forever, you will feel better when you look better. Stretch the budget to purchase some new clothing. You will look slimmer in clothing that fits while you s l o w l y shrink to your former size.

- Camouflage "twin skin " or extra pounds by wearing overblouses, tunic tops, sweaters, and blazers over slacks or skirts. When you tuck a shirt in, lift your hands over your head to loosen material around your waist. Dark clothing makes most women look trimmer than pale colors. Avoid horizontal stripes that make anyone look wider.

- Combining resistance exercises with aerobic exercise can help you get back in shape and is a good way to release tension while recharging energy stores. Jogging, jumping rope, or briskly pushing a 10 to 20 pound stroller filled with multiple babies (while possibly wearing one in a baby carrier) are good forms of aerobic exercise. Stroller aerobic groups are popping up in many urban areas. Group exercise routines may be available on video or DVD when there is no local group.

- If you ever have second thoughts about spending money on yourself for new clothing, supportive nursing bras, a practical yet stylish haircut, etc., remind yourself of all the money you are saving by breastfeeding your multiples. You are worth it! The entire family benefits when you feel good about yourself.

Nursing Bras

Depending on your build, you may consider your breastfeeding bustline a blessing or too much of a good thing during the early months of frequent feedings. Most department stores, maternity clothing shops, and major retail catalog chains carry nursing bras. The best ones can be opened easily with one hand when a baby wants to breastfeed. It is difficult enough to juggle two babies at once without having to undo tricky clasps.

- Nursing bras should fit well and provide proper support, but finding such bras can be a challenge for the well-endowed. There are specialty bra catalogs and breastfeeding equipment companies that sell bras designed for larger-breasted women. (See Resources.)
- When choosing a nursing bra, be sure that it fits properly. There should be no pressure from elastic or an underwire on breast tissue; pressure on breast tissue may contribute to plugged milk ducts.
- Some mothers buy a supportive, standard bra or elasticized sports bra and cut circles in each cup large enough for the nipple and areola to protrude for easy feeding. If you try this, cut the circles large enough so that a baby can latch on deeply and also allow for skin-to-skin contact during feedings. Stitch around the circle to reinforce the material.

Weight Loss and Dieting

After waiting a few months for their bodies to shed the extra weight naturally, some mothers reach a point where they want to do something more about losing weight. Weight loss programs can be compatible with breastfeeding when: 1) a mother waits until she has recuperated physically from pregnancy and birth, usually at least 12 weeks after giving birth; and 2) weight loss is gradual–weight loss goals are confined to 1 to 2 pounds (0.45 to 0.9 kg) a week or 4 to 5 pounds (1.8 to 2.3 kg) a month.

- Women breastfeeding multiples should be aware that research studies related to weight loss during lactation looked at women breastfeeding single-born infants. Because multiple pregnancy and birth are more physically stressful and producing milk for multiples uses more physical resources, get your health care provider's approval before beginning any weight loss program.
- Avoid crash diets that result in too rapid weight loss. Also avoid fad diets or diets that recommend eliminating or severely restricting a major food group–no-fat and no-carbohydrate diets are not for the lactating woman!
- Breastfeeding women who combined gradual weight loss with regular exercise lost more weight and were more likely to keep it off.
- Be sensitive to changes in babies' breastfeeding patterns or your milk production after beginning a weight loss program.

Physical Challenges

If your multiples' combined weights were high, you may find you suffer from what has become known as "twin skin"–also referred to as "seersucker skin." A new mother of multiples tests "positive" for twin skin if: 1) her stretch marks have stretch marks, producing an interesting seersucker pattern, 2) her abdomen looks like it has been accordion pleated, or 3) her abdominal skin can be pulled out several inches and folded/rolled up to be tucked into the waistband of her slacks or skirt!

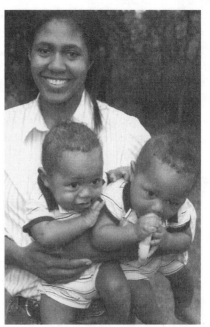

Multiple pregnancy can stretch the abdominal skin covering the over-distended uterus beyond the usual limits, and the overstretched skin loses some of its elasticity, like a balloon blown beyond capacity or a rubberband stretched too wide.

A mother of multiples needs to take good care of herself so she can take care of her babies.

- When uterine distention causes a separation of the vertical abdominal rectus muscles, it is called a *diastasis recti*. The separation can be followed down from the breastbone through the umbilicus (belly button) to where the pubic bones join. Some degree of diastasis is common with pregnancy, but an extreme diastasis gives the abdomen a pendulous, or "potbelly," appearance. If not corrected, diastasis may lead to lifelong back pain and poor posture.

- To test for diastasis: 1) lie on your back with knees bent and feet flat on the floor. 2) Lift/roll your head and shoulders forward and slightly off the floor. 3) At the umbilicus (belly button), press in with the fingertips and feel for the harder muscle to either side of center/midline. 4) Measure the softer space in the middle that is between the muscles. If that space is greater than the width of two fingers, it is considered *diastasis recti.*

- Exercise can improve rectus muscle tone, and there are books and Web sites that target postpartum fitness and include information about resolving *diastasis recti.* Get your health care provider's approval before beginning any exercise program.

- Avoid exercises, such as sit-ups and abdominal crunches or curls that cause bulging or a band-like appearance down the midline until the diastasis resolves, unless supervised by a fitness expert familiar with postpartum physiology.

- Recommended exercises strengthen all muscle groups in the abdomen and spine, allowing them to work together.

- Learn to "hold in" the abdomen when exercising, changing position, lifting, coughing, or sneezing, etc. To do this, "pull" the umbilicus (belly button) up and in as if trying to get it to touch the backbone. Practice maintaining this while breathing out.

- Postpartum fitness experts recommend that a woman with a postpartum diastasis recti "splint" the abdomen during exercise and other activities that require lifting, supporting babies in slings or carriers, etc. Abdominal support is needed to "hold" the recti muscles together during activity and healing exercise. Support aids which are designed specifically for postpartum diastasis recti are available. (For exercise and abdominal support aids information, see Resources.)

- Tummy tuck surgery or abdominoplasty, a less extensive variation, may be recommended to repair extreme cases of diastasis recti or twin skin. Both versions are major abdominal procedures. As with any major procedure, these elective surgeries are not without risks or side effects. Both require a significant post-surgical recovery period. Generally, a tummy tuck is not recommended for anyone contemplating a future pregnancy.
  - ❏ Wait if considering such surgery. Give your body time to recover from the multiple pregnancy; it often takes at least a year for recovery. Do not expect surgery to magically transform your abdomen to its prepregnant condition. Although surgery generally leads to some improvement, it is no panacea.

Litter Phenomenon

You are not alone if you sometimes feel like some other mammal feeding a litter when breastfeeding multiples. Many, if not most, mothers of multiples experience this litter phenomenon during the early months of breastfeeding. Initially, it usually is considered to be a negative feeling until a mother recognizes its humorous side.

- Most human mothers of multiples could learn a lot from fellow mammal mothers. These mothers are able to relax and simply accept the intense, but brief, period of their babies' simultaneous demands for frequent feedings.

- If you have experienced the litter phenomenon but have not yet found another mammal to identify with, consider the she-wolf that fed Romulus and Remus, the mythological founders of Rome. In many sculptural renditions, the wolf's expression as she feeds the human twins captures the conflicting wonder and weariness human mothers of multiples often feel with the frequent breastfeeding during the first months.

Isolation

Mothers of young multiples can easily become physically and emotionally isolated. To "get up and go" with infant and toddler multiples takes much more preparation and management than for a single baby. Taking infant multiples out requires carrying around a lot of extra baby paraphernalia, and mothers often worry about what they will do if everyone gets hungry or fussy at once.

Few homes are as childproofed as homes with multiple toddlers. Mothers may stay home because the pleasure of getting out is easily lost when keeping track of two or more unconfined toddlers in an unfamiliar environment. In addition, many mothers find the number of invitations to come and "play" dwindle after someone experiences a visit or two by curious multiples.

Not only do some mothers of multiples feel physically isolated, they often feel emotionally isolated and alone. Have you ever felt no one else understands–not even your life partner? Your feelings probably are valid. Unless a relative or friend has had multiples (or the same number of multiples) and been the one responsible for their around-the-clock care, it probably is difficult for anyone to understand.

- Do not allow yourself to become isolated. Make yourself go out. Make yourself take the babies. (See Chapter 23, "Getting Out and About.") It gets easier every time you do it.
- You may feel more comfortable taking multiples out or having others visit you in your home once you learn to breastfeed one or two babies discreetly. Two-piece outfits are most convenient for discreet feeding. Simply lift a shirt up, or unbutton a blouse from the bottom up, just enough to allow one baby to latch on. Clothing specifically designed for discreet breastfeeding is also available. (See Resources.) To decrease possible exposure and gain confidence while you and the babies learn to breastfeed with others around, you could drape a baby blanket, shawl, poncho, towel, or diaper (or two) from your shoulder across each baby's body. Repeat the process on the other side if feeding two at once.
  - ❑ Discreet simultaneous breastfeeding may be more difficult to achieve, but many mothers have found a way. The babies' styles and adeptness with breastfeeding influence the ability to do this.
  - ❑ Many find the cradle-football (cradle-clutch) combination or the double football (double clutch) positions lend themselves best to discreet simultaneous feeding with young babies. As babies grow older and latch on without help, you may find the double cradle position allows the three of you to be less conspicuous.
- Grab 30 to 90 minutes for yourself and walk, relax in a bubble bath, or go to a mall alone when babies are sleeping. (You know you have been in the house too long when a 10 PM trip to the all-night grocery store seems like a grand adventure!)

- Nothing replaces communication with other mothers of multiples. Find someone who does understand because she has been where you are now. Contact an organization for mothers of multiples and find out if a local chapter holds meetings. (See Resources.) Asked to be "matched" with a mother who has breastfed the same number of multiples. Attend La Leche League meetings with your babies.
- If you or your babies are not ready for meetings or there is no group nearby, the telephone and email or Internet group discussions are wonderful ways to stay in touch. Long distance phone calls with another mother of multiples are relatively inexpensive mental health morale boosters when a mother is feeling alone.

Beating the Blues: Postpartum Mood Disorders

It is important to distinguish the postpartum blues and the ongoing merry-go-round ride of the postpartum adjustment period with multiples from true postpartum mood disorders (PPMD), because these disorders often have lasting effects on an entire family. If untreated, PPMD takes a horrendous toll on a mother and it can result in poor mother-infant(s) attachments, disruptive infant (and older child) behaviors, or a marital crisis. Early intervention can save weeks or months of anguish and years of dealing with potential consequences.

Postpartum Blues

It is believed that as many as 80 percent of new mothers experience the mild depression-like symptoms of the *postpartum/baby blues* during the first two to three weeks after giving birth. Many mothers report feelings of sadness, irritability, and anxiety. They have difficulty concentrating. A few have trouble falling asleep even when their babies sleep. Many suddenly find themselves with tears in their eyes or actually crying, and they often are not sure why. The symptoms of the "blues" usually appear within days of giving birth and disappear by the end of the second or third week.

Postpartum Depression (PPD)

Postpartum mood disorders can have lasting effects on an entire family; early intervention can save weeks or months of anguish.

The Greek physician Hippocrates, the "Father of Modern Medicine," was the first to record the symptoms of women affected by postpartum depression (PPD) when he practiced medicine in 300-400 BC. Mothers of twins accounted for a number of these early PPD cases. Two thousand years later research indicates that mothers of multiples still are at higher risk for PPD.

Although depression is related to a change in brain biochemistry, other factors associated with PPD are often magnified for mothers of multiples. These include the double (triple, quadruple, etc.) demands of child care, stressful changes in routine and lifestyle, and a lack of social support. A history of a prior depressive episode also puts a new mother at a higher risk.

Unlike the postpartum blues, PPD lasts for weeks or months instead of days. It often seems to begin as a case of the blues, but it does not go away by two to three weeks postpartum and the symptoms often intensify. PPD can occur months later–at any point in the first year or two after a multiple birth.

The signs of PPD are similar but worse than those for postpartum blues. When depressed, several of the following symptoms are experienced on most days, and much of each day, during a (consecutive) two-week period (or longer):

- Frequent tearfulness or loss of emotional control;
- Insomnia–difficulty sleeping even when babies sleep or hypersomnia–sleeping too much and at inappropriate times;
- Extreme fatigue or lack of energy;
- Appetite changes–lack of/poor appetite or overeating;
- A lack, or loss, of enjoyment in the babies and in pleasurable activities;
- "Foggy" thinking–difficulty concentrating or making decisions;
- Intense or excessive feelings of hopelessness, loneliness, emptiness, worthlessness as a person or a mother, anxiety, insecurity, guilt, or fear of "going crazy";
- Obsessive thoughts of harming oneself (suicidal thoughts), the babies or other(s).

A mother experiencing PPD may be able to go through the motions of child-care tasks. She may be able to feed, change, and bathe her babies. However, the depressed mother often feels detached–unable to love and interact with her babies although she truly wants to. Multiples may be cared for assembly-line style and treated as a unit instead of as individuals.

In addition to PPD, other postpartum-onset conditions have been identified in the last century. Sometimes symptoms of one condition overlap with those of another.

Postpartum Onset Panic Disorder

Mothers suffering from a postpartum panic disorder experience episodes of extreme and unexpected anxiety, apprehension, or intense fear that occur in conjunction with a panic attack. Symptoms of this condition usually arise in the first weeks to months after giving birth. It occurs more often among women with a history of an anxiety disorder. This condition may occur alone or as a component of PPD.

Every mother of multiples is different; their responses are different, too.

During a panic attack, the affected mother feels several of the following symptoms develop rapidly:

- Racing or pounding of her heart,
- Tightening of her chest or throat,
- Shortness of breath,
- Trembling or shaking of extremities, which begin to feel numb or tingly,
- Sweating accompanied by hot or cold flashes,
- Nausea or stomach upset,
- Faintness, lightheadedness, or dizziness,
- A sense of unreality or detachment,
- A sense of losing control, doom, or of "going crazy,"
- A fear of dying.

Panic attack symptoms may last a few minutes or for more than an hour, and the frequency and intensity of attacks vary. Attacks may occur rarely or several times a day. Concern about having an attack in public often results in an affected mother staying home, increasing her feelings of isolation.

Postpartum Obsessive-Compulsive Disorder (OCD)

With postpartum obsessive-compulsive disorder (OCD), intrusive and inappropriate thoughts or images plague a new mother. The obsessive thoughts generate feelings of anxiety and distress as the mother tries, but is unable, to "turn off" or ignore them. To minimize anxiety or prevent a dreaded situation, this mother repeatedly or excessively performs certain behaviors or mental acts–behaviors or acts that do not have a realistic relationship to the feared situation.

Affected mothers have experienced all kinds of obsessive thoughts. The most frightening obsession, yet one that is fairly common with postpartum OCD, involves horrendous thoughts or images about harming one or all of the babies. Although women rarely carry out such actions, a mother having these thoughts may become afraid or panicky about being left alone with her babies. An "excessive" response may be acting overprotective of the babies, bathing or changing them over and over, or calling the pediatric care provider several times a week with superficial questions and concerns.

Getting Help

Medications considered compatible with breastfeeding are available for most postpartum mood disorders.

Women affected by postpartum mood disorders frequently say they knew something was wrong shortly after giving birth. However, many new mothers delay seeking treatment, because they find it difficult to discuss symptoms of depression, extreme anxiety, or obsessive thinking with others.

A mother may be afraid to face her feelings, or she may be afraid that her children will be taken from her if she discusses her feelings with anyone. Sometimes a mother's feelings and concerns are dismissed when she finally does mention them to a friend or family member. Yet some "gut" feeling usually keeps surfacing that tells her she must do something about this problem.

A mother may think seeking help will take more energy than she has at the moment, but constantly ignoring a gut feeling takes as much or more energy than taking action. If your mental or emotional state is interfering with how you want to live your life, trust a gut feeling that will not leave you alone. Get professional help.

Discuss your feelings and concerns with a mental health professional. Ignore any friend, relative, or health professional who says you are fine when you know you are not.

Talking to your obstetric care provider is a good place to start. Ask for a referral to a mental health professional specializing in postpartum disorders. If you do not have the energy or feel afraid to make calls, ask your partner or a close relative or friend to dial the phone for you. Sometimes it is necessary to interview more than one therapist, but keep calling or looking until you find a comfortable fit.

You may feel less alone and get ideas for coping if you speak with a mother who has recovered from a postpartum mood disorder. Large support organizations often have local chapters that meet regularly, and a member may be available by phone. Members may also know of good therapists in your area. (See "Resources.")

Gaining coping skills through psychotherapy may be all that is needed in some situations; however, psychotherapy alone is not always enough. Sometimes medication is necessary to "fix" brain biochemistry. Medications considered compatible with continued breastfeeding are available for most postpartum mood disorders. A La Leche League Leader or a lactation consultant usually has references about such medications. Let your babies' pediatric care provider know what medication(s) you are taking, including any plant/herb antidepressant or anti-anxiety preparations.

In addition to standard health care treatments, evidence indicates that taking supplemental omega-3 fatty acids, such as those found in pharmaceutical-grade fish oil, and/or B-complex vitamins, particularly B-6 and B-12, has been helpful in lessening depressive feelings. Regular exercise, such as brisk walking for at least 20 minutes several times a week, has also been found to help relieve symptoms of depression. See Resources for links to information on alternative or adjunct treatments.

Get help. Get it today. Please. You deserve to feel your best. Your family needs you–and they need you to be your best. The earlier you get help, the sooner you will be on the road to recovery.

KEY POINTS

❑ Postpartum–the first months after the birth of a baby–is always a time of adjustment.
  • The adjustment period lasts longer after the birth of multiples.

❑ A new mother of multiples must get to know each baby and learn to care for all of them while recovering from a more difficult pregnancy and birth.
  • A mother's feelings may go up and down with little in between for several months.

  • Learn to ask relatives or friends for help.

❑ Mothers with young multiples often say they feel better when they:
  • Make time for themselves each day–even if only 10 to 30 minutes.

  • Exercise regularly.

  • Eat extra calories in the form of nutritious "healthy" foods.

  • Drink water, 100% juice, or another healthful beverage whenever thirsty.

  • Keep a snack and something to drink next to their favorite breastfeeding spot.

  • Wear comfortable clothing that fits and opens easily for breastfeeding.

  • Get a stylish easy-care haircut.

❑ Postpartum mood disorders (PPMD), such as postpartum depression (PPD), are more common after a multiple birth.
  • Contact a doctor immediately if feeling depressed, blue, "down," or anxious for more than 2 or 3 weeks. Early treatment is the key to feeling better sooner.

  • Treatment for PPMD, including taking medication, rarely interferes with breastfeeding. A lactation consultant or a La Leche League Leader can provide specific information.

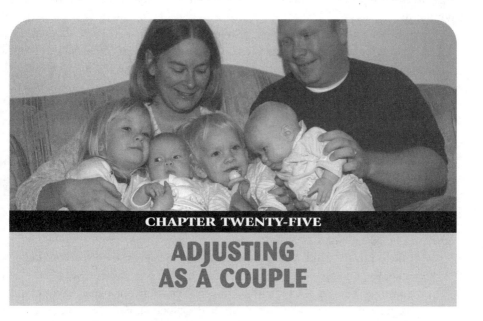

CHAPTER TWENTY-FIVE

ADJUSTING AS A COUPLE

Becoming parents always affects a couple's relationship. Whether the new baby is a couple's first or their tenth, its arrival changes the family. Partners must often postpone meeting their needs as a couple in order to meet those of the baby and any other children. The birth of multiples creates greater change and the adjustment period lasts longer. It takes a great deal of maturity on the part of both partners to put aside their own needs for those of the babies.

Breastfeeding

When expectant parents discuss breastfeeding one baby, they often ask whether the new father/other partner will feel left out. Few expectant parents of multiples raise this question. There is always plenty for both parents to do.

Most mothers of multiples say their partner's support and encouragement are more influential during the weeks, months, or years they breastfeed their babies than anyone or anything else. The new mother feels most supported when her husband or partner recognizes that it takes longer to recuperate after a multiple pregnancy and birth and expresses appreciation for the time and attention the mother gives their babies through breastfeeding.

Supportive words mean the most when followed by supportive actions. Assuming more care of an older child and taking over more household tasks are ways to show support, since they free more time for the new mother to nourish and nurture the babies.

Encouragement often helps both parents maintain perspective on days when babies hold a breastfeeding marathon, an older child "paints" the hallway with colored markers, and the supper hour is fast approaching but the menu is still in question.

Time Together

Both partners still need time together as a couple. It is crucial to keep the lines of communication open, but keeping lines open requires creativity. Of course, "creative thinking" is a stretch for parents who rarely have a moment to spare during the daylight hours and are waking several times at night.

If you and your mate are too tired to be creative, try some of these ideas that other parents of multiples have found helpful.

- **Take a family walk.** When constantly busy meeting the needs of young multiples, finding even five minutes to talk with one another can be a challenge. Enjoy a relaxed, adult conversation as the changing scenery occupies the babies' and any older child's attention.

- **Plan a romantic dinner at home** every one to two weeks. Even a sandwich seems special when it is accompanied by candlelight and soft music. Who cares if each of you is holding a baby as you whisper sleep-deprived "sweet nothings" in each other's ear?

- **Invite good friends to share the candlelight and soft music occasionally** when babies are young and social activities are curtailed. If you tell them the cuisine will be simple or that you are calling for take-out because you are unlikely to have time to cook, they probably will offer to bring at least one course. Better yet, simply ask an invited couple to contribute to the meal rather than wait for them to offer. And let friends know that you, your spouse, and the babies are free to return the visit almost any time. Some friends even may be willing to plan a dinner around your babies' bedtime once one is established.

- **If you or your partner feels the need for time alone together,** also keep in mind the babies' need for your presence. Ways to meet your partner's and your babies' needs may include:

  ❑ Going out during the babies' naptime or after their bedtime once either sleep period is fairly predictable.

  ❑ Leaving briefly during a predictable daily "calm" period, especially if babies do not nap at the same time or they do not go to bed early enough.

  ❑ Going out does not have to mean hours away; an hour or two together at a nearby restaurant is often enough time alone to feel refreshed. For

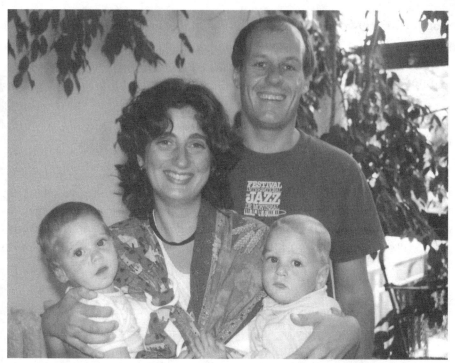

The arrival of multiple babies challenges the relationship between husband and wife.

example, one couple planned a weekly date at a nearby restaurant for Saturday breakfast–the only calm time of the day–after settling in at home with their second set of twins. A couple with triplets occasionally rented a motel room for an hour. Where there's a will....

❑ If going out without the babies, be certain that any babysitter is mature enough to manage more than one baby. Since sitters may find it difficult to physically handle two babies, many couples hire one sitter per multiple and then "assign" the care of any older child depending on the sitters' abilities.

> **Most mothers of multiples say their partner's support and encouragement are more influential during the weeks, months, or years they breastfeed their babies than anyone or anything else.**

❑ Carry a cellular phone or digital pager, so you can be contacted quickly if babies need you before your planned time of return. You probably will feel more relaxed if you can be called or paged when a sitter has a question or problem at home.

❑ Many mothers arrange couple outings around babies' feeding times. They leave soon after one breastfeeding and plan to be home in time for the next. Remind sitters not to feed babies if you will be home to

Supportive words mean the most when followed by supportive actions.

feed them. Leave expressed milk in the refrigerator and directions for warming it if you may be late. Missing a feeding can have more consequences when producing milk for two or more babies. (See Chapter 16, "When Mother Has a Breastfeeding Difficulty.")

A new father of multiples also needs to feel encouraged and supported in his new role. There are many ways to offer support.

- Go out of your way to do something special for your spouse each day. Ask him what one (realistic) thing he would most like to see accomplished around the house. You may not be able to do it every day, but the effort usually is appreciated during multiples' early months. Develop an alternate plan if you are not able to accomplish that one thing yourself. If appropriate, put it at the top of the household helper's list. During a period of chaos, the important thing is to let him know you care.
- Acknowledge the adjustments your spouse must make and the responsibility he may feel after multiples arrive. Not only is his lovely and adoring partner busy caring for babies 24 hours a day, but he may feel a very real financial burden providing for this baby bonanza. "Two for the price of one" definitely does not cover multiple babies!

Many couples are told to avoid certain sexual intimacies and intercourse during the last weeks or months of a multiple pregnancy. Within several weeks of the babies' births, there is usually no physical reason that interferes with making love. However, many women find their interest in the sexual relationship is at an all-time low. Whether due to physical recuperation, hormonal influences, fatigue and sleep deprivation, a feeling of being "touched out" after holding babies all day, or some combination of these is not important. Patience and understanding by both partners is important.

- Both parents are likely to feel tired when caring for multiples, but the male libido, or physical sex drive, usually is less affected. Generally, a couple's physical relationship improves as babies get older and require less intense time. In the meantime, it takes communication if each is to understand that the other is sensitive to their differing needs for physical intimacy. Be honest about your sexual needs, and encourage your partner to be the same.
- Tell your spouse often that you love him and appreciate his understanding even if you do not feel able to express it as often physically.
- Think creatively and let go of old expectations in order to meet each other's current physical needs. Babies in bed with you much of the night? Who cares? A creative couple can find lots of other romantic spots in their

home. And who says a couple can be intimate only at night? Both partners can enjoy making love when neither is too tired, which is more likely to occur at some time during the day. Naptime may work. Your babies do not yet have a reliable naptime? Ask a friend or relative to take them, or just the one(s) that does not sleep, for a long stroll. No need to tell that person your plans. Involve older children in an interesting project that will hold their attention. Perhaps they could join the babies for the stroll.

- You might say to your spouse, "I've got 10 minutes free; meet you in our bedroom in two minutes—and be ready!" He knows what you mean, and he will be! Because the male sex drive tends to be more physical, try a physical rather than an emotional approach when time is limited and you want him to respond more quickly. Use your imagination!

> **Go out of your way to do something special for your spouse each day.**

- There may be times when you can offer your partner a choice between completing a household task or lovemaking. Many, if not most, men would happily fold a load of laundry if it freed up time for lovemaking.
- Even when not built like a Hollywood starlet prior to multiple pregnancy, a woman may feel self-conscious if her abdominal skin looks like loose seersucker afterward. If this is an issue, let your spouse know that you do not feel as physically attractive because of "twin skin." In all likelihood, you will find it bothers you a lot more than it does him.

It is important to let your spouse know if you feel overwhelmed or exhausted at times. He needs to know why you may need some time alone to unwind once the babies and any other child finally are sleeping, since he may think this would be the perfect time to spend together. Just as you want to meet his physical and emotional needs, he should accommodate your needs as well.

- Let your partner know if you want to express your affection for him, yet you do not always have enough energy for physical intimacy. He needs to know if you ever avoid holding, kissing, or telling him how much you love him because you think he will consider those actions to be a prelude to intercourse.
- Let your husband know if your ideas about romance have changed. In the past flowers, a romantic card, and dinner out may have seemed the ultimate aphrodisiac. Most mothers with young multiples find it much more arousing to discover a basket of washed and folded laundry, clean dishes in the cabinets, or the toilets scrubbed without ever having to say a word.

Many new fathers of multiples expend energy and relieve tension by participating in sports and other healthy activities or outlets. A busy new mother may begrudge the time needed for an outside activity, considering it as time that could be spent helping with babies. Communication is the key. Let your partner

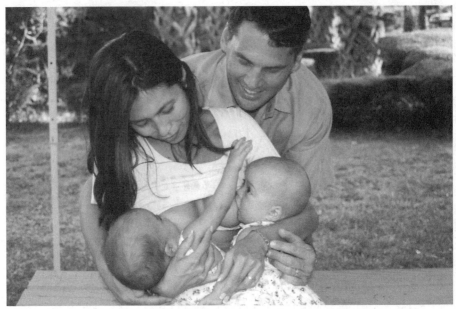

A breastfeeding mother needs and appreciates the support of her partner.

It takes communication if each is to understand that the other is sensitive to their differing needs for physical intimacy.

know how you view the time invested in such activities and how it affects the family. Balance his need for an energy outlet with your need for his help. Negotiate with him to arrive at a mutually satisfactory decision. Your spouse is more likely to recognize your need for time to recharge, and help you make time for you, when you recognize his need for an outlet.

There are no two (or more) ways about it. Multiple babies impose stress on the couple relationship. However, a commitment to communicating with one another and learning to cope together can enhance a good relationship with mutual growth. Both appreciate one another more for the sacrifices each makes for the good of the children and for one another. It takes maturity to act lovingly in spite of the more intense adjustment of integrating multiples into a family. And, whether it seems believable or not during multiples' early years, the intense investment of time it takes to meet the needs of multiple infants and toddlers lasts a brief time in a committed relationship. The increased caring that comes from sharing this intense experience can last the rest of your lives.

KEY POINTS

❏ Multiple babies impose stress on the couple relationship.
  • Continuing to communicate with one another is the key to a strong relationship.

  • A new mother needs her partner to tell her and show her that he is supportive of her breastfeeding and the way she mothers their babies.

❏ There are ways to make time as a couple.
  • Some activities could include babies, such as a family walk.

  • Time for couple activities may be brief, but more time will be available when multiples are a bit older.

  • Both emotional and physical needs should be openly discussed so that a couple can develop a plan for meeting those needs.

❏ Do one special thing for your partner each day–and let your partner know what you would most like him to do for you.

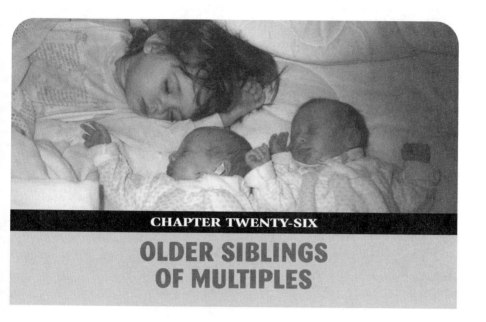

CHAPTER TWENTY-SIX

OLDER SIBLINGS OF MULTIPLES

The life of an older child is turned upside down when multiples join the family. The free arm that would have been able to hug an older child when caring for one new baby now holds a second baby. Mother is occupied with babies around the clock, which means she is not getting much rest so her level of patience probably is lower.

Sleep deprivation can lead to a build-up of tension. Everyday child-related occurrences that once were considered only mildly annoying may now loom as major catastrophes. What previously was a minor aggravation, such as a child spilling a glass of milk, may now produce tears in a mother coping with the needs of multiple infants and an older child or two. Fitting in a clean-up may seem too much to add to an already overfull day. The older child who accidentally tipped the milk glass may wonder what happened to the "old" mother who would never "cry over spilt milk."

Instant Celebrities

Multiples are instant celebrities, attracting attention wherever they go. An older sister or brother is often completely ignored. It can be very difficult to watch an older sibling's face as the minutes tick by and the person gushing over the babies never even thinks to acknowledge an older child.

Many mothers of multiples say the hardest thing for them to deal with is the anguish they feel because of the abrupt loss of "mother time" that leads to so many changes for their older children. When feeling sad for an older child, it can help to

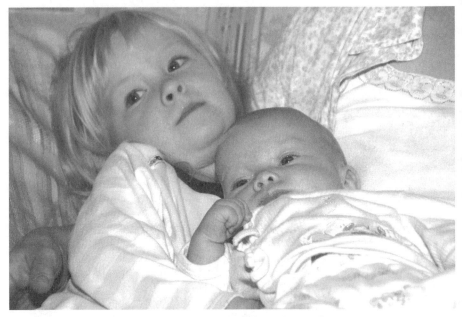

An older child needs to know that he or she is still important.

Older children often surprise parents with how well they adapt.

remember the firm foundation already developed with each. As an infant, each older child never had to share their mother as the multiples always will. Each multiple now needs that same time and attention to develop a similar foundation.

Meanwhile, older children often surprise parents with how well they adapt. Mothers often report that the older siblings not only survive, they often develop self-confidence by having to learn for themselves how to clean up that spilled milk. Of course, an older child still needs help while adjusting to life with multiple siblings. And there will be more time for all the children as the months go by. In the meantime, there are ways to provide attention and ease the period of adjustment.

- Free hands are not needed to say to an older child, "I love you." Say it often throughout every day.
- Five minutes of time when an older child needs it is often more beneficial than an hour when it is more convenient. When even five minutes is impossible, there is usually time for a hug and kiss.
- No matter who now performs the bedtime ritual with an older child, make time each evening to give each a brief backrub before the child falls asleep. It helps the two of you reconnect, which is important on days when a child managed to spill five glasses of milk, or you said "wait a minute" (and a minute turned into five or ten or twenty minutes) a hundred times. It is a hands-on way to say, "I love you." It is an "I care

about you" in spite of any mischief-making or loss of time and attention.

- Dad becomes even more indispensable to an older child and to you. As an older child depends more on him for time and attention, the bond between Dad and that older child grows stronger. It is easier to enjoy the time caring for the babies when Dad and an older child are enjoying time together.

> **Five minutes of time when an older child needs it is often more beneficial than an hour when it is more convenient.**

- An overnight or weekend vacation with grandparents, relatives, or special friends often allows an older child to enjoy time as the center of attention again. These quick trips also take some responsibility off your shoulders for a day or two. However, the older child's age and stage of development should be considered. One toddler or preschool child might feel "grown up" going away for the weekend, but another may be able to handle only a few hours away. Also, do not push such visits when a child says he does not want to go or his behavior indicates feelings of being "shut out." The idea can always be brought up again later.

Once the babies develop a dependable naptime, ask your husband, friend, or relative to stay in the house with them while they sleep, or hire a babysitter. This allows you to take an older child somewhere special. An outing may be as exciting as a trip to the zoo or as simple as a walk around the block. Another option is to have a friend take the babies for a walk, so you can read a story or sit in a rocker with an older child without interruption. In either case, take advantage of the opportunity to spend time and talk with an older child.

- If you have more than one older child, you may choose to take all of them on an outing while the "poor" babies stay home and sleep or you may want to take turns with one older child at a time. Most mothers have children take turns for some outings and take everyone on others.
- Outing time may be limited when the multiples' naps or calm periods are brief. Fortunately, most children are not clock-watchers. The older child is more aware of being on a special outing and having your undivided attention–whether it is for 15 minutes or a couple of hours.

Downplay the fact that family outings may occur less frequently for awhile. It is harder to get up and go with two or more babies. Yet an older child might come to resent the babies if the babies are blamed for any curtailment in social activities. "I'm sorry, but we can't go. Maybe we can go some other time," sounds much different than, "I'm sorry, but we can't go now because of your baby sisters. Maybe we can go when they get bigger."

> The older child is aware of being on a special outing and having your undivided attention –whether for 15 minutes or a couple of hours.

Behavior Problems

With all of the attention multiple babies receive, who wouldn't want to be a baby? An older child may feel jealous of a new sibling or sad about the loss of his mother's time and attention. When children must cope with the addition of two or more new siblings, it seems understandable that their feelings might be exaggerated. This may lead to "acting out" and regressive behaviors. An older child may release tension through sudden outbursts of anger, thumb-sucking, nail-biting, and so on. Some children go out of their way to find mischief while mother breastfeeds the babies. Regressive behaviors, such as wetting or soiling pants long after toilet learning has taken place, or waking during the night again are not uncommon.

Although most behaviors associated with the adjustment to new babies occur within the first months of bringing the multiples home, some siblings seem to have a delayed reaction. It may be more difficult for these children when multiples start moving around and "invading" their private spaces. It may be months before a child can put feelings into words. What appears to be a sudden acting out or blurting of thoughts and feelings may have been building for months.

- Let older children know you understand it is not always easy getting used to two or more new babies. It is important to acknowledge their negative (and positive) feelings. Open a discussion by tying the child's behavior to a related feeling. You might say, "Wow, you looked really angry when you threw the ball so hard it hit the table. What made you feel so mad?" or "You're holding your doll really tight and your face looks kind of sad. What happened that you look sad?"
- Take out the family photo albums, baby books, DVDs and videos. Point to photographs of the older child as a baby. Describe what you remember about that child's infancy. Let each child know how you met his or her needs and how much time it took. Then gently remind the child that there are two, three, or more babies needing you, and each needs you as much as the older child did as a baby. By preschool age, many children can talk with you about what it must be like to be a baby who does not have to share his mother and what it must be like for multiples to have to share her. If you let a child look at the photo albums, DVD, or video while you are breastfeeding babies, it may cut down on mischief by an older child who is so inclined! (But keep an eye on photo albums that can be taken apart.)
- Try to stay calm. Change the wet pants. Comfort the night-waker. Do it without making negative comments or punishing the regressive behavior. However, if the child's behavior is having a negative effect on you, link your response to the behavior. For instance, you may say, "When I have to

get up a lot at night I feel tired during the day and I act more grumpy."

- Emphasize all the things a "big boy" or "big girl" can do that the babies cannot. At times an appropriate consequence of acting like a baby can be the temporary loss of a "big" boy or girl privilege. Of course, the reverse also is true; increasing privileges may be an appropriate consequence of acting one's age.

- If an older child seems to be doing a lot of acting out, reach for a book that describes general growth and normal development

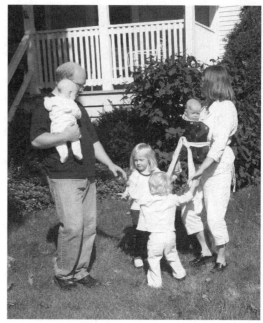

Spending time together as a family builds special memories.

of children. Many parents worry that the new babies are responsible for all the negative behaviors an older child displays. However, some behaviors simply may be typical for the child's age and stage of development. Often, behaviors that usually would be given little consideration seem problematic because the parents are also trying to figure out the behaviors of two or more babies.

Breastfeeding Activities

Mothers often find it helpful to provide special activities for an older child during breastfeeding times.

- Sometimes a mother gives an older child a gift of multiple dolls so the child can breastfeed and care for his or her babies while mother breastfeeds and cares for the new family members.

- When a child is able to manipulate a tape recorder, mothers can record the child's favorite stories. The child enjoys listening to mother reading those favorites while he or she follows along in the book.

- Many mothers create childproofed play space in the room where they usually breastfeed the babies, so an older child can stay busy while babies eat. They keep toys, books, puzzles, etc., there, but most avoid stocking

Let older children know you understand it is not always easy getting used to two or more new babies.

the area with "messy" activities. Some find it helpful to use a room with a television and video/DVD player, so occasionally everyone can watch a favorite program.

When an older child still also breastfeeds, developing balance within the breastfeeding relationships may take time. Often the older child asks to breastfeed more frequently, which may be related to the increase in milk production, the adjustment process, or a combination of factors. If any multiple has a feeding difficulty after birth, a mother may feel relieved that the older child's frequent breastfeeding will help boost milk production. However, when multiples breastfeed well, which means they breastfeed frequently, a mother may find it necessary to place limits on the older child's breastfeeding.

Some mothers feel guilty about introducing limits because they know the adjustments the older child is already coping with. Yet limits may be necessary to meet babies' nutritional needs. Also, frequent breastfeeding by an older child sometimes strains a mother's ability to cope with so many little ones at once.

Some of the ideas in Chapter 28 about "Weaning" may help if setting some limits are crucial to coping. You will also appreciate the book, ADVENTURES IN TANDEM NURSING by Hilary Flower (LLLI). (See Resources.)

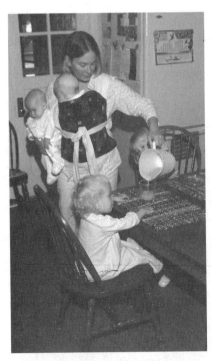

Mothers of multiples find a way to meet everyone's needs!

Sibling Reactions

Discourage activities that can divide the family into "the (multiple) babies" and "any other child." Within reason, let older siblings hold and cuddle the babies. (Of course, no one can explain why big brothers and sisters always have to cuddle the new family members as soon as the babies finally drift off to sleep and mother has a moment's peace.)

Involve an older child in the babies' care. A sibling can fetch diapers, get a snack for you to eat while you breastfeed, or tell a baby that "Mommy is coming soon" when you are busy with another. Watch out for unrealistic expectations, however, when it comes to the amount of help an older child can give. A child's interest in helping will vary depending on age, stage, and personality. Acting as "mother's helper" can quickly lose a lot of its glamour if expectations are too high.

An older child may develop a preference for one multiple. As the babies grow, that preference often changes. If it does not and the preference causes difficulties in the family, you may want to provide opportunities for an older sibling to interact with the "less" preferred multiple(s) alone at times.

> **Avoid activities that bring attention to your multiples at the expense of an older child.**

Avoid activities that bring attention to your multiples at the expense of an older child.

- Remind visitors that older children are going through a period of adjustment. When arranging a visit, ask them to notice any older child before they ask to see the babies. Post a sign at the door with this request if drop-in guests are a common occurrence.
- Bring attention to an older child when people stop and ask about your multiples. You might share something special about each one. An older child may enjoy assuming the role of the spokesperson who answers questions about the babies. (See Chapter 23, "Getting Out and About" for other ideas.)
- There may be days when you hope strangers will stop and ask you about the babies. People often express admiration for the parents caring for multiple infants while they ogle the babies. Let's face it, most parents of multiples need a pat on the back at times—but not if it comes at the expense of an older child. When you could use some well-deserved attention, take the babies for a stroll but do it when an older child is not a part of the entourage.
- If multiples become extended family celebrities, you probably will have to remind relatives that an older child is in need of special attention, too.
- Without a doubt, "group" photos of multiples are adorable. However, be sure to include an older brother or sister in some of the group shots and in photos with each baby.

Do not be afraid to talk to an older child about your feelings. It is all right to let them know you sometimes feel overwhelmed with two, three, or more new babies. Even a young child will understand the emotion, if not always the words. If you find yourself crying, that's all right too. Crying while talking about feeling overwhelmed seems to go hand in hand. Fortunately, no one understands a good cry better than a child. You will probably find yourself on the receiving end of some much needed hugs and kisses and an "I love you" from the older child, which will make you and the older child feel better.

Although the lives of older children change suddenly with the birth of multiple siblings, there can be many positive aspects to that change. Look forward to the ways they will grow through the experience of having multiple siblings. In the meantime, liberal doses of physical contact, a frequent "I love you," and the passage of time usually eases the adjustment for older siblings.

KEY POINTS

❑ The birth of multiples changes the lives of older children in many ways. Parents can help the older child adjust:

- Listen and accept a child's feelings. Also, share some of your feelings about the changes in the family when it seems appropriate.

- Not more than a few seconds are needed to give the child lots of hugs and kisses and tell him "I love you."

- Give the child a backrub at bedtime to reconnect and let him know how much you care.

- Let the older child help with the babies in ways that "fit" the child's age and abilities. Tell the child what you remember about his/her infancy.

- Don't "blame" the babies if it is more difficult to spend time with the older child or do some of the things you did with him/her before the babies were born.

❑ Use gates to keep an older child nearby while you breastfeed the babies. Be sure there are toys, books, and other interesting things on hand while you are busy.

❑ Be sure others understand that the older child is going through an adjustment. Ask them to talk to or spend time with the older child.

❑ The passage of time usually eases the adjustment for older siblings.

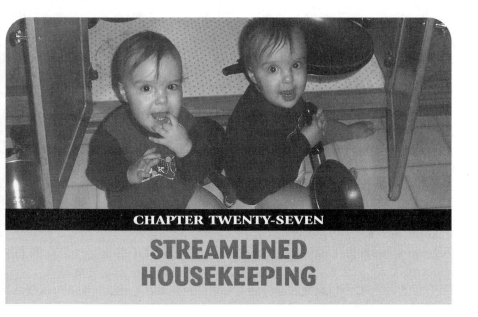

CHAPTER TWENTY-SEVEN

STREAMLINED HOUSEKEEPING

A mother of multiples becomes efficient because she has no other choice! Her time is at a premium. One mother of twins expressed it this way, "It's as if you used to have a whole ship load of time, but now you're in a small lifeboat. You have to throw everything overboard that there isn't room for."

You do not have to be "Supermom" simply because you gave birth to multiples. The arrival of two or more babies is bound to disrupt any family's routine for quite a while. Forget about the "back to normal" you daydreamed of during pregnancy. That pre-multiples "normal" is gone for good, but eventually, you and your family will find a new "normal." A new household routine does not miraculously appear. Give it a few months, and allow additional months for every additional baby. In the meantime, a few things may help the process along.

- *Set priorities* in order to meet your babies' needs and those of the rest of the family–including your own! Ask yourself, "What truly has to be done around the house? What can wait?"

   The babies cannot be expected to compromise their needs, so caring for them is top priority. Other family members are right behind them on the list. Of course, your family will need to eat, and it's nice to wear clean clothes. Beyond this, little is actually essential.

- Most mothers of multiples rely on some type of *household help and convenience services.* Never forget that your time is money! When concerned that investing in some household convenience may put a dent in the family budget, remind yourself that such items or services give you invaluable extra time for your babies, other family members, and yourself. Often the cost of the item or service is more than made up for by the cost savings of breastfeeding.

Meeting Infant Developmental Needs

When time with babies is used wisely, babies receive the stimulation they need without creating additional baby care stress for parents.

Meeting babies' developmental needs is a priority, but creative parents of multiples combine infant stimulation with routine baby care and household tasks. Research has shown that multiples do not get the physical and mental stimulation parents give single-born infants. There is no question that the time of parents of multiples is stretched to the limit, but there is also no question that each multiple still needs this kind of attention. When time with babies is used wisely, babies receive the stimulation they need without creating additional baby care stress for parents. Some ideas to accomplish this include:

Play with each multiple while accomplishing baby care tasks. There are numerous opportunities every day for interaction when changing diapers or clothing, bathing, or feeding each baby. Play is possible whether you are handling only one baby or accomplishing a task assembly-line style.

Make eye contact with one baby at a time–if only for a few minutes. Ideas for play once you have made eye contact may include:

- Call that baby by name.
- Talk to that baby. Explain what you are doing as you change, bathe, or feed her.
- Exercise little arms and legs. Sing to that baby–babies don't care whether you actually can carry a tune.
- Smile in response to that baby's smile; repeat verbal sounds in response to the sounds that baby makes.

Place one baby in a carrier or sling just before you vacuum, do laundry, prepare a meal, etc., and let him/her "help" you. (Take turns with the babies so each often gets to "help.")

- As you walk through the house, describe the rooms and the objects in them. Explain the job you are doing and what you think about it. Although the babies cannot yet understand what you are saying, talking to them now is the beginning of later speech development. Each baby learns how language works and eventually learns words by listening and "participating" in conversations with you and others during infancy.
- Sing, dance, clap hands, etc., to make task time "special" for each, providing each with a variety of sensory stimulation.

- Take only one baby to the market or on errands with you. (Again, take turns so each baby gets to go on special outings.) You may be surprised to find how easy and enjoyable it is to get out with only one baby, and each baby is being exposed to a whole new world of sights, sounds, and smells—stimulation most single babies experience often.
  - ❑ Talk to the baby as you shop. Point to items on shelves or racks, naming the items. Describe different shops and the kind of business each does. Talk, talk, talk! Babies love to hear your voice!
  - ❑ Talk as you drive. If you stop to use an automatic teller machine (ATM) or pick up dinner at a fast-food restaurant's drive-through window, describe what you are seeing, hearing, and smelling.

Household Management

Mothers of multiples have shared the following suggestions for keeping up with the household while still having time to spend with family members.

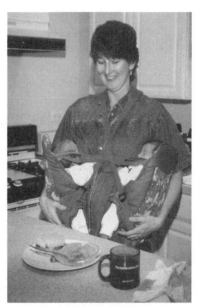

Find someone to help with the household. When you have two, three, or more times the number of young babies than the typical new mother, it is unrealistic to think you can meet the needs of the babies and those of other family members without help. Chapter 7, "Getting Ready: Preparing for Multiples," includes ideas for finding help. Evaluate honestly any prospective helper's ability to fulfill household needs.

- You will want someone who frees you to get to know and to frequently breastfeed your babies. A helper should understand that the duties may

Preparing simple nutritious meals can be a challenge for a mother with multiple babies.

include physical care of any older child, food preparation or cooking, laundry, cleaning, etc., rather than most of the babies' care. Of course, extra hands to help with the babies are also appreciated at times.
- Let any helper know you are breastfeeding and interested only in positive comments.
- When full-time help is no longer needed, you may still require part-time help—for years! Scheduling a regular housecleaning service may still be a sanity saver when two or more toddlers or preschoolers are finding creative uses for household items. You may also want to have a mother's helper help with older children or babies for a few hours several times a

> Forget about the "back to normal" you daydreamed of during pregnancy; eventually, you and your family will find a new "normal."

week. Junior and senior high school students are often excellent. Because you would be there to supervise, a younger student may be an option.

Everyone loves to see multiples, but *limit visitors* during the first weeks or months at home. Be frank when you would rather not have someone over. Let guests know if you feel tired and want them to cut a visit short.

- Let guests know that performing the role of "perfect hostess" is low on your list of priorities. Actually, they should wait on you when babies are young–not the reverse. If you want to offer a snack, direct them to the proper spot in the kitchen, and ask them to bring an extra plate and napkin for you. Remind them to pour something for you to drink when they are getting something for themselves.

- If drop-ins become a problem, you could hang a sign on the front door asking them to call first. For example, one mother posted, "Mom and babies are napping. Call at 3 PM to see if we're having a good day for company." You might need to record a similar message for voice mail or the phone answering machine.

- Holding family gatherings at your home may be more relaxing than going to someone else's home. This is especially true once multiples are mobile, and two or more toddlers are constantly headed in opposite directions.
  - ❏ After explaining why you prefer to host the party, ask each household to contribute a dish. Another suggestion is for the host home to supply the beverages and bread while everyone else divides the meal courses.
  - ❏ Simplify gatherings by using sturdy paper goods in festive colors or patterns that decorate the table while minimizing clean-up. Bring the good china out later when your multiples are older.

Never turn down an offer of help! Never deprive someone of the opportunity to perform a good deed. Relatives and friends wouldn't ask if they didn't mean it. And if they did not mean it, they should have known better than to ask someone with multiples. When someone does not follow through with an offer to help, it is often because the person did not know what kind of help to provide. Share specific ideas about the kinds of help you need. Also, ask for a specific "delivery" date.

- A friend willing to grocery shop or run errands can lift what sometimes may feel like an extra weight of responsibility. If the friend separates your items from her own at the check-out counter, the cashier can subtotal one order and then add the other or she may ring each individually–either way you know how much to reimburse a shopping helper.

- Visitors often are willing to run the vacuum, wash and fold a load or two of laundry, clear out a sink full of dishes, or do any other small household jobs. Let them. If a visitor does not think to ask if she/he could help, do not feel shy about asking them.

It is unrealistic to think you can meet the needs of two, three, or more babies and those of other family members without help.

If mothers of multiples awarded a *"favorite babies gift,"* the complete meal that arrives after the excitement dies down or the full-time helper has returned home would likely be named the winner. This gift is appreciated whether multiples are a few weeks or several months old.

- A "drop off" schedule relieves the stress of having to think about meal preparation on a given day, but a call from a friend with a last-minute offer of a meal can be a nice surprise–one that always seems to arrive on just the day it is needed.
- Suggest that meals be delivered in disposable containers, so you will not have to think about returning any dishes.
- Having friends bring ingredients and prepare a meal in your kitchen can be an enjoyable option. Or plan a dinner party, but ask each friend to bring a prepared dish. Either way you have the pleasure of adult company, and perhaps a few extra arms to help with babies as well. Include clean-up as part of the cooking process, so you are not left with a mess when everyone leaves.

There are many ways to cut corners on routine baby care. (A discussion about diapers and clothing needs for multiple babies is included in Chapter 22, "What You Will Need.")

- Wash laundry less often by borrowing or buying extra (secondhand) items of baby clothing. When borrowing clothing, ask each lender to mark each item, by placing an initial on a tag.
- Wash secondhand items before using. It is less expensive, less time-consuming, and most babies are just as happy when you launder their clothing with the rest of the family wash.
  - ❑ Cloth diapers are an exception; diapers should be washed as a separate load.

Young babies do not need daily baths. If each baby's face and diaper area are kept clean, most babies can get by with one or two weekly baths. Some mothers bathe a baby (or two) every day, alternating babies so that each is bathed every other day. An occasional baby does seem to get grimy enough to need a daily bath. Other babies seem to find a warm bath so relaxing that they drift to sleep soon after the bath and stay asleep longer. In either case, simply bathe these babies more often, which may not be every member of a set of multiples.

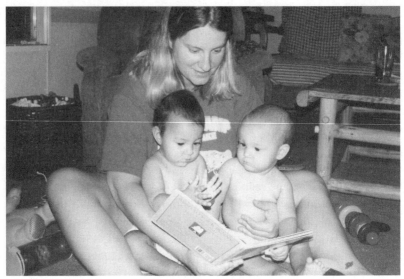

You may have to let go of your previous standards of neatness while you give your babies the attention they need.

Meal preparation can be a challenge when multiple babies request round-the-clock time and attention. The following hints have helped other multiple-birth families continue to eat well.

- Collect recipes that can be prepared in stages and prepare different parts of a meal when convenient. Casseroles are a good example. Thaw meat in the refrigerator and chop vegetables during a calm period in the morning. Prepare and add a sauce to the meat and vegetables during naptime. Then wait to heat the ready-to-go dish during the hectic late afternoon or early evening. For other meals, organize the ingredients early in the day and throw them together just before supper.

- Look for recipes that eliminate steps. For instance, one recipe might list several ingredients for the casserole sauce mentioned above. Another version asks only for a can of soup and a little water or milk, and voilá—a casserole sauce. The second version saves preparation and pot-scrubbing time. You can go back to the gourmet version when multiples are older.

- Teach a household helper to prepare ingredients, such as chop vegetables, hard-boil eggs, or form meat patties to store in the refrigerator or freezer for later use.

- In many areas, items such as chopped fruits and vegetables, salad greens, meat patties, and so on are available at a market salad bar or in prepackaged bags or boxes. Buying already prepared fresh or frozen foods can save hours of work in the kitchen and are still less expensive than fast-food options.

- Use household appliances, such as a food processor, blender, crockpot, and microwave to save valuable time. One of these appliances may be a good investment of some of the money saved by breastfeeding the babies.

- Even when old-fashioned ways of cooking and baking are a passion for you, these methods may have to be put on hold until multiple babies need and want less of their mother's time and attention.

> **Let guests know that performing the role of "perfect hostess" is low on your list of priorities.**

❑ Drive the route your husband takes to and from his place of employment, and write the names of the markets and restaurants he passes. Have him call early every afternoon to see how things are going at home. If it has been a hectic day, give him the shops' names and ask him to stop for groceries or to pick up a ready-to-eat supper.

❑ Plan at least one night out of the kitchen each week. Keep numbers posted near the phone and order a meal for carryout or delivery. You may feel more relaxed all day when you know you don't have to think about meal preparation later.

You may have to let go of old standards of neatness–at least for a while. However, *there are ways to control some of the clutter.*

- Keep a laundry basket or two in well-used rooms. To achieve a tidy look quickly, collect clutter in one basket and throw soiled clothing or other laundry in another. Later, when it is convenient, put items away or take them to the laundry area for sorting.
- After taking a shower, clean the bathroom when everything is steamy by simply wiping fixtures, a shower door, tiled walls, etc., with an already damp towel.
- Soak dirty dishes in the sink in hot, soapy water. The kitchen will look cleaner when countertops are empty, and you can wash dishes when time allows. (If the water gets too cool for effective dishwashing, drain the sink and refill it with more hot, soapy water. Repeat as necessary on any given day!)
- Cut down on the number of dirty dishes by using paper plates, bowls, and cups. Then throw the mess away.
- To minimize ironing, read clothing labels for laundry instructions before purchasing clothing. Since there may not always be time to fold clothing straight from the clothes dryer or line, choose items made of easy-care, wrinkle-resistant fabrics.
- Look for delivery, drive-through, or Internet delivery services. A grocery, laundry/dry-cleaner, or restaurant may add a delivery charge, but you save time, energy, and the fuel needed for a round trip to the shops. You are also saved from dressing two or three babies and older children and then strapping them into car seats–not to mention figuring out how to get all of

> **Never turn down an offer of help or deprive someone of the opportunity to perform a good deed.**

them into the store, managing everyone once inside, and getting babies and purchases back into the car again. That effort is worth the delivery charge any day!

• Be a catalogue shopper for the next few years. You can clothe your family, buy groceries, or have holiday gifts ordered and delivered to out-of-town relatives from the comfort of your home. All it takes is a telephone or a computer and a credit card!

Cut household chores to the bare minimum and get the help you need. You cannot do everything, so you will have to decide what household tasks are most important–after taking care of the babies, other family members, and yourself. Housework will be with you always, but your multiples will not be babies for long. (Really!)

KEY POINTS

❑ Mothers of multiples become more efficient and organized because they have to!

❑ It takes time for a new household routine–a new "normal"–to develop.

❑ Set priorities. Babies' needs come first, followed by other children and your own needs.

  • Food and clean clothing are the only essentials. Let go of the rest.

  • Breastfeeding saves money. Spend some of the savings on household help, services, or appliances that save you or your partner time and energy. These are not luxuries when you have young multiples.

❑ To meet babies' needs for stimulation, take turns playing and talking to each whenever you feed, change, bathe, or care for them in some way.

❑ Find household help. It is unrealistic to have twice or more the usual number of new babies without household help and extra hands.

  • Good helpers should free you to care for and get to know your babies.

  • Never turn down an offer of help.

❑ Limit visitors. Those who do come should wait on the new mother!

❑ Plan for simple meals that you can prepare at more convenient times durng the day.

  • Buy ingredients that are ready to go.

  • Take advantage of drive-thru or delivery services when you need a break.

❑ Use a laundry basket to collect clutter until there is time to put items away.

❑ Keep family or social events simple. Think paper plates, ready-made menu items, and catalog or online-shopping for gifts.

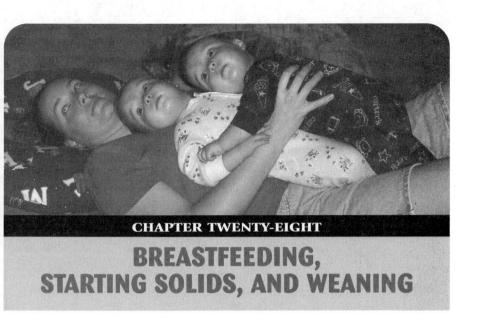

CHAPTER TWENTY-EIGHT

BREASTFEEDING, STARTING SOLIDS, AND WEANING

The breastfeeding routine changes during the second half of multiples' first year with babies' introduction to solid foods. By their first birthday, these foods often provide much of the babies' diets. Babies begin to join the family at the table for meals. Gradually, they drop a breastfeeding here and there, or they begin to shorten the time spent at the breast for feedings. As babies become toddlers, they may breastfeed more often for comfort than for a meal.

Eventually, one, and then another, multiple stops breastfeeding altogether. The process often occurs so gradually that a mother cannot point to a specific day or moment when a baby weaned completely. The process begins, however, when babies first indicate readiness for and later gain more interest in solid foods.

Starting Solids

Mothers of multiples may be tempted to offer solid food earlier than a mother breastfeeding a singleton. During a particularly overwhelming period, a mother may feel that anything is worth a try. It is often due to pressure from family or friends. Occasionally, a pediatric care provider suggests starting solids before babies are at least four months. However, it has been shown that introducing solid food before about six months offers no nutritional benefits, does not prolong babies' sleep, and may interfere with babies' intake of appropriate nutrients. This is the reason that associations for pediatric care providers, including the American Academy of Pediatrics (AAP), the Canadian Paediatric Society (CPS), and the World Health

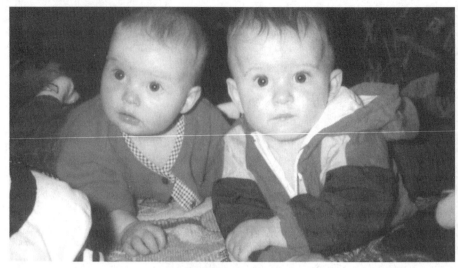

When babies are around six months old, they usually indicate readiness for solid foods.

Organization (WHO) recommend waiting until the middle of babies' first year.

Because so many sets are born preterm, multiples may not be ready for solid foods until a later age than many single-born infants. Babies may experience intestinal upset when their digestive tracts are still too immature to handle solid food, and the nutrients in solid food may not be absorbed or used well by babies' bodies if introduced too early. Plus, when babies fill up on solids, they take in less human milk—a food containing the most suitable and easily digested nutrients.

Most babies are close to six months, and many are over seven months, before they indicate readiness for solid foods. The multiples in some sets may be ready to begin experimenting with solids at about the same age. However, each multiple may signal readiness for solids at a very different time during the second half of the first year. Pay attention to the individual baby's signals. There is no reason to offer solids to all babies when only one is ready.

Signs of Readiness

> Because so many sets are born preterm, multiples may not be ready for solid foods until a later age than many single-born infants.

One mother said she knew when each multiple was ready for solids because that particular baby started grabbing at the food on her plate and tried to put it in his mouth while sitting on her lap. This definitive behavior often coincides with the appearance of the first teeth. Increased drooling at about four to five months is thought to be a sign of readiness for solids by some, but it is more a sign that a baby is "getting ready to get ready" for solid foods.

Many babies experience signs of a breastfeeding frequency spurt at about five to six months, and if a frequent feeding spurt at that age lasts beyond a week, it may be time to offer that baby a little solid food. (For a description of a frequency spurt, see Chapter 13, "Effective Breastfeeding.") When a disruption in routine or an infant illness coincides with signs of a frequency spurt, chances are continued requests for frequent feedings are in response to the stress of the change in routine or illness. Wait until the problem resolves and see what happens.

Some have suggested that when multiples reach some arbitrary combined weight they should be given solid food. However, mothers have reported their babies' combined weights as anywhere from 15 to 45 lb (7 to 20 kg) before one or more of the babies showed signs of readiness for starting solid food.

How to Begin

When any baby first begins to take solids, consider these early meals as "practice." Start slowly when introducing solid foods. Solid foods replace some of the perfect nutrition of mother's milk rather than offering additional nutrients. When introducing solid foods:

> **Pay attention to the individual baby's signals. There is no reason to offer solids to all babies when only one is ready.**

- *Breastfeed first.* By breastfeeding before offering babies the solid food, a mother prevents a drop in milk production, ensures that her babies continue to receive adequate nourishment, and avoids babies who are too hungry to be interested in this new experience of taste and texture. Too much solid food too soon not only is a shock to babies' digestive systems, it can also be a shock to your milk-making system. If two or more babies suddenly breastfeed less because they are stuffed with solids, a plugged duct or mastitis for their mother may not be far behind.

  ❑ Initially offer one or two teaspoons of a single food, like mashed ripe banana. Mixed foods, such as soups or stews or even mixed grain cereals, should wait.

  ❑ Let each baby's response be the guide when deciding whether it is time to offer more. Offer more when any baby requests it, and do not ignore cues, such as head-turning, spitting food out, pushing the spoon away, and so on that say a baby has had enough.

  ❑ Some babies need a few practice sessions before they can use their mouths differently to take food from a spoon. However, when a baby consistently pushes food back out of her mouth as fast as it is spooned in, she may not be quite ready for solid food. Take a break from introducing solids to this baby for now and try again in a few weeks.

- Introduce only one new food at a time to be certain that each baby is not sensitive or allergic to a particular food. Wait a week before offering the next new food, and keep the "old" food(s) in a baby's diet, too.

❑ Be particularly cautious about introducing new foods if either parent or a close relative has a history of allergies.

❑ Avoid foods associated with allergic reaction, such as cow's milk, eggs (whites), nuts and nut butters, smoked or pickled fish, shellfish, and citrus fruits or juices. Wait until babies are at least a year, based on full-term due date for birth, before slowly introducing any of these foods.

❑ Common allergic reactions include rashes on the skin or around the diaper area, hives, wheezing, and diarrhea.

❑ Do not offer honey to babies less than a year old. Honey may contain botulism spores, which can make babies extremely ill.

It usually is unnecessary to buy commercial baby foods if babies are older than six months (adjusted for full-term age) when they begin to eat solids.

- To make "easy" early foods, use the flat of a fork to mash: banana, avocado, other soft fruits or cooked vegetables, baked sweet or white potato, tender pieces of meat, tofu, etc. Smash peas between clean fingers and offer directly from your finger.

- Because of the protein and iron it contains, meat is often recommended as an early solid food for breastfed babies of six months or older.

- Depending on babies' age, puree or grind single foods using a blender, food processor, or baby-food grinder.

- Mothers sometimes express/pump a small amount of milk or thaw some frozen human milk to dilute or soften foods for younger babies.

- Avoid canned and processed foods that tend to be high in salt (sodium) or sugar (or other sweeteners).

If commercial baby foods make life easier with multiples, look for jars containing a single food. *Read labels carefully.* Choose brands that offer a food without added sugar, salt (sodium), preservatives, etc.

- Mothers who have used commercial baby foods suggest skipping pureed "first foods" and moving directly to single-ingredient "second foods." These foods are more economical and offer babies more texture, which six to seven month old babies often prefer. Because the jars are slightly larger, mothers say one jar tends to be the perfect size to split between two babies, so there is less waste.

- At about 9 months (age-adjusted for full term) each baby begins to use her thumb and index finger to form the "pincer" grasp to pick items up. She probably will enjoy finger foods that allow her to practice this new skill. Most of these foods also have more texture, which she will find interesting. Unsweetened, dry breakfast cereal in the form of little Os, cooked peas, whole-grain bread cubes, or slivers of stewed or well-cooked meats are examples of such foods. Each multiple is likely to have her own favorite finger foods.

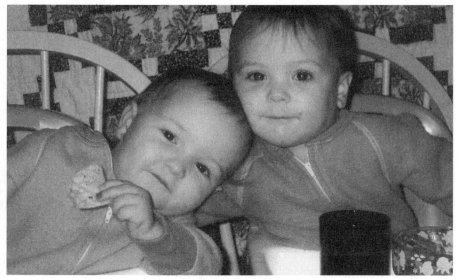

Toddler multiples enjoy "sharing" their meals.

- If breastfed multiples are receiving supplementary formula, it may be possible to wean them from infant formula as solid foods are added to their diets. The nutrients in human milk and solids will provide the calories they need to grow and develop.

Ask a La Leche League Leader for books or pamphlets containing additional ideas for introducing solid foods. THE WOMANLY ART OF BREASTFEEDING contains an entire chapter on this topic. (See Resources for information.)

Vitamin and Mineral Supplements

Supplemental vitamins or minerals are unnecessary for most full-term, fully breastfed single-born infants. With only a couple of exceptions, the content for vitamins and minerals in mother's milk is fairly stable and in a form that a baby's system can easily absorb and use.

- Mothers on vegan diets may need to take a vitamin B_{12} supplement while fully breastfeeding to avoid producing milk that is deficient in this vitamin.
- Infant and adult bodies require sunlight to process adequate vitamin D. A supplement may be warranted for those babies more at risk for vitamin D deficiency. Risk increases with inadequate exposure to sunlight, which may occur if all of the babies' body parts are constantly covered by clothing or sunscreen when outdoors or for geographic areas having long, cloudy winters that result in minimal sunlight. Babies with darker-skin tones are more at risk than light-skinned babies.

> If breastfed multiples are receiving formula supplements, it may be possible to wean them from infant formula as solid foods are added to their diets.

As with their singleton counterparts, supplemental vitamins or minerals are unnecessary for many full-term, fully breastfed twins. However, even when full term, an iron supplement may be recommended at some time during the first year if prenatal conditions were less favorable for one or more of the multiples, such as with intrauterine growth restriction (IUGR) or twin-to-twin transfusion syndrome (TTTS). An iron supplement is also likely to be recommended when multiples were born preterm, because babies' bodies store iron during the last weeks of pregnancy, which is then available during babies' first several months. Multiples often miss out–to varying degrees–on this important prenatal development.

- When their iron stores are limited because of multiples' preterm birth, usually all of the babies are affected. Only the affected multiple(s) would require iron supplementation when babies are term but intrauterine conditions caused one to store insufficient iron.
- Most pediatric offices are equipped to test an individual baby's blood if there is a concern that any baby may be anemic. A normal, but borderline low, or an actual low test result may indicate a need for supplemental iron for an individual multiple. (Some mothers prefer to follow up with more in-depth testing if initial results are in the borderline range.) If supplemental iron is recommended, it may be needed until that baby can get enough iron from solid food sources.
  - ❏ Iron supplements and iron-enriched formula or foods are not as well absorbed as the iron in a mother's own milk. Also, some babies' digestive systems are sensitive to an iron supplement, and iron supplements may lead to fussing, crying, or other symptoms similar to colic for these babies. (See Chapter 20, "Comforting a Fussy Baby x 1, 2, or More!")

Organizing Mealtime

The introduction of solid foods heralds a new phase in babies' development. Breastfeeding is still babies' primary source of nutrition and comfort but, with a little organization, the introduction of solid food meals can decrease at least a little of the intensity.

- Dad can help with feeding solids so involve him as soon as any baby "requests" solid food. Plan at least one of their meals for a time of day when he can take over. Handling babies' solid food meals is a great opportunity for dad to get to know each multiple better while learning to deal with all of the babies at once.
- Once two or more babies are taking food from a spoon, place them side by side in infant-seats, high chairs, or their stroller. Use one bowl and one spoon, and feed them assembly-line style, alternating bites and babies.

Meals Are a Social Time

The family is each baby's first and most important social group, and mealtimes are traditionally a time for family socialization and sharing. Breastfeeding provides babies with their first lesson in being part of a social relationship, and this is especially true for a multiple who often breastfeeds simultaneously with another in the set. Family meals offer the next lesson. Let multiples participate at family mealtimes by bringing them to the table as their feeding skills improve.

Use one bowl and one spoon, and feed babies assembly-line style, alternating bites and babies.

Any baby who sits well in a high chair or a booster seat with tray, and uses his thumb and index finger in a pincer grasp to pick up particles of food, is ready to take part in family meals. (This occurs by about nine months for full-term babies.) At first it may be easier to place their high chairs side by side at the table and offer them some solids before the rest of the family sits down. Then everyone can enjoy the meal while the satisfied babies experiment with a finger food. Some parents divide multiples at the table, letting dad supervise one (or two) while mother watches the other(s).

Older babies often discover that throwing bits of food at one another is great fun, especially if another family member laughs at their antics. Parents and siblings may think it is less funny if it becomes a regular occurrence. Separating babies at opposite ends of the table with a parent or older sibling to intervene before any food is thrown usually halts this behavior fairly quickly. If early intervention does not do the trick, remove the food from in front of the babies. You may have to remove the babies from the table, too. If a parent responds consistently to food-throwing for several meals, these solid food fights generally end quickly, as most babies do not want to miss out on family interaction during mealtime. Occasionally, it may be necessary to feed one baby at a time or return to spoon-feeding for a brief period.

Picky Eaters

Toddlers are notoriously picky eaters. One of the advantages of having multiples is that one often encourages another, so that all toddlers eat at least a little of a wide variety of foods. Still multiples are not exempt from picky eating. The picky eating stage tends to coincide with increased interaction for multiples and they may not always want to interrupt a joint activity for mealtime. Some babies simply are too physically busy to take the time to sit still in a high chair or booster seat to eat a meal. "Picky" eating usually is not a problem. If the foods the babies do eat are nutritious and each continues to grow and develop at an appropriate rate, there usually is no cause for concern.

Because of their genetic differences, dizygotic (DZ/fraternal) multiples are more likely to have very different appetites and grow at very different rates, yet all may be growing appropriately. It is important to look at the individual growth patterns rather than at the set. Monozygotic (MZ/identical) multiples may also have different appetites or they may take turns flip-flopping picky and hearty eating periods. Their eating patterns and growth rates also should be examined individually. Interestingly, MZ multiples often continue to grow at similar rates even when they seem to have different appetites and eat different amounts.

Since anything and everything seems to find its way into the mouths of older babies and toddlers, some mothers take advantage of this behavior. They place finger foods on a clean plastic cloth on the floor to encourage their multiples to eat a variety of solid foods. (If any pets roam the area, this strategy obviously would not be helpful.)

Breastfeeding Older Babies and Toddler Multiples

In some Western cultures women have been given the idea that breastfeeding benefits only young babies, so there is no reason to breastfeed beyond a year. Not true. There are many good reasons to continue to breastfeed as babies develop into toddlers. Although the number and length of feedings may decrease, a mother's own milk continues to provide multiples with important nutrients and disease-fighting antibodies for as long as they breastfeed. Breastfeeding continues well beyond a year in most cultures, because the benefits for older nurslings have been recognized over time.

Mothers are often surprised to discover new or different benefits of breastfeeding as their babies become more mobile. For instance, breastfeeding is better than a Band-aid® to calm an active toddler who has fallen down or bumped into something, which is a regular occurrence with multiple toddlers. When an older baby or toddler becomes ill, breastfeeding is often the only way a baby will take food. Once past any cultural barriers, most mothers say breastfeeding their single-born older baby or toddler is a personally rewarding and special period in the breastfeeding relationship.

Breastfeeding multiple older babies and toddlers is different, yet it is equally rewarding and special. The relationship(s) between or among multiples develops rapidly as they enter toddlerhood. Their ongoing interaction creates a dynamic multiples' "entity" that affects the individual mother-child breastfeeding relationships in many ways.

Finding ways to balance the "give and take" between two persons is an aspect of every human relationship. Breastfeeding offers toddler multiples a unique opportunity to explore this aspect of their growing relationship(s) in positive ways. Nothing compares with the emotion a mother feels while observing toddler multiples as they drift off to sleep side by side at the breast, each stroking a cheek, an ear, or an arm of the other. Being part of this circle of comfort fills a mother with a sense of wonder.

Although there are new or different benefits of breastfeeding older babies and toddlers, there also are new and different challenges that may arise when breastfeeding older babies and toddlers. Most of them are rooted in multiples' developing relationship(s). These challenges, plus ideas for dealing with each, are described below. Fortunately, consistent handling resolves most difficulties, and a sense of humor sees most mothers through the rest.

> **Nothing compares with the emotion a mother feels while observing toddler multiples as they drift off to sleep side by side at the breast.**

Changing Breastfeeding Patterns

About midway through their first year, babies become very efficient and effective at breastfeeding. Nature apparently knew they would be easily distracted by all the exciting stimuli around them at this age, since this change in breastfeeding behavior coincides with babies' "nosiness" about everything in the environment. Older babies can become so efficient they often may finish breastfeeding within five minutes, give or take a couple of minutes.

- Mothers sometimes worry that briefer feedings signal a decrease in milk production. Usually, this is not an issue. If concerned about milk production, consider whether there has been any significant change in each baby's diaper counts since babies take less time to breastfeed. Although the number or consistency of stools may change over time, a decrease in the number or length of breastfeeding should not result in a sudden or significant change and each baby should continue to produce about 6 wet diapers in 24 hours. Contact a La Leche League Leader or a lactation consultant if you have questions or diaper counts are a concern.
- Increased variation in the babies' breastfeeding patterns is common as multiples reach their first birthday, especially among DZ multiples. One may request to breastfeed only one or two times a day; another may want to breastfeed six or seven times.
- Many mothers find one of toddler multiples frequently requests to breastfeed only because another wants to breastfeed.
- You may notice that babies seem to breastfeed more for comfort than for food as they move into toddlerhood. Many toddlers ask to breastfeed at sleep-related times, such as just before going to sleep for naps or bedtimes and when they first wake up. Breastfeeding also may serve as their cure for illness or injury.

Biting

Breastfeeding-related biting seems to be more common with multiples than for single infants during the second half of the first year. It rarely is necessary to discontinue breastfeeding if one or more begins to bite. In most instances, biting is easily overcome by: 1. becoming sensitive to changes in older babies' feeding cues and 2. dealing swiftly and consistently with the act of biting.

Babies do not bite during actual breastfeeding. The two actions cannot occur simultaneously. In a typical scenario the baby, who has become a more efficient breastfeeder, has finished her meal. Mother has not yet realized that this baby now knows how to get a good meal in a much shorter amount of time, so the mother tries to keep that baby at the breast when the baby is no longer interested. It is at this point–at the end of a feeding as far as the baby is concerned–when a baby tends to bite.

A baby also may bite if feedings are delayed. Mothers often increase household or outside activities during the second half of babies' first year. As a mother becomes busier with other activities, she may not realize if one or more babies frequently must wait to breastfeed while she gets "just one more thing" accomplished, or a delay in breastfeeding one or more may be part of an effort to get all the babies on a certain schedule. In either case, some babies balk and begin biting if this occurs without "consulting" them or if it has caused milk production to decrease.

To put a quick end to a baby's biting, first review that baby's breastfeeding routine and fix any problems. For instance, is the baby breastfeeding more quickly or does a baby seem frustrated if there is a delay in response to his cues to breastfeed? Biting often can be prevented once a mother becomes aware of the early signs preceding the behavior.

- Pushing away or increasing fussiness after breastfeeding happily for several minutes may be behavioral cues that baby has become more efficient at breastfeeding and has removed enough milk. Usually sucking stops and there is a shift in the baby's jaws or the way a baby is latched on prior to biting.

- Do not ignore any baby who tries to tell you via his breastfeeding behavior that he has become a more efficient breastfeeder. Let him know you believe him by ending feedings when he signals he is finished. Otherwise, a biter will bite to remind you that he really meant it when he let you know he had had enough!

Beyond reexamining a biter's breastfeeding behavior, consistent handling of biting is crucial. Do not ignore biting one time and get upset the next. This is confusing for a baby; he does not have the ability to figure out what you want.

Ignoring biting is not a good strategy if it bothers you for any reason, including that biting usually hurts! Ignoring this behavior merely reinforces it, so it is more likely to be repeated and become a more persistent problem. Biting usually is not a difficult behavior to change. To end biting, try the following.

1. Stop the feeding immediately *every time* a baby bites.

2. Without scaring another multiple who may be nursing, firmly but quietly say, "No," or "Ouch!" (Neither expression requires much thought!)

3. Remove the baby from the breast and put him down. If several minutes

later he indicates he would still like to feed, offer the breast again.

4. Repeat the procedure *any time* he bites whether it is five minutes, five hours, or five days between bites.

- Some mothers find it is less disruptive to a multiple still peaceably breastfeeding if they stop the feeding by quickly pulling the biter closer into the breast, covering this baby's nostrils so he cannot use his nose to breathe. The biter lets go of the breast in order to open his mouth and breathe and the mother removes that baby without disrupting the breastfeeding of the other.
- Other mothers report more success if they use a simultaneous breastfeeding position that leaves them with a free hand. They can then insert a clean finger between the biter's jaws if they feel the beginning of a bite and remove him.
- With either alternative method, the mothers then proceed with steps 3 and 4 as above.

It may be necessary to breastfeed multiples separately while resolving this uncomfortable predicament. A firm, "No!" may also startle the "innocent bystander" baby. It can be difficult to put one baby down and supervise when he begins to breastfeed again a few minutes later if feeding two simultaneously. However, individual feedings may be difficult to accomplish since biting often coincides with the debut of "jealous" breastfeeding behavior. (See "Jealous Breastfeeding" below.)

Don't be surprised if about the time multiples learn you won't let them bite you, they begin to bite each other.

Nursing Strikes

When a baby abruptly refuses to breastfeed, it is called a *nursing strike*. A nursing strike is more likely to occur during the second half of the first year, although an occasional four to six month old baby will stage a strike. Nursing strikes seem to be more common among multiples than single-born breastfeeding babies, but generally only one multiple in a set—often a more patient multiple—ever goes on strike.

Because a baby suddenly refuses to breastfeed, a mother may think this baby is weaning. Complete weaning from the breast is very unusual in a baby younger than 12 to 15 months. Think nursing strike rather than weaning if any multiple suddenly stops breastfeeding.

An observant mother usually can help her affected baby resolve a nursing strike within several days.

- If a strike occurs, first *try to determine the cause*. The multiple that has been willing to wait for feedings, or the one who has been more agreeable when rushed through a feeding so that another multiple can be put to the breast, may finally put his foot down by "striking." Frequently, an illness affecting a baby's ability to comfortably breastfeed precedes a nursing strike. Sometimes the discomfort of teething leads a baby to strike. A baby may strike if mother has been doing too much lately and milk production is lower as a result.

- *Combine breastfeeding with extra skin contact* to help a striking baby return to the breast. Feed this baby in a quiet room away from distractions when possible. Take baby's shirt off and take yours off and breastfeed skin to skin. Take this baby into a tub of warm water with you. The bath is relaxing and the breast is available. Put this baby to the breast while he is in a light sleep state, before he realizes he's been "tricked" into breastfeeding.
- If this multiple *prefers a certain breast,* assign that breast to him for now.
- *Try to stay relaxed and calm.* At least with multiples there is another baby or two to help out with frequent breastfeeding so that you remain comfortable and milk production is not affected.

A La Leche League Leader or a lactation consultant will have additional ideas to help you and any multiple weather a nursing strike.

For Multiples Only

Breastfeeding often gets caught in the middle of multiples' jealous behaviors even in the first year.

Although biting or nursing strikes may occur among breastfed multiples, dealing with either issue is no different for one of multiples than for a single baby. However, there are breastfeeding behaviors that are unique to multiples during later infancy and the toddler years. To cope with these behaviors, mothers sometimes employ solutions that seem to contradict a "baby-led" breastfeeding philosophy. The reality of multiples may require the use of strategies that could conflict with a "baby-led" philosophy, yet such strategies still can remain "babies-sensitive."

Jealous Breastfeeding

According to child development experts, jealous behavior, or "an awareness of and desire for" another's possessions, is not supposed to occur until some time during a child's toddler years. However, many mothers of multiples report how they seemed to become the object of babies' jealousy as early as four to six months. For example, a mother may describe that if she interacts with one multiple, the other(s) quickly lets her know he does not approve of another baby receiving her individual attention. Then when her attention shifts to the other(s), the baby originally interacting with her begins to protest.

Breastfeeding often gets caught in the middle of multiples' jealous behaviors during the second half of their first year. This scenario is typical. One baby "asks" to breastfeed because she is hungry or needs comforting. Although the other(s) seem perfectly content playing with a toy or an older sibling, the other multiple(s) soon demand to breastfeed, too. Before a mother knows it, she is never "allowed" to breastfeed only one.

Some mothers are not bothered when jealousy appears to be the motivation for many breastfeedings, but other mothers find this behavior very frustrating. Most mothers have looked forward to a time when they may enjoy the luxury of interacting with only one multiple while breastfeeding. That time seems almost at hand when the number of babies' solid food meals increases and the number of breastfeedings start to drop.

When most of older babies' or toddlers' simultaneous breastfeedings are a result of the competition for mother's attention, a

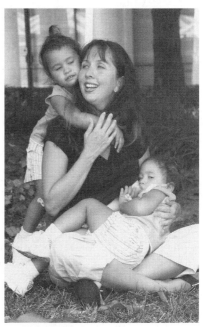

Breastfeeding may become the focus of a toddler's jealousy.

mother may begin to resent the double breastfeedings that helped her survive the early months. Few mothers enjoy being the center of this kind of attention if it means they rarely, or never, are "allowed" to breastfeed one without another multiple demanding the same attention at the same time.

There is no easy answer to help mothers cope with multiples' jealous behavior, although it is important to remember this behavior is not deliberate. Most babies and toddlers do not have to share their mother with another child of the same age and developmental stage; it is normal for a baby or toddler to want the primary caregiver for himself. Multiples tend to become more conscious of one another and the attention each receives throughout the toddler and preschool years, so this behavior may escalate or change in how multiples express it. Mothers have found a few ideas to be helpful.

- Some mothers purposefully choose to change their attitudes when they find feelings of resentment sneaking up. Although the other multiple(s) may not seem to "need" to breastfeed when one requests it, these mothers redefine their notion of "need" and breastfeeding for comfort. Competing for mother's attention may leave a baby or toddler feeling jealous or insecure, and his requests to breastfeed with another multiple may be a source of comfort and a way for him to cope with his feelings.

- Many mothers encourage slightly different wake-up or go-to-sleep times before or after naps and bedtime, so they may enjoy breastfeeding one at a time. Some mothers say they cherish older babies' or toddlers' night feedings, because these feedings allow for individual "cuddle" time with each multiple.

- When one multiple needs to breastfeed after hurting himself, which is extremely common with increased toddler mobility and the punching, pulling, and poking that often characterize multiples' interactions, many mothers breastfeed that baby/toddler while standing. (Standing does not always work well, since a mother usually finds the other[s] soon stuck to her legs like human Velcro®.) Another option is to take the injured party and retreat to an area separated by a doorway gate.

Food Fights

Mothers of multiples are likely to find themselves the center of food fights, or breastfeeding brawls, as multiples grow in size. Food fights may erupt when a mother's lap decreases in proportion to babies' increasing sizes. Jealousy may trigger some brawls. Also, an initial enthusiastic interaction between multiples often escalates to a slugfest.

Growing babies take up extra space on a mother's lap, and their movements during feedings may become more restless once their mobility increases. Competing for lap space as well as for mother may lead to a shove here and a kick there. Gentle physical requests to move over soon give way to more vigorous reminders.

Mother may not be the only one who sometimes resents a second multiple demanding to breastfeed. The older baby or toddler multiple who hoped to have mother to herself may not take kindly to another's intrusion. She may then feel compelled to let the interloper know of her displeasure–physically.

The closer multiples move toward their first birthday, the more aware each becomes of the other(s). The babies spend more time interacting, and relationships between, or among, the members of the set really begin to bloom. Since young toddlers have limited verbal ability, interactions during this early phase of their relationship tend to be very physical. Each generally continues to interact physically with the peer(s) while sharing mother's lap for a breastfeeding. Mother tends to become the forgotten figure as their enthusiasm of learning about each other grows.

Breastfeeding brawling is fairly easy to halt. If your lap becomes a battleground, don't be alarmed. Many multiples behave this way as they approach toddlerhood. On the other hand, you do not have to accept this behavior. You are a member of the breastfeeding relationship, too, and you deserve to be treated with respect during feedings.

- Distracting each baby with another activity during feedings often ends food fights. For example, a mother may tie a small toy to each end of a scarf and then drape the scarf around her neck so that a toy is within reach of each breastfeeding baby. New toys may be substituted when any baby becomes bored with the current distraction.

- Individual feedings are a short- or long-term solution for many. Babies or toddlers are told they must take turns. If a multiple is waiting in line for her turn, it may be necessary to repeat the message several times. However, individual feedings may be an unrealistic expectation if jealous breastfeeding is an issue.
- Treat food fighting as you would biting if multiples rate physical interaction higher than any distraction, or jealous breastfeeding interferes with feeding multiples separately,

  ❑ Stop the breastfeeding if you become uncomfortable with babies' physical interactions. You might say, "No, you may not punch or kick during breastfeeding," or "No, I will not be a part of a fight." (Keep explanations simple for older babies and toddlers.)

  ❑ Remove each baby or toddler from a breast and then put both down. Allowing either to continue to breastfeed may come across as "taking sides."

  ❑ If several minutes have passed and one after the other indicates she would like to feed, offer the breast again.

  ❑ If another food fight erupts, repeat the procedure whether it is five minutes, five hours, or five days between brawls. Consistency is crucial.

Feeding Frenzies

Sometimes multiples "progress" from jealous breastfeeding where every multiple demands to breastfeed as soon as one indicates the need to what some mothers dub "feeding frenzy" behavior. Instead of waiting for one to signal a need to breastfeed, toddlers descend on mother en masse to request to breastfeed. It is as if each anticipates that another might soon ask to breastfeed, so all skip the first step and automatically proceed to the next step of vying for mother's attention.

You are a member of the breastfeeding relationship, too, and you deserve to be treated with respect during feedings.

No matter how busy each toddler acts or how happy each seems, as soon as mother sits down anywhere in the vicinity, she is (or feels) "attacked" by every multiple demanding to breastfeed. Frenzied behavior usually involves toddlers who push and punch one another and their mother in order to be first in position to breastfeed.

This behavior differs from "food fight" behavior, because the toddlers act frenzied from the outset of the breastfeeding. Food fights are more likely to erupt after multiples have begun feeding. Also, feeding frenzy behavior rarely develops before multiples are of toddler age, whereas food fights are more common during the second half of the babies' first year.

As a member of the breastfeeding "team," a mother has rights that deserve to be respected by the other members. Breastfeeding should be comfortable for all involved, but it is difficult to feel comfortable when toddlers' breastfeeding behavior turns one's lap into a battleground. A mother does not have to "put up" with this kind of behavior simply because it involves breastfeeding; toddlers can learn breastfeeding etiquette. Mothers of multiples shared the following ideas for coping with toddlers' feeding frenzies.

- Stand up–a lot–during multiples' second and third years, to avoid feeding frenzy behavior. When mother sits down, multiple toddlers see it as an invitation to swarm!

- A consistent refusal to participate often limits or puts an end to feeding frenzy behavior. If multiples begin shoving or slapping as they approach you to breastfeed, simply stand up and announce, "No breastfeeding* when there is hitting and kicking." Then walk away and wait several minutes before sitting near any multiple. Repeat the action as necessary.

- When feeding frenzies continue frequently after trying other strategies, some mothers limit breastfeeding to a specific area of the house or to certain feedings that seem the most meaningful to the toddlers.

(*Insert whatever word you use for "breastfeeding.")

Weaning

Weaning is a slow process rather than an abrupt event. It actually begins the first time a baby is offered something other than mother's milk. When multiples are partially breastfed, the process may begin within days, weeks, or months of the babies' birth. The weaning process does not begin for fully breastfed multiples until they are introduced to solid foods. Complete weaning may occur on a similar timeline for multiples whether they were fully or partially breastfed during early infancy, although early weaning is less likely among the fully or almost fully breastfed groups.

When babies are the ones to set the pace, the process of weaning generally occurs gradually over a period of many months or years. There is no natural "rule" specifying that complete weaning must occur by a designated age. Some societies seem to have developed such rules, but complete weaning is unusual at or before one year of age. Children do not wean completely until at least two to four years of age in most cultures. There are good reasons to let each child set the weaning pace.

Gradual weaning is easier for mother and for babies. Only each baby knows when she no longer needs the breastfeeding relationship–when other foods and other forms of maternal attention are preferable. Gradual weaning allows babies' bodies the opportunity to slowly mature and assume the tasks of digesting "foreign" foods and developing an immune system more capable of fighting diseases.

Many mothers also prefer to have breastfeeding gradually taper off, as this allows a mother time to adjust to changes in each mother-multiple relationship. Also, a mother's body adapts easily to a slow decline in milk production, whereas an abrupt weaning often results in engorgement with the potential for plugged ducts and mastitis.

Multiple older babies or toddlers affect the entire breastfeeding process, including weaning. The increasing interactions and growing relationships between or among multiples, their differing individual needs for breastfeeding, and jealous breastfeeding are a few of the factors that influence the way a mother of multiples views and responds to the weaning process. (See Resources for books about weaning and toddler breastfeeding.)

Baby- or Child-Led Weaning

The need to breastfeed varies for older babies and toddlers just as it does for newborns and young babies. Most babies or toddlers tend to ask to breastfeed less often as they grow older and more of their diet consists of solid foods. The wise mother does not offer breastfeeding as a distraction or a way to quiet the older baby or young toddler, but also does not refuse the child when he indicates the need to breastfeed.

Baby-led weaning is realistic with many sets of multiples. It seems to work best with fraternal multiples having different temperaments and very different breastfeeding needs. When multiples' approaches to life are dissimilar, jealous breastfeeding tends to be less of a factor and individual breastfeeding is more the norm. As with many other behaviors, different gender (opposite-sex) multiples also seem to vary more in their approaches to the weaning process.

Although two multiples occasionally stop breastfeeding within days of each other, the time when each completely weans usually varies by weeks to years. The difference(s) in ages is a reflection of their differing needs for breastfeeding and the respect a mother has for each multiple as an individual.

Mother-Guided Weaning

Many mothers of multiples find their toddlers' jealous breastfeeding behavior or the development of feeding frenzies affects their desire for, or their ability to go along with, individual baby-led weaning. Although a mother of multiples may do her best to let each baby set the pace for weaning, a mother may sometimes find it necessary to refuse one toddler who seems to want to breastfeed simply because of the behavior of the other(s). Also, she may impose more restrictions, or "rules," on breastfeeding in order to limit the effects of her multiples' jealous behaviors, which in turn often limits each child's requests for breastfeeding.

When a La Leche League Leader with toddler twin daughters found she had to place some limits on their breastfeeding, she dubbed this weaning process as

Some breastfeeding generally is better than none for toddlers not yet ready to wean completely.

"mother-encouraged, baby-led" weaning. The limits she set acknowledged each multiple's individual needs yet also recognized that her multiples had formed a twin "entity" that affected their breastfeeding behavior.

Mothers who agree with the concept of baby-led weaning, especially those who have enjoyed this process with an older child, may feel ambivalent about implementing a modified mother-encouraged approach. Even if it has become obvious that a baby-led weaning plan of "don't offer but don't refuse" must be modified due to a set's "entity" behaviors, a mother may feel guilty that she cannot figure out a way to meet each toddler's individual needs. She also may think there is something wrong if she feels resentful of entity behaviors that interfere with the enjoyment of breastfeeding each.

Weaning "guidelines" that are ideal for most single-born toddlers may not work for sets of multiples. When baby-led weaning is not realistic, accept the differences that may be inherent for breastfed multiples and accept the feelings that probably are normal under the circumstances. Then move forward accordingly. Do your best and let go of the rest.

For some, "mother-encouraged" means beginning to set flexible limits on certain aspects of breastfeeding when toddlers begin to understand spoken language. This usually occurs by about 15 to 18 months for full-term babies. Toddlers who have developed this "receptive" language ability are able to follow simple directions, and their behaviors show an understanding of words, such as "wait until we get home."

- One of the first limits that mothers of toddler multiples tend to impose addresses breastfeeding in public or breastfeeding at another person's home when strangers are present. Breastfeeding older babies or toddler multiples simultaneously easily turns into a "spectacle" that may become uncomfortable for a mother as well as for those nearby. Multiples' interactions are attention-getting under any circumstances. No words adequately describe the same situation when jealous, frenzied, or food fight behaviors occur in conjunction with simultaneous breastfeeding. Therefore, some mothers limit breastfeeding to home or to situations where everyone is familiar and comfortable with toddler multiples' breastfeeding behaviors.

- Some mothers find they reduce the amount of jealousy-inspired breastfeeding when breastfeeding is designated to a specific room in the house—one that is quiet, dark, and boring—one that requires leaving the scene of family activity. A toddler who truly wants or needs to breastfeed will be willing to walk to the less stimulating environment. A multiple that asks to breastfeed only because another wants to is less likely to make the move to the assigned room.

- Imposing a rule that limits breastfeeding to a certain position, such as lying down, may encourage toddlers to limit requests. Except for sleep-related feedings, many toddlers quickly lose interest if they must lie down to breastfeed.
- An idea that has worked for many mothers is to tell multiples they may breastfeed but only to the count of a certain number, such as "20." When a mother has time, she may count aloud very slowly. She may count more quickly if certain behaviors or interactions escalate and when she has other things she needs to do.
- Offer all multiples a distraction when one signals a desire to breastfeed. You might read a favorite story to them or ask each if she would like a cup of juice or water instead. Often suggesting an activity with another multiple is the best diversion.

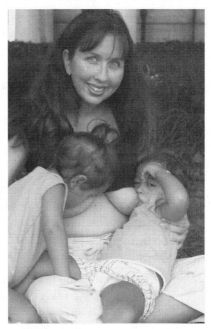

A mother has a right to "set limits" on toddlers' breastfeeding behavior.

Toddlers are more likely to completely wean within days or weeks of one another when using a "mother-encouraged, baby-led" approach. Whether the shorter time span is related to a mother-encouraged approach to weaning or the behaviors that warranted its use, it is difficult to say. Either possibility seems likely.

Partial Weaning

Sometimes a mother is more ready than her babies or toddlers to wean completely. It may be due to her multiples' breastfeeding behaviors, a perception about the age when weaning should occur, a feeling a mother has that she will never get her body back, a belief that multiples will sleep longer without waking, and so on. A mother may think her only option is to completely wean each baby or toddler, but many mothers have found partial weaning to be an alternative.

Partial weaning has allowed many mothers to meet a personal need to decrease the number of breastfeedings while continuing to meet the needs of their babies or toddlers for breastfeeding to some extent. Although partial weaning may be more restrictive than a "mother-encouraged, baby-led" approach, it still is more gradual and easier physically and emotionally for both multiples and their mother than abrupt weaning.

- Several suggestions listed for "mother-encouraged, baby-led" weaning may apply to toddlers when partial weaning or very limited breastfeeding is the goal. Counting to 20 to restrict the length of feedings or limiting breastfeeding to a particular room or to a certain feeding position often is enough to make breastfeeding enjoyable again for all concerned–including mother.

- Night weaning is a form of partial weaning, since any nighttime breastfeeding is halted rather than changing the conditions in which it may occur, but some mothers say they could not have continued breastfeeding at all if unable to wean their multiple older babies or toddlers at night.

  ❑ Many mothers have successfully night-weaned with little apparent distress or tears for their multiples. Many say it did require several nights of patiently coping with each one's night-waking by extra cuddling, giving them drinks of water, etc. (For more discussion, see "Night Waking" in Chapter 30.)

  ❑ Mothers who implement night-weaning generally stress that they would not have considered it prior to at least nine to ten months and many found it better to wait until multiples were toddlers and understood more language. Then they prepared their toddlers for the night change by explaining in simple sentences what to expect if they woke during the night, which they repeated several times throughout the day and at bedtime.

  ❑ If night-weaning includes skipping more than two night breastfeedings, watch for signs of engorgement, plugged duct, and mastitis. A sudden halt of all nighttime breastfeeding for two or more multiples may be asking too much too quickly of a mother's body. To avoid these problems, some mothers breastfeed each sleeping baby just before the mother goes to bed if different from babies' bedtime; others keep a breast pump available to pump just to comfort before mother's own bedtime or during the night if she wakes and is uncomfortably full.

- When the suggestions for "mother-encouraged, baby-led" weaning do not meet a mother's needs, some mothers limit their multiples' breastfeeding to the one or two daily feedings that appear to be most important to them. For most multiples this would be a sleep-related feeding, either immediately preceding sleep or following waking.

Sometimes limits are imposed temporarily; a mother lifts restrictions slightly when the situation has changed. For others the more limited breastfeeding is a permanent change until all babies completely wean. Whether a mother-guided weaning approach is "loose" or more restrictive, some breastfeeding generally is better than none for toddlers not yet ready to wean completely.

Abrupt Weaning

Abrupt weaning, or suddenly stopping all breastfeedings, is a difficult way to end the breastfeeding relationship due to the physical and emotional implications for babies and mothers. Unavoidable abrupt weaning, such as for a maternal health condition requiring immediate treatment with one of the few medications that are incompatible with breastfeeding at any time, rarely occurs. When possible, it is better to try other weaning options first. Gradual weaning over a period of several weeks is usually easier for babies and mother's milk-producing body!

Mother-Initiated Weaning

A mother may wean older babies or toddlers abruptly due to a health condition, but more often weaning occurs after a mother-guided approach has not had the desired results. If a mother has considered the options and still decides to wean her multiples abruptly, she will want to go out of her way initially to offer other forms of comfort and attention. Each multiple should be watched closely for any adverse physical or emotional effects. A mother must reevaluate when any multiple has real difficulty with the loss of breastfeeding.

Abrupt Baby-Initiated Weaning

It is unusual for a single-born older baby or toddler to abruptly stop when still breastfeeding several times a day. Although multiples typically follow their single-born counterparts and wean gradually, a "natural" abrupt weaning seems to be somewhat more common with multiples at about 10 to 15 months of age; weaning may involve one or more in a set of multiples. This type of weaning takes mothers by surprise, since the babies usually had been breastfeeding happily at least two or three times a day prior to abruptly stopping. Also, it often occurs before a mother imposes limits, such as ones for "mother-encouraged, baby-led" weaning.

> Imagine how secure a baby must feel and the amount of confidence it must have taken for him to suddenly stop breastfeeding.

A nursing strike is the most likely reason for a baby younger than 15 months to suddenly stop breastfeeding. (See information about nursing strikes in a previous section of this chapter.) If multiples abruptly wean, they tend to behave somewhat differently than a baby on a nursing strike when breastfeeding is offered. Still, the possibility of abrupt baby-initiated weaning should be considered only if none of the factors commonly associated with a nursing strike is present or when interventions for a nursing strike have had no effect after several days.

The reason that abrupt baby-initiated weaning may be more common among multiples is unknown. Perhaps the subtle limitations imposed by the situation of breastfeeding more than one, the same limitations that may be associated with an increased number of nursing strikes among multiples, also lead to earlier and abrupt weaning more often. Multiples' growing interest in each other at one year may diminish the need to breastfeed for some of them.

In spite of its abruptness, this type of weaning is baby-led. Since the baby chose to stop breastfeeding, the weaned baby is unlikely to experience negative physical or emotional effects. A mother may develop engorgement or a plugged duct, but this is less likely if another multiple continues to breastfeed. Mothers often express a feeling of emotional "shock," since the decision to wean was sudden and taken out of their hands. Many mothers also feel a profound sadness, because they were not yet ready for an ending to any of the breastfeeding relationships with their multiples. Also, some are concerned that they somehow caused the abrupt weaning, or they worry that they may feel closer to any multiple(s) that continue to breastfeed.

To paraphrase an old saying, you can lead a baby or toddler to the breast but you can't make him drink–even if you would still like him to. Imagine how secure a baby must feel and the amount of confidence it must have taken for him to suddenly stop breastfeeding. Allow yourself to feel sad, but also celebrate what you've given this baby or toddler through breastfeeding and your milk. You still have every right to enjoy breastfeeding any other multiple, but find other ways to enjoy skin contact and one-on-one time with the baby who weaned. Back rubs and cuddle time should not be limited to the period when a baby breastfeeds.

Mother-Related Implications of Abrupt Weaning

A mother may be surprised at the amount of milk she still is producing if she suddenly stops all breastfeeding of older babies or toddlers or if any multiple(s) choose to do so on their own. Although physical problems for mothers are usually less severe with abrupt weaning of older babies or toddlers, they can and do occur. Intervene immediately if breast engorgement or a plugged duct develops. One option for mother-initiated abrupt weaning is to let multiples breastfeed again until the problem resolves, and then reintroduce steps toward complete weaning, but take the steps more slowly.

- Because *engorgement* also usually leads to swelling in surrounding breast tissue, options include applying cold compresses or ice packs to breasts for 20 minutes every 60 to 90 minutes to reduce swelling. A mother could pump her breasts when they begin to feel overfull–pumping only to the point that relieves breast fullness. Some mothers find herbal anti-galactogogues help decrease milk production more quickly; a lactation consultant should have information on such products.

- For a *plugged duct* use massage to "move" a plug downward, starting above the plug and then firmly massaging over it, repeating several times. Sometimes it helps to pump the affected breast during or just after breast massage. When engorgement and swelling are not an issue, mothers may use hot or cold compresses over any plugged duct, depending on which feels more comfortable. (For abrupt weaning of young babies, see "Early Weaning," in Chapter 18, "Full and Partial Breastfeeding.")

Breastfeeding multiples continues to differ from breastfeeding a single child as multiples grow and develop into busy toddlers. Many of the joys, benefits, and problems of breastfeeding older babies or toddlers are similar whether you have one or several toddlers; yet many joys, benefits, and problems are unique to this special situation. As with younger babies, breastfeeding easily becomes confused with issues related to parenting multiple toddlers. A mother who breastfed her multiples into toddlerhood, a La Leche League Leader, or a lactation consultant may be able to give you new ideas and a fresh perspective about breastfeeding even as your babies grow and develop into fast-moving and independent children.

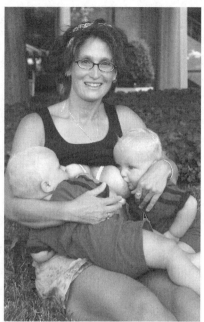

Older babies find a way to nurse in a variety of positions.

KEY POINTS

❑ Breastfeeding multiples gradually changes during their second six months, as they begin to eat other foods, become more mobile, and interact more with each other.

❑ Babies let mother know when any is ready to begin eating solid food. Signs of readiness may include: a longer "frequency spurt," the ability to sit, grabbing for an adult's food, etc.

❑ When starting to give solid food: 1. Always breastfeed first; 2. Offer one to two spoonfuls and watch how each baby responds–don't "force" any baby to take more than he wants; 3. Offer only one new food a week; 4. Use one bowl and one spoon to feed both/all babies.

❑ Move babies' high chairs to the table for family meals once they can pick up food with the thumb and index finger (pincer grasp).
  • Separate multiples at the table if "food fights" become an issue.

❑ As multiples grow, they play with each other more, which affects the breastfeeding relationship. Certain breastfeeding-related issues occur more often with multiples:
  • Nursing strikes and biting.
  • Jealous breastfeeding, breastfeeding "food fights," and feeding frenzies.

❑ In most parts of the world, children breastfeed for 2 to 4 years. The breastfeeding relationship changes as children gradually get more nutrition from other foods.

❑ Weaning is a gradual process–it was not designed to be a sudden event.
  • Most multiples would choose to continue to breastfeed into their toddler years.
  • Complete weaning is likely to occur at different times for each multiple.
  • Some mothers find they must set some limits on multiple toddlers' breastfeeding.

❑ Abrupt complete weaning may be the idea of a mother or one of her babies.
  • Abrupt baby-led weaning is slightly more common among toddler multiples.
  • When weaning is a mother's choice, doing it gradually, over a period of weeks, is easier for babies and mother.

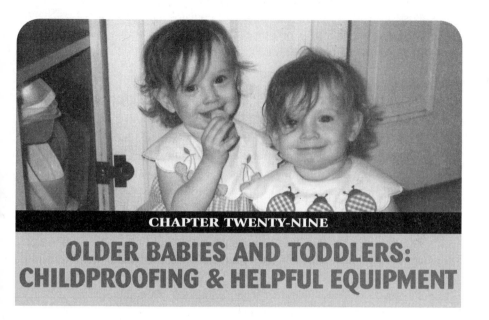

CHAPTER TWENTY-NINE

OLDER BABIES AND TODDLERS: CHILDPROOFING & HELPFUL EQUIPMENT

Older babies need room to practice new motor skills. They also become curious about the environment and want to explore everything within reach. By the time they are toddlers, multiples can figure out ways to explore everything–including places or items that parents think are far out of their reach. It is crucial for the development of their minds and bodies that multiples be given room to roam and to discover the exciting qualities of everyday objects. At the same time, safety is a priority when multiples are in the vicinity.

Safety and Childproofing for Older Babies
Basic Safety

Injury prevention involves anticipating the unanticipated. For parents of mobile multiples, childproofing is the first intervention to protect babies and toddlers from physical injury. However, no matter how thoroughly parents childproof, injuries sometimes do occur. Are you prepared? Have you:

- Taken infant-toddler cardiopulmonary resuscitation (CPR) and first aid classes?
- Posted a personal phone pad on or near all phones for writing the number where you can be reached if away from home?
- Programmed ICE ("in case of emergency") numbers in home or mobile/cell phones with address book capability? Emergency workers are now being

trained to check phones for ICE numbers.

- Posted the number for your children's pediatric care provider?
- Posted emergency (911 or police, fire, emergency medical transport, etc.) and poison center numbers on or near all phones?
- Bought syrup of ipecac (to cause vomiting) and stored it in an identified, safe location in case you or a sitter is instructed to give it to any multiple by someone at a poison center or your children's pediatric care provider? (*Never* give syrup of ipecac unless instructed to do so by an appropriate health care provider. Inducing vomiting may produce more physical damage after the swallowing of some toxic substances.)
- Created a first aid kit and shared its whereabouts with any helper or sitter?
- Placed smoke detectors and carbon monoxide detectors in/outside bedrooms and other appropriate locations in your home and routinely check the working condition of each?
- Developed a household fire emergency plan?
- Interviewed any helper or sitter for their level of knowledge of safety and first aid?
- Reviewed with any helper or sitter the childproofing and safety interventions you've established in your home?

Childproofing

By the time they are toddlers, multiples can figure out ways to explore everything– including places or items that parents think are far out of their reach.

Parents have a responsibility to make their home as physically safe as possible for babies, toddlers, and older children. This is called "childproofing." Childproofing the home begins before babies actually develop the ability to move themselves from place to place. Since injury prevention is the major theme of childproofing, it begins even before babies arrive home from the hospital. Expect to take more intense precautions for multiple explorers. Adapting a home for this higher level of environmental safety is dubbed "twinproofing" or "multiples-proofing."

Some parents consult with professional childproofing experts for help, as they are trained to see potential dangers that parents are more likely to miss. For information about professional childproofing services, check the yellow pages of a nearby city, ask someone in the parent education department of the nearest children's hospital, or search the Internet for "childproofing experts or services." (Check Resources, "General: Equipment and Childproofing," for online distributors of childproofing devices.)

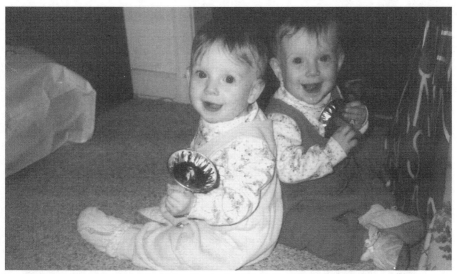

"Twinproofing" describes the higher level of childproofing required for toddler multiples.

Pre-mobile childproofing

The word "never" applies to few situations in life, but most existing applications probably pertain to caring for children—whether newborns or toddlers.

- *Never leave a baby of any age on a surface off the floor.* This would include changing tables, beds, sofas, etc. Babies' movements can cause a shift in their positions so that a fall can occur long before they are able to roll over or crawl. And the baby who could not roll yesterday may suddenly develop the ability today. Leaving a toddler alone on a high surface is the same as daring her to jump or climb higher, or fall.

- *Never leave any baby or toddler in a tub with any amount of water* for even a moment. Do not depend on sponge rests, seat rings, or other "in tub" seats to keep any baby safe in water. Babies' and toddlers' heads weigh proportionately more than the rest of their bodies, so babies and toddlers are top heavy. Should any baby find herself on her tummy in even a minimal amount of water, that baby is in danger of drowning because she may have difficulty keeping her head up in that slippery tub.

- *Never trust that faucets actually are out of babies' or toddlers' reach.* A determined baby will find a way to get to them one unexpected day. As an extra precaution to avoid accidental burns, check the temperature on the hot water heater to be sure it is set no higher than 120°F (approximately 45°C).

Childproofing for the Newly Mobile

Older babies are compelled to explore with their eyes, their hands, and their mouths. This compulsion is a vital step in learning about the wider world. Once multiples begin to crawl, their home becomes the original new frontier. To each baby it is virgin territory just waiting to be explored and conquered. Until parents of multiples are issued extra eyes for the backs of their heads, they must anticipate the movements of little explorers who are likely to wander off in different directions. To make your home ultra-safe:

- *Get down on the floor yourself and view it from the babies' level* before any of the babies takes off rolling or crawling across the floor. If anyone can find the proverbial "needle in a haystack," it is a marauding multiple! Look on the floor and under any sofa, on carpets, through any bordering fringe, under chairs and tables for coins, crumbs, and other mouth-size odds and ends.

- *Conceal electrical outlets with childproof caps or plugs* so that older babies or toddlers cannot stick fingers or other objects into them. Covers to place over an entire outlet may be needed for explorer multiples who often find a way to remove individual socket or outlet safety caps. If removed by a toddler, these caps also become a potential choking hazard.

- *Eliminate wires dangling from lamps and other electrical items,* as electrical wires may be bitten or pulled and babies may be shocked or injured when hit by a falling object.

- *Apply childproof window blind cord roll-ups.* Parents may use the blinds normally, but these safety covers prevent babies from getting tangled in any cords lying on or close to the floor or hanging near a crib.

- *Move to higher ground any expensive stereo and television equipment, remote controls, breakable or heavy knick-knacks, etc.* Plastic control panel guards designed to protect such items from older babies are unlikely to stop multiple curious toddlers. Moving these items now may save you from saying the word "no" a lot, and you are much less likely to someday find an item in pieces.

- *Keep printed materials, such as newspapers, magazines, and books in an out-of-reach basket or on a high shelf.* Babies love almost anything made of paper. Paper makes a great noise when wadded in the hand, and most babies seem to think it tastes good. Unfortunately, the ink used for some printing may be toxic and a small wad of paper can lodge in a baby's throat and cause choking.

- *Ban all ashtrays or any other tobacco-related items such as cigarettes, cigars, pipes and tobacco, matches, lighters, etc.* Avoid any possibility that older babies and toddlers may be burned, eat a tobacco-containing object, or start a fire because of such paraphernalia. Create a family policy if a parent or frequent guest smokes or uses tobacco, since adult smoking is not an appropriate behavior in any home with children. Children exposed to secondhand smoke have much higher rates of respiratory illnesses, and children of smokers are more likely to smoke later in life.

> **In the blink of a father's eye or the turn of a mother's head, toddler multiples will run in opposite directions to investigate different fascinating objects.**

- *Move all toxic substances to higher ground.* Start in the kitchen by looking in cabinets and the pantry. Move any "occasional use" toxic substance out of the kitchen, and lock these items in the highest cabinet or in a container on the highest shelf in the laundry area or garage. Place dishwasher soap or powder, medications, vitamin and mineral supplements, and alcoholic beverages inside a high, locked kitchen cabinet, since all can be toxic.

- *Inspect cabinets and move items with the potential for injury or illness,* such as plastic garbage bags, dishwashing soaps, heavy cans or pans, breakable bowls, and so on to higher, locked cabinets or containers on shelves. Open kitchen drawers and inspect each as closely as you did the cabinets. Silverware and cooking utensils may look like toys to toddlers, but these items have the potential for causing stab injuries, so they should be kept in a impossible-to-reach drawer that even inventive climbers cannot access. (Never underestimate the word *impossible* as it applies to multiple explorers!)

- *Move items that are not necessarily harmful but could create a mess* you would rather not have to clean!

- *Attach specially designed childproof guards or locks to cabinet doors and drawers* to prevent children from opening them after you have moved dangerous or risky materials. *Never depend* on such guards, however, to keep like-minded multiples from getting into cabinet doors or drawers. Sooner or later they will combine their brains and brawn to figure out how to manipulate such locks.

  ❏ *Skip a few drawers when attaching safety guards.* Many mothers fill lower drawers with unbreakable items, such as small pots, pans, plastic storage containers, and plastic lids to keep babies busy when mommy is working in the kitchen.

- *Measure the space between spindles on a stairway, balcony, or deck banister.* Older babies could wriggle through and fall or get their heads trapped if there is too much room. It is best to use a gate to limit access to stairways or outdoor decks so babies or toddlers do not have the opportunity to become trapped in banisters.

Until parents of multiples are issued extra eyes for the backs of their heads, they must anticipate the movements of little explorers who are likely to wander off in different directions.

Helpful Equipment

Infant equipment assumes a new role as babies become mobile and begin to explore. Different items can help or hinder your efforts to keep multiple babies or toddlers safe. Certain items can also help or hinder babies' development.

Infant Seats for Younger Babies

Babies often outgrow *infant seats and automatic swings* between four to six months (based on full-term birth). At this age babies begin to arch their backs in a way that can propel them out of such seats or cause a lightweight seat to tip over. Therefore, babies must be carefully supervised when in such seats.

As babies gain the ability to sit more erect, it may be necessary to readjust *car seat placement* and car seat safety belts or harnesses. The same may hold true for the positioning of some *stroller seats* and the placement of stroller safety belts. No matter how contented a particular multiple may seem when in the stroller, *always* secure all babies with safety belts before using a stroller.

Walkers and Play Seats for Older Babies

It may be tempting to put one or more multiples in individual walkers, especially when it seems to keep any or all busy for a while. Yet walker use is associated with one of the highest rates of emergency room visits among older babies, which has led to bans on walkers in some countries.

- *If using walkers with multiples, use only a type with locking wheels.*
  Wheels should be locked if an adult is unable to walk directly alongside a baby. The average baby moves three feet (almost one meter) per second in a walker. Never mind that yesterday a baby could not move it or could only move backward in the walker; today that same baby suddenly may figure out how to move forward and toward the stairs.
  ❏ *Walker wheels easily catch on uneven spots* or breaks in a floor, grass, or pavement, causing many tip-over accidents every year.

- *Safety is not the only problem with walkers.* The overuse of walkers is also associated with problems or delays in proper growth and development. Walkers may become a substitute for more appropriate opportunities for infant mobility. When babies are in walkers, they are not learning to move their bodies themselves.
  Walker use may interfere with babies learning to walk properly. Babies in walkers move forward by shuffling their feet, which may prevent babies from learning "alternate stepping," or placing one foot forward and then the other as with a normal walking gait.

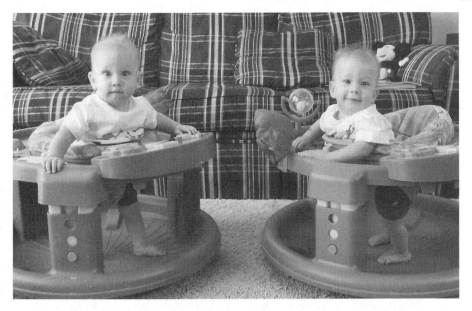

These saucer type play seats can keep babies entertained for short periods of time

- Any type of play seat in which a baby is virtually suspended in a sitting position, including most walkers, may create undue stress on the structures in a baby's pelvic area. To avoid problems with growth or development, babies should not be left in walkers, saucer seats, or jumping seats suspended from a doorway for more than 20 to 30 consecutive minutes.

High Chairs

High chairs, booster seats with trays, or seats that attach onto the adult table become useful once babies are able to maintain an erect sitting position. Because most high chairs are exactly that–high off the floor–they should be used only during mealtimes or when babies can be watched constantly.

- *Always secure each baby by fastening the seat or shoulder belts that are built into the high chair.* Never turn away from or leave babies unattended in high chairs or other types of seats. A large number of babies and toddlers are seen in emergency rooms for falls from high chairs every year.
- *For visiting relatives or friends or for enjoying a family meal at a restaurant,* many parents invest in portable cloth restraints designed to hold baby in a secure sitting position in adult dining chairs. Some slings and harnesses are also designed to secure older babies and toddlers in straight-back chairs, grocery cart seats, etc.
- *Investing in multiple high chairs can be a big expense.* For cost-savings and more versatility, some parents purchase multiple booster seats with trays or seats that attach to the adult table. These seats often are easier to

clean than high chairs and either type saves space in the dining area. Toddlers often prefer these seats, because they enjoy sitting at the table with the rest of the family. Since most brands take up little space in the car, these seats can travel to grandparents' house or a family restaurant.

❏ If booster or table-attaching seats sound like a good option, look for a brand that has safety straps to restrain a child in the seat. Booster seats should have safety straps that attach it securely to a chair, and trays should be easy to use. Look for brands that adjust in height to accommodate a growing child.

Play Yard

A standard play yard is a fairly dull place to play, especially once babies begin to crawl or pull themselves to a standing position. The standard play yard is soon outgrown when it is shared by two or more budding explorers. *Expandable play yards* make more sense for multiples. These play areas provide more functional space—enough space to practice new physical skills as well as create a safe space to play indoors and out. Look for play yard pieces that link together and form play yards of varying sizes. (Avoid purchasing an older model with crisscrossing slats, however, as children's heads and fingers have been caught in them.)

Doorway Gates

To create larger indoor play areas, use gates to block doorways or stairways and to keep babies in or out of rooms and other household areas; extra-wide gates are available for hallways or room entryways. A gated area provides more of the space babies need to practice new physical skills and a wider expanse to roam. Properly used, gates meet the babies' needs for exploration and parents' need to safely contain their multiples' curiosity.

To save money long term, purchase gates with toddlers' increased mobility in mind. A less-expensive, standard 24-inch (60 cm), pressure-mounted gate may work fine for a singleton toddler, but multiple toddlers often find ways to crash through or climb over them.

- Look for gates that are several inches above standard height.
- For gate stability consider the wall-mounted rather than the pressure-mounted type. Safety experts say pressure-mounted gates should not be used at the top of stairways.
- For reasons of safety, choose gates with vertical slats. Little body parts can become trapped or pinched when slats crisscross. Gates with a mesh panel are usually safe for older babies, but the mesh can provide toddlers with a toehold for climbing up and over. When blocking stairways, some mothers leave a few (two to four) stairs open for climbing practice. By carpeting any exposed stairs and the foot of the staircase, there is little risk of injury when babies take the inevitable tumbles.

Out and About

One of the pleasures of older babies is their ability to sit upright in stroller, car, or grocery cart seats. They are able to enjoy the world from a new, more visual perspective. Their newfound preoccupation with all they can see from a sitting position usually makes it much easier to take them out. As babies move into toddlerhood and develop new physical skills, they may be less content with merely viewing the world from a sitting position.

Toddlers love to go outdoors, and most parents welcome opportunities for multiples to expend energy.

- Older babies and toddler multiples may be able to climb (or fall) out of some stroller or grocery cart seats. Harnesses that fasten in the back and have straps that attach to the stroller or cart frame will safely "hold" multiples in their seats. In addition to preventing falls, harnesses restrict multiples' ability to reach items on store shelves.

  ❏ Harnesses also may be used with leashes when taking two or more toddlers for a walk. Although some people find it offensive when they see toddlers wearing harnesses while linked to a parent by a leash, these people probably do not have multiple toddlers who tend to run in opposite directions. Using harnesses with leashes is a safety strategy. Rather than restricting multiple toddlers, harnesses with leashes often allow for out-of-stroller walks and play that would not be possible without them.

- If multiples frequently move in different directions or one always runs ahead while the other lags behind, harnesses with leashes may not result in a workable walk. Use harnesses in the stroller and, perhaps, try again later.

- You may be able to carry one curious older baby or toddler in a baby sling on your hip longer than in a backpack. Some mothers find multiple toddlers become too heavy or simply too difficult to manage when one "rides" on mother's hip while shopping. However, some mothers are able to crisscross slings and hold two multiples–one on each hip–for their first several years. (The way a mother's and her toddlers' bodies "fit," plus her toddlers' activity levels, influence this ability or lack thereof.)

- Many stores now provide carts with double child seats. If you find one, grab it! (Be sure to let the manager know why you have just become a regular customer.) The shape of these seats and the attached safety belts may deter some climbers, but don't depend on these features alone. The seat shape may interfere with harness use, but it may be possible to use extra safety belts.

- If you use two standard carts, form a train–push one and pull the other–so at least two multiples ride in individual cart seats. Avoid putting two or more multiples in one cart.

Warning Never let any child stand in the body/basket of a shopping cart. Most cart accidents occur when a standing child reaches to touch some item on a nearby shelf and then leans too far forward.

❑ Multiples standing in one cart present an additional danger. If two or more children rush to the same spot, the cart could become unbalanced and tip over.

❑ Never leave any child alone in a shopping cart for even a moment.

❑ When forming a two-cart train, don't forget to make "choo-choo" noises to keep multiples entertained.

• Many mothers find the train is easier to manage when they put heavier items in the cart they are pulling. The ability to form a two-cart train may depend on a mother's fitness level. After walking miles pushing a multiple-stroller, most mothers are up to creating a shopping cart train. However, toddlers' changing weights and physical abilities may also affect its use for a particular family.

Toddler multiples are notorious for figuring out how to get out of *car safety belts.* The safety belt systems of newer car seat models are more difficult to release, but "difficult" does not necessarily mean impossible. Older, pre-owned seats may not have newer safety features.

It is crucial that each multiple learn no one is going anywhere until everyone's safety belts are in place and remain in place. This requires consistent handling by parents if any multiple aspires to a career as an escape artist. Any time a child releases the safety belt, immediately pull off the road and stop the car. Refasten the belt and resume the drive. Repeat this action each time one releases the belt system no matter how many times it occurs. When parents are consistent, multiples rarely continue this behavior for long. It may be aggravating, especially if it takes a few car rides, but stopping this behavior now will make for safer and saner car trips long term.

Your toddlers are watching you, so *be sure to buckle your own seatbelt* every time you get into a car.

Childproofing for Very Mobile Toddler Multiples

There is nothing quite like rediscovering a familiar world through the eyes of a toddler, unless it is rediscovering the world from multiple new viewpoints. For many parents it seems only minutes before multiples progress from crawling to walking to running and climbing. Older babies' increasing mobility offers only a peek at both the excitement and the challenge two or more toddler explorers provide.

Individual safety becomes the major issue as active multiples become even more mobile toddlers. In the blink of a father's eye or the turn of a mother's head, toddler multiples will run in opposite directions to investigate different fascinating objects. Count on all of them to pop those different objects into their mouths or a toilet as a crucial aspect of their investigations.

Together two can do what one toddler could not, such as drag a chair so they can climb onto a shelf or cabinet to reach a knife or that jar of vitamin tablets. Three or more multiples contribute even more interest to the pool of toddler ideas and escapades. Perhaps this explains the response of one mother of toddler twins when asked the question "What do you do for a living?" "I save lives–all day, every day," she said with a straight face.

Basic Safety

Keep first aid skills fresh, those emergency numbers posted, and the syrup of ipecac in a high but convenient cabinet. Update an emergency fire plan regularly to adjust for children's changing sizes. Toddlers are heavier and taller than infants, and preschoolers are larger still. Even if no longer using a sling or backpack carrier for outings, it may be a practical means of carrying an extra child if it becomes necessary to leave a home in a hurry.

Basic Childproofing
Home

Whether your multiples' activity levels are best described as *sightseers, wanderers, trailblazers,* or a combination of two or more, it can only make family life easier to childproof as if all are trailblazers. Trailblazers constantly explore. The higher or more out of reach an object is, the more compelled they seem to attain it. Trailblazers seem to relish the challenge of finding ways around, over, or under every childproofing barrier their parents erect to keep them safe. (See Chapter 30, "Parenting Toddler Multiples," for toddler activity level descriptions.)

Multiple trailblazers and trailblazer-wanderer combos frequently work as a team. Together they can execute actions that a single trailblazer has neither the strength nor range to even attempt. Two wanderers or a wanderer-sightseer combination may also gain confidence together and engage in risky trailblazing behaviors, although they tend to do so less often. In spite of close parental supervision, the following escapades are common and frequent occurrences for trailblazing multiple toddlers, are regular occurrences for wanderers, and may happen occasionally with sightseers.

- Multiples can help one another drag a chair alongside a shelf, the stove, or the dining table, and then stand on it to reach objects formerly out of reach. A well-placed chair also makes it easy for them to climb onto countertops and other furniture.

- With one on either end of a bureau or chest of drawers, each can grasp a drawer pull or knob to open it. Both then use the drawers as a stepladder–usually after they have already emptied the contents. Once on top of the furniture, they will likely use it for jumping practice. A greater danger occurs when climbing toddlers cause a heavy chest of drawers to become unbalanced so that it topples forward, which can crush the small children using it for a ladder.

- Multiples learn to stack pillows from beds, a sofa, or outdoor furniture against doorway or hallway gates, stairway banisters, or deck rails in order to climb over. Or they will simply climb on available furniture if a piece of furniture is near or against something any would like to see better.

- Two will find a way to open almost any kind of door–to different rooms, the refrigerator, the oven, the dryer, a basement stairwell, and doors leading outside.

- Knobs of any kind draw toddlers like magnets. To multiples, knobs are irresistible. There are knobs to adjust stovetop burners, turn the oven on, and control the stereo, television, or other electronic equipment. Water–cold or hot–goes on and off with the turn of a knob in the bathroom and kitchen. And of course, once doorknobs are mastered, toddlers can open doors to rooms someone probably did not want them to go into. Also, many knobs may be used to gain a toehold when multiples are moving vertically.

- A toilet may be the only thing multiples seem to find more compelling than a knob. Water play is always fun, but multiples also like to top one another by finding interesting items to flush. This is not only a plumbing problem; every year toddlers drown because their heads become trapped after they fall forward into a toilet bowl.

- If an item can fit in a toddler's hand, chances are another multiple will encourage him to eat it or drink it. It does not matter how inedible or unsafe that item is. Toddlers do not think of choking or poisoning as possible consequences when they pop interesting objects into their mouths.

- Most multiples will at some point use a wall or one another's body as a canvas for their artwork. (Some clever parents have attempted to curtail their multiples' artistic efforts by rolling paper over, and taping it to, the walls at toddlers' arm level. Their multiples quickly learned to draw above and below the paper.) In addition to such standard mediums as pens, pencils, colored markers, crayons, etc., many sets have helped one another remove diapers and then used the contents as fingerpaints.

- Most parents can count on one multiple to run ahead and another to dawdle behind during any walk out-of-doors. The parent is left wondering whether to first stop the multiple who appears to be chewing the mysterious berries he just pulled off a neighbor's shrub, grab the one balancing on the stone retaining wall, or tackle the one who is running toward the street.

- Almost all parents with trailblazing multiples have stories of the time a neighbor found their toddlers wandering up the street after they had escaped the safety of their home. To reach the street, multiples have done such things as pushing a screen out of a window (and not always one on the first floor), figuring out a deadbolt lock or scaling a six foot fence. Usually their parents' heads sported several new gray hairs immediately after the episode.
- Older toddlers or preschoolers may become intrigued with fire. Many parents have a frightening tale of the day their multiples stumbled onto a pack of matches or suddenly decided to prepare a meal on the stove while their mom took a quick bathroom break. Likewise, older toddlers and preschoolers may become more and more interested in any firearms that a parent may keep in the home.
- Besides climbing and investigating areas where they don't belong, toddler multiples can become frustrated with one another's behaviors which often leads to pushing or punching. Multiples may be injured in a fall from some perch on a countertop or from hitting a body part, usually one's head, on the floor or a corner of a wall after being pushed or punched.

Indoor Solutions

Assuming the childproofing interventions for older babies are already in effect, what can parents do to make homes even safer–short of emptying one's home of all furniture for several years? Once again, get down on your knees to look at your home from your toddler multiples' perspectives. Afterward, you may decide removing some furniture is a good idea, especially if the items in question have any sharp edges, pointed ends, or protruding pieces. Books, electrical equipment control panels, electrical wires, window blind cords, lamps, knickknacks, etc., that were out of reach for babies crawling on all fours, may now be within the reach of toddlers who move vertically as well as horizontally.

- If possible, find or create an even higher place for potentially dangerous, breakable, or valuable items. However, many parents choose to store such items and any unsafe furniture out of sight in a locked attic, cellar, storage closet, or rented storage area.
- Medications, certain cosmetics, cleaning solutions, and other toxic substances are a greater danger with toddler climbers in the house. These items should be far out of reach from both the floor or if standing on a countertop. If no shelf is safe enough, consider keeping these items in locked storage containers.
- To avoid injuries, keep electrical equipment, lamps, and other objects with wires to a minimum. Be certain there are no wires or cords dangling from a shelf or table and that none are out in the open on a floor.

- It may not be possible to eliminate all edges and corners, but cushioned strips are available that can be applied to the sharp edges and corners of tables, a fireplace hearth, and so on. If investing in any new furniture, purchasing pieces with rounded edges may save on trips to the emergency room for stitches.

- If possible, empty one room completely of "grown-up" items and designate it as a playroom. Choose a room that is carpeted, easily gated, and one that is either near, or actually is a part of, the center of most family activities. Toddlers like to be near Mom or Dad, so a playroom in a distant part of a home is unlikely to be used.

  Warning No matter how well parents "multiples-proof" a room, two or more toddlers still require adult supervision when in a playroom.

- To give young artists an appropriate outlet for their talents, some parents paint all or part of one wall with "chalkboard" paint. The fact that the chalk used on this wall washes off more easily when multiples decorate one another may be considered an added benefit.

- Trailblazers and wanderers usually enjoy practicing large motor skills. To keep these multiples busy, happy, and off the furniture, many parents purchase durable, hard plastic indoor-outdoor gym equipment, such as seesaws and slides with attached steps and platforms.

- Toddler multiples have devised all sorts of uses for small toys or for pieces of such toys. Their parents have to examine small toys for aspects that may not occur to most parents of single-born children. For instance, parents should look at toys for:

  ❑ The number of parts or pieces. Stock multiples' playroom with toys having the least number of removable, and therefore swallowable or flushable, parts.

  ❑ A toy's weapon potential. In the hands of active multiples, many toys easily become weapons. Avoid any having sharp or pointed edges. Rubber or spongy toys are less likely to cause an injury when used as weapons by one multiple to hit another. However, not all spongy toy materials are equal. Avoid spongy materials that are easily bitten and swallowed. (A parental taste test rarely is necessary. A pinch test usually will do!)

  Warning Toddler multiples generally maintain a "non-discrimination policy" when it comes to eating, choking on, or flushing small toys or related parts that happen to belong to an older sibling. If a toy (part) fits inside a cardboard tube for toilet paper or paper towel roll, consider it a potential choking or flushing hazard that should be kept in a restricted area, such as the sibling's "off limits" locked bedroom.

- Never trust toddlers in a loft area or on a deck. Open banisters on indoor stairways or outdoor decks pose a danger for toddlers, since they are associated with a significant drop to the ground. Banisters on cellar stairways may be little more than open holes. Some toddlers may be able to squeeze through smaller banister spaces, others could get their heads trapped between slats, and many are likely to give climbing over banisters a try. Also, toddlers may use the space between slats as a hole to drop things through to the floor or ground below.
  ❏ In addition to wall-mounted gates that already block access to stairways or decks, consider attaching banister shields designed for this purpose across open banisters. **Caution:** Net or mesh varieties may provide toddlers with a toehold that could help rather than hinder climbing.

Toddler multiples consider an open door as an invitation to an older sibling's or parents' bedroom, the cellar, any bathroom, or the outdoors. Slamming a door to slow another multiple or an angry sibling hard on one's heels can be great fun—unless someone gets hit in the head or gets fingers pinched in the process. Closed doors are the safest doors, but keeping them closed yet accessible to other family members can be a problem.

- Childproof locks that fit into the space at the top of a door may work perfectly for doors that lead to a cellar or the outside, since most mothers also want to know if an older sibling has gone through these doors. These locks may be less practical if parental help is required to open doors when an older child wants to use a room, such as a bathroom or the child's bedroom.
  ❏ Another solution is to install a surface bolt or small barrel bolt, which are types of slide locks, into these doors at a height that is too high for a toddler but within reach for an older child. When in the locked position, these locks are difficult for toddlers to manipulate, although a pre-school sibling can easily open them. For cellars with an open banister on the stairway, consider installing a slide lock plus a childproof lock at the top of a cellar door to provide additional safety.

  Caution: Hook-and-eye locks may seem to be an inexpensive option. However, many sets of toddler multiples have figured out how to use a pole, such as a broomstick or mop handle, to open hook-and-eye locks within an hour of installation, even when the locks were set high on doors. Low placement of these locks is a breeze for them to figure out!
  ❏ Check installed locks routinely to be certain other family members are remembering to use them.

Toilet-seat lid locks provide extra insurance for keeping small objects or a multiple from falling in. Lid-locks may be opened easily by adults or an older sibling.

To avoid injuries from tipping furniture, install *childproof braces/brackets* to help protect multiples from furniture pieces they may use as steps. These braces/brackets may be installed on all chests of drawers, bookcases, shelves, and so on.

A space heater or a wood-burning stove may be an economical way to warm a drafty room, but either can be extremely dangerous when curious multiples are in the vicinity. Due to the obvious potential for burn injury from touching a wood-burning stove and many types of space heaters, parents must weigh the risks versus the benefits of using such appliances.

- In addition to the potential for contact burns, there is a danger that one multiple could push another into a space heater or wood-burning stove. A child could be burned more extensively or a heater or stove may tip over, creating a greater threat of fire.
- Installing a wood-burning stove in an out-of-reach spot may be difficult or impossible to do, so parents must always treat it as the fire and burn injury hazard it is.
- Certain brands of space heaters are safer than others. Any type that requires fuel, emits fumes, or produces a flame adds an element of danger.
  - ❏ If using a space heater that is hot to the touch, check it daily for safe, out-of-reach placement and treat it as the fire and burn injury hazard it is.
  - ❏ If a space heater requires some type of fuel, be sure to store fuel in an inaccessible, remote area of the home where curious children can never reach it. The storage area should be vented properly so children are not exposed to fumes.

Having firearms in a home with older toddlers and preschool multiples can be extremely dangerous. Any type of firearm, whether hand held or rifle, should be kept in a locked cabinet or closet. No firearm should be kept loaded. Store ammunition in a separate container in a locked cabinet or closet. Play-acting preschoolers *will* pick up a firearm to incorporate into "make believe" play if it is available.

Warning: Never clean or load any firearm in the presence of one or more young multiples.

Multiples' Bedroom

Whether multiples spend a lot or only a little time in a room designated as their bedroom, it usually is a room that requires extra childproofing effort since parents may not always be in the room supervising. Many parents view a nursery or bedroom for toddlers as a decorating project. Care must be taken to ensure that safety and style work together.

- To confine their energy when it is time for them to sleep, many parents use a higher gate to remind multiples where they are. Some parents have found it more helpful to cut the multiples' bedroom door in half, creating a Dutch door, or they insert an actual Dutch door in the frame.
- One or more of multiples may still sleep in a crib, but often the first one to climb out quickly teaches the other(s) how to do it, too.
  ❏ Once two are climbing out of cribs, multiples could share a mattress. To increase safety, place their mattress directly on the floor and away from a wall with a window. Be certain window screens are intact and locked in place on any bedroom windows. **Warning:** Do not install bars or anything else that could block access or escape through a bedroom window; this is a dangerous fire hazard and in some areas it may be illegal.

  ❏ Many parents strip their multiples' bedroom of chests of drawers, curtains, window blinds, artwork, and so on to create a safe and less-stimulating sleep room once any toddler is able to climb out of a crib. (See "Night waking," in Chapter 30, "Parenting Toddler Multiples.")

Kitchen

A kitchen is a room of both wonder and danger for active toddlers. Kitchen appliances and equipment pose particular dangers for multiple toddlers.

- Kitchen doorways are often open passages without a door that can be closed, so many parents install a higher gate to block multiples' uninvited access to this room.
- To keep multiples from opening refrigerator, oven, and dishwasher doors, parents can install special latches and locks designed for these specific appliances. Some parents have used bungee cords across dishwasher or oven doors, and some installed padlocks on refrigerator and freezer doors to keep multiples from opening them. (Yes, they carefully drilled holes in these appliances to install the locks.)
- Many parents store all knives, scissors, food processor blades, pointed tools, matches, etc., in a locked chest, such as a standard tool chest. **Caution:** Be sure to hide an extra key to open any padlock or chest—one is bound to get lost.
- Childproof stove shields and knob covers or locks help prevent toddlers from reaching stove controls or touching burners or hot pots and pans. Some parents are able to remove control knobs. They use only one knob for all the burners or they replace the knobs only when a burner is to be used.
  ❏ All family cooks should be instructed to use only back burners when possible and always turn pot handles away from the front; pots are less likely to be tipped when facing the middle or the back of the stove.

- To minimize multiples' use of chairs as stepstools to climb onto tables, large appliances, and countertops, some parents eliminate most or all lightweight chairs in their homes for a year or two. They store their dining or kitchen chairs in an attic, cellar, or rented storage space. In place of typical dining chairs, they use folding chairs during meals, which they fold and place on top of a dining table or in a locked closet between meals.

Outdoor Solutions

Toddlers love to go outdoors, and most parents welcome opportunities for multiples to expend energy by playing on gym equipment, scooting around on wheeled carts, or splashing in a small pool. The following strategies have helped other parents of multiples supervise two or more active toddlers.

- Fence in any open yard directly connected to the house, but purchase fencing material with older toddlers and preschool multiples in mind.
  - ❑ When multiples realize there is more to explore beyond the fenced yard, they are likely to try climbing over the fence. Many sets have succeeded in scaling a standard-height fence after getting a toehold in the fencing material. To minimize this problem, many parents buy fencing higher than the norm.
  - ❑ If a fence has no gate, access in and out of the yard is possible only via the house entry (or by climbing over the fence). However, a gate may increase the long-term usefulness of a fence so many parents install a padlock or combination lock to keep a gate securely closed. One mother wore the key to a gate's padlock on a chain around her neck. Her inventive toddler twins once gently removed it when they noticed her resting on the sofa with her eyes closed. She let them know she was not actually sleeping before they could leave the room and head for the back door.
- In addition to preventing falls through banisters or over railings on outdoor decks, falls can also occur on steps or through stairway banisters leading from the deck to the yard. A gate mounted at the top and bottom of an outdoor stairway may be necessary to keep toddlers where a parent can watch them. Netting or protective shields on stairway banisters may also prevent injuries, although netting is more likely to provide a foothold for climbers.

Most toddlers relish any type of *water play* but pools, ponds, and fountains of any kind and any depth are particularly dangerous outdoor hazards. No matter what kind of safety devices are used to keep children out of the water, there are many who have managed to get past such devices before drowning or being injured by a fall into a pool, pond, or fountain. Also, child drowning often occurs during supervised pool time due to moments of caregiver distraction. When monitoring multiple toddlers or preschoolers, opportunities for distraction only increase.

> **There are no childproofing interventions that will ever replace constant parental supervision.**

- It is extremely important to install tight pool covers and pool alarms on any nearby body of water. Alarm bands are available that fasten around each child's wrist and sound an alarm if a child enters the water; however, these wristbands were intended mainly for use during supervised pool time. To use them otherwise can create a false sense of security for parents.
- A separate fence should surround any pool, pond, lake, or fountain; its entry gate should self-close and then self-lock. Ideally, the fenced body of water is inaccessible from the main play zone.
- Keep furniture away from a fence surrounding water, as multiples have used furniture to climb over a fence.
- Do not leave toys near a pool when no one is (safely) using it, as toys may attract toddlers to the water.
- It may be necessary to drain a pond, lake, or fountain if fencing is not a feasible option.
- Current certification in the resuscitation skills used for drowning is crucial for parents, and any other care provider, if there is a pool, pond, or fountain in the vicinity. Parents should know how to use related lifesaving equipment, which should always be within reach at poolside.
- Parents must become aware of, and make certain that safeguards are in place for, any body of water that is in the vicinity–whether in a public area or in the yards of neighbors, relatives the family is visiting, etc.

Many toddler and preschool multiples have escaped outside through a *door left partially open* by an older sibling, or they have pried or pushed a loose screen and climbed outside. Escaping young multiples have led to more than a few parental gray hairs! To avoid becoming prematurely gray, many parents have tried:

- Installing alarms on all doors leading to the outside–even to areas enclosed by a fence. The alarm emits an audible signal anytime someone passes through a door.
- Making it a habit to regularly monitor window safety by checking windows the same day of each week. Parents look to see if window screens are locked in place and whether any have been exposed recently to wear-and-tear by multiples. (See "Indoor solutions" above for other considerations regarding window safety.)
- Asked neighbors to call immediately if they see any or all multiples out of the fenced play zone. If multiples have wandered from the yard, neighbors should be advised to ensure the toddlers' safety before calling.

Warning: No matter how high the fence or how many safety devices are in place, there is no substitute for constant parental supervision when multiples play outdoors.

Providing a stimulating yet safe environment for mobile older babies and toddler multiples can be a challenge for parents. Each multiple has the same need as any single older baby or toddler to explore the environment, but multiples often combine brains and brawn to explore in ways that would not be possible for a single child. Many of the challenges to babies' or toddlers' safety are due to the multiples' interactions. Thoroughly multiples-proofing the home and yard does help so that older babies and toddlers can explore and parents can relax–but only a little. There are no childproofing interventions that will ever replace constant parental supervision.

KEY POINTS

- A baby's home is the baby's world. As older babies begin to crawl, they naturally begin to explore that world.
- Babies learn by touching and tasting. A baby "gets into things" and puts things in her mouth because that is how she learns about her world.
- By childproofing the home, parents provide a safer home (world) for older babies or toddlers to explore while these young children gradually learn what is safe to touch and taste.
- The idea of childproofing is to prevent accidents or injuries when possible and be prepared to handle any accident or injury that a parent was unable to prevent.
- Childproofing for really active young multiples may be more challenging, because multiples often work together to explore areas that a singleton could not reach.
- It is important to recheck and change childproofing to fit multiples' new skills as they grow.
- The childproofing that worked well for older babies is not enough once toddler multiples begin to run and climb. Now they can reach dangerous places or items that they could not get to earlier.

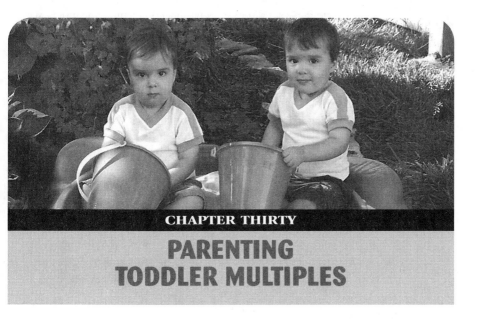

CHAPTER THIRTY

PARENTING TODDLER MULTIPLES

So much to discover in every direction they look! So many internal light bulbs blinking on at once that parents can almost see in their multiples' faces as the switches flip "on" inside their toddlers' heads. With newly developed mobility and a growing sensitivity to each other's cues, there isn't any direction that appears uninteresting–whether they set off to explore together or separately. There isn't anything they wouldn't investigate together–no matter where or how high its location. There isn't anything they cannot reach when they are of like mind, which they frequently are. Surely parents of multiples must have coined the phrases "two heads are better than one," "all for one and one for all," and "divide and conquer."

Guiding multiples through toddlerhood can be a challenge, but it is never dull. Multiples' social situation is unmatched by any other setting or circumstance, since each is constantly interacting with an exact age-mate(s)–a peer(s) of precisely the same developmental level. This leads to unique situations for parents–some of which are great fun and others that are extremely frustrating.

Multiples' Interactions

Most parents anxiously wait for the time when their multiples will begin to play together. Multiples often notice one another and they sometimes interact during their first year, but it is during the toddler years when the bonds between multiples seem to cement. Because of the closeness they share, multiples often seem to be both the best of friends and the worst of enemies. Most multiples appear to share a

The dynamic of multiple, same-age children affects the process of discipline.

special bond, but temperament also plays a key role in the degree of closeness experienced by the individuals within any set.

A bond is more likely to develop between *pairs of multiples.*

- Twin multiples are a custom-made pair.
- Among higher-order multiples, pairings may take different forms. Parents of odd-numbered multiples often say there really is something to the adage "two's company, but three's a crowd."

❏ Two may get along so well that once bonded they are inseparable throughout childhood.

❏ Others may interact more with another particular multiple for awhile, but days, weeks, or even months later the pairings shift so that each multiple now spends more time in the company of a different multiple. In time the pairings shift again. What this can mean for odd-numbered sets, such as triplets and quintuplets, is there can be an "odd one out"–briefly—when pairings shift often or long term if two develop a closer bond.

- Multiples have been constantly in each other's company since sharing a womb, and during toddlerhood many sets develop mutually understood *verbal and nonverbal cues.* These cues allow multiples to communicate long before they express themselves through language.

    This communication cueing is not the same as *idioglossia*–the development of a special language by multiples. It is more similar to the repetition of certain phrases and the unspoken signals used by two adults sharing a close relationship.

- A toddler multiple actually plays with a fellow multiple, not merely alongside another as two single-born toddlers tend to do in parallel play. Parents of multiples report social behaviors between, or among, their toddlers that child development books generally list as more typical for preschool children.

    Multiples often treat other children as they treat one another, and they expect these children to understand the interactive cues they have developed for the set.

Multiples often demonstrate a *deep caring* for one another.

- *Each will comfort the other(s) when one is upset.* Multiples hug and pat one another affectionately, establish eye contact to send a look of reassurance to another, or whisper soothing sounds in another's ear. If one is injured, the other(s) often cry harder than the one who is hurt.
- *Multiples share with one another.* When mother hands a treat to one, that multiple often points to the other(s) and waits until mother has handed

over a treat for each. (However, that multiple probably will be smart enough to inspect each treat and take the largest piece!)

- *Multiples often defend one another* if an older sibling or an outsider bothers any of them–often by physically or mentally ganging up on the offender.
- *If any multiple is in trouble with mother or dad, the other(s) may become angry or upset* if a punishment is involved–even when the one being punished is in trouble for biting or hitting the one now complaining about the consequences.

> Because of the closeness they share, multiples often seem to be both the best of friends and the worst of enemies.

Multiples may express *hostility* toward one another, too. Imagine how frustrating it would be to have shared everything with the same person(s) since in the womb. Who wouldn't feel hostile at times?

- If one multiple is enjoying a toy, a snack, or some individual time with mother or dad, it may lead to a display of *jealous behavior* by the other(s). There could be 100 red balls in a room and every multiple in the set would want the same red ball.
- Multiples *may compete* to take possession of a toy, be the first to reach the countertop, or gain mother's attention. (About the time parents are able to treat each multiple as an individual, multiples reach a developmental stage when they demand equal time and attention.)
- Many multiples fight. Since most toddlers do not yet have the vocabulary for verbal sparring, *disputes are often settled physically.* Unfortunately, toddlers cannot grasp the concept of a "fair" fight. Most do not appreciate their own strength. With a gentle but purposeful nudge or poke by one, another is pushed into a piece of furniture or a wall, or onto the floor with one more scrape, bump, or bruise.
- *Biting is extremely common among multiples.* Most sets have at least one biter. Often it occurs apart from brawling behavior. The combination of toddler frustration and minimal coping skills may lead to this aggressive behavior.

Multiples' individual temperaments and related activity levels influence whether they interact more by reassuring or wrestling one another.

Toddlers' Temperaments

Temperament refers to an individual's behavioral and emotional approach to situations. An individual's temperament has a genetic basis, so it is something a baby is born with. When a young baby is described as being calm, average, or high need, adults are actually referring to behaviors that reflect a baby's inborn temperament.

As babies become mobile and begin to explore the environment, temperament is reflected in a child's level of activity and approach to exploration.

Toddler Activity Levels

Many so-called discipline problems in toddler multiples actually are related more to their interactions and combined energy-activity level.

Toddlers come in a variety of normal activity, or exploration, levels. Since behavioral styles and activity levels have a genetic basis, it is not surprising that monozygotic (MZ/identical) multiples usually share a similar level of activity. The activity levels of dizygotic (DZ/fraternal) multiples may range from very similar to completely opposite ends of the spectrum, and different-gender boy-girl multiples tend to be the most different.

A toddler's level of activity tends to fit in one of several basic categories. However, the lines between the categories are blurred because level of activity progresses along a continuum. The majority of a multiple's characteristics may place him in one category while a particular aspect of her activity level fits better with another category. One way to describe toddler activity level categories is to use an analogy for different types of tourists.

- Toddler *sightseers* are usually content to go along with the tour guide's agenda. They seem able to learn about their environment by observing the persons, places, and things they encounter all around them. Although sightseers sometimes engage in more active exploration, they tend to stick to the designated route. In fact, they will reverse course if a recommended activity requires too much exertion or some element frightens them.
  ❏ Sightseers actually take hold of mother's or dad's hand when told to do so and stop doing something when a parent says "no." Many sightseers focus more on fine motor skills development than on the large motor development used for advanced physical exploration. These children are first to build tall towers of blocks, use a spoon to transport food into their mouths without losing one pea, and figure out how the pieces fit together to solve a puzzle.

- *Wanderers* generally enjoy the guided tour, but they also experience a bit of wanderlust. They feel drawn toward the horizon and the discovery of what lurks just beyond. One moment nothing seems able to distract the wanderers working on a block tower, but in the next moment they are off to investigate some new sight or sound. Although they may balk at holding mother's hand or being attached by a wrist cuff when out and about, most will settle down or save exploration for items within easy reach.
  Nonetheless, a parent must expect the unexpected walk-about from these mini-adventurers.

- *Trailblazers* cannot merely observe something of interest in the environment. Constant touching and tasting are crucial aspects of learning for them, and they let nothing come between them and any item they consider worthy of investigation. When no obvious path exists to reach the object in question, they forge ahead and create their own roads. They will break away when holding a parent's hand, find a way out of a wrist cuff, or climb out of a stroller if something catches their eye–and something always does.

Few trailblazers are satisfied only in attaining out-of-reach objects. Compelled to master large motor muscle coordination, they seem to enjoy the challenge of testing the limits of their newly achieved mobility. Trailblazers quickly abandon quiet projects for more active pursuits. Most seem as comfortable moving vertically as horizontally. Excellent climbers, these toddlers see almost everything in their home as a mountain. Impulsive exploration lands them literally in one scrape after another. To identify the trailblazers, look for toddlers with several bumps and bruises on their foreheads and scrapes on their knees.

Whether a multiple is more an observer or a participant, all definitely are aware of and enjoy one another's exploits. Multiple sightseers sometimes encourage each other to roam a little farther on, or off, the designated path. The combined courage of two or more wanderers easily propels each to discover what is waiting around the next bend. With the slightest support from fellow trailblazers, all are ready to run faster and climb higher!

One multiple's activity level affects the other(s). Usually a less active toddler takes direction from one who is more active. Often each member of the combined duo or trio then behaves at an increased level of activity, and the combined energy of the duo or trio forms a multiple entity with its own separate activity level.

Typically, a *trailblazer* inspires a *wanderer* to pick up the pace and follow his lead–frequently right into mischief or danger. Sometimes a *wanderer* encourages a *sightseer* to explore farther afield. Such influence does not appear to work in reverse. A more active multiple rarely decreases activity to join in the calmer play of a less active one. Apparently, a mover's got to move.

Are They Hyperactive?

When caring for more than one trailblazer or a trailblazer-wanderer combination, parents may wonder if their toddlers are hyperactive. Also, a trailblazing multiple may seem hyperactive when compared to a set's sightseer. Although parents should discuss this concern with the toddlers' pediatric care provider, multiples' combined activity level does not necessarily mean one is truly hyperactive. When parents have an opportunity to spend several hours with only one multiple, they may be

> One multiple's activity level affects the other(s)

surprised to find that a single trailblazer is not as difficult to watch as two. Also, many trailblazers settle down when alone and act like more easily supervised wanderers.

- When multiples' activity levels are extremely different and parents are tempted to compare, a book that discusses the ranges in normal toddler development should be within easy reach. Frequent review is often reassuring.
- Ask the pediatric care provider about a referral for an in-depth assessment if concerns about hyperactivity for any multiple persist, especially if behaviors persist into the preschool period.

Dominant vs. Passive

Many parents express concern when the dynamics within the multiples' relationship(s) seem to be uneven. They may worry when one toddler is a show-off, directs the set's activities, gets his way every time, starts–or at least ends–most of their disagreements, etc. On the other hand parents feel equally troubled if one multiple goes along with anything another initiates, gives up easily when the other(s) demands it, rarely or never defends himself, etc.

Some parents observe a different form of dominance between multiples. In this instance none is passive and parents report a physical or mental struggle, or competition, for dominance. Their struggles often play out in jealous behavior and the strong desire for the same toy, treat, or parent's attention. It seems to occur more often among MZ multiples and same-gender, similar-temperament DZ multiples.

Depending on the direction each multiple's dominance or passivity takes, parents may feel confused as to whether or when to get involved.

- *Avoid the temptation to intervene.* In many sets, multiples take turns or "flip-flop" taking the dominant or passive role every few weeks or months. Whether one or another's dominance or passivity lasts briefly or for years, multiples are testing these characteristics within the confines of their developing relationship. Allow them the freedom to build that relationship on their own terms. Their relationship belongs to them–not to their parents. For better, and perhaps for worse at times, multiples need lots of time to learn when to give and when to take in that relationship. It is not always easy, but avoid rescuing or saving them from each other. They can handle their relationship even as toddlers. Really. They can.
- *The increased verbal ability of one multiple is often a factor in one's dominant behavior.* The more verbal multiple becomes the set's spokesperson and sometimes continues to assume this role long after the other(s) is speaking well. Generally, girls lead boys in verbal ability, and many parents have described how the girl takes charge of boy-girl sets' activities.
- *Think positive!* The words "dominant" and "passive" both have a positive

and a negative connotation in American culture. When parents are concerned about a multiple's dominance or passivity, they often focus on the negative aspects of those words. A dominant toddler may act bossy, but that bossiness may reflect self-confidence, assertiveness, and the beginnings of leadership. That passive multiple may be more flexible, more easygoing, or more self-assured. Look at the positive sides of both traits.

High Need Flip-Flopping

Many toddlers go in and out of periods when one (or more) sticks to mother like super-glue as each vacillates between the quest for independence and the familiar security of the mother's arms. For each multiple, this is part of the normal process of learning one is a separate individual. What may be a surprise is the way in which this behavior can flip-flop between or among multiples. Often a multiple that had been the "needier" baby becomes a more independent toddler, and one who had seemed more easygoing or woke less during the first year begins to cling and wake more at night as a toddler.

Dealing with this flip-flop can be difficult. A clinging toddler often has a much different "feel" than a clingy, high-need baby. Mothers often expect high-need behaviors to decrease during toddlerhood, as multiples play and interact more. When a mother has less patience for the toddler who has waited more than a year for his turn as the higher need one, she may feel guilty about her response and sad for that multiple. Ideas for coping are included in several of the following sections. Related information about toddler breastfeeding is discussed in Chapter 28, "Breastfeeding, Starting Solids, and Weaning."

Discipline of Multiples

Babies usually begin to learn that their family "society" has rules once they become mobile and their adventures take them into unsafe territory or they discover another family member's private property. Since dangerous activities can have life-threatening natural consequences and because each family member is entitled to personal possessions, parents must impose certain limits or boundaries on their

In spite of any challenges, toddler multiples still want and need limits on their behaviors.

older babies' or toddlers' explorations. Setting physical limits is the beginning of discipline, and parents must now assume a more active role in guiding their children toward safe and responsible behavior. Self-discipline is the eventual goal, but many years will pass before each multiple achieves it. Expect multiples to test the limits and push all boundaries for at least a couple of decades!

As their children's guide on the road to self-discipline, parents explain the behaviors they expect, reinforce and reward appropriate behaviors, halt inappropriate behaviors while diverting a child to appropriate ones, and identify the consequences of inappropriate behaviors. Consequences may be a natural result of an action or behavior, but sometimes they may be in the form of a punishment imposed by parents (and later by society). Whether parents use the term *punishment, consequences,* or *corrective measures,* this is only one small aspect of discipline.

After months of parenting multiples, it should come as no surprise to discover the dynamic of two or more same-age children affects the process of discipline. Just as multiples-related issues may have gotten confused with actual breastfeeding problems during their early months, many so-called discipline problems in toddler multiples actually are related more to their interactions and combined energy-activity level.

Parental guidance will be more effective, and parents will feel less frustrated, when the rules/limits they set and the ways they choose to reinforce them reflect their multiples' current stage of development and individual temperaments. Of course, this assumes that parents have learned about the capabilities and the limitations of the normal toddler's thought processes, which is referred to as cognitive ability. It is too easy to label the toddlers' behavior as "purposeful" or "willful" when multiples simply got caught up in the "thrill" of the moment and acted, or reacted, impulsively.

In spite of any challenges, toddler multiples still want and need limits on their behaviors. Defining and continually reinforcing the limits that have been set is a serious parental responsibility. Reinforcing rules often requires parental action. It is not enough to remain seated on the sidelines and merely remind toddlers about a rule or the consequences of breaking it; parents must be ready to get up and physically intervene when toddlers push the limits. This is not an easy task day in and day out, as multiples may work individually in different areas of the house, work together at other times, and frequently may disagree on which activity may be the most fun at the moment.

Models of Behavior

Parents are their children's first, and remain their most important, models of appropriate behavior. From birth, infants constantly observe their parents. They listen to what parents say and how they say it long before they understand the actual words. An older sibling also provides an example for a younger one. The behavior of an older child provides a younger one with the opportunity to see what happens when someone with a little more experience follows or breaks a rule.

Multiples have a built-in buddy, and unless they have very different temperaments, toddler multiples tend to model their behaviors on each other. And who can blame them? Another toddler's ideas are usually more interesting–and definitely a lot more fun–than those that mommy, daddy, or a big brother or sister may come up with. They happily guide one another into all kinds of mischief.

Reinforcement from one's fellow multiple(s) often seems to have more meaning than any positive or negative reinforcement from parents. In spite of the creative benefits for the multiples, modeling another toddler has major drawbacks!

The parental interventions that usually are effective for reinforcing behaviors with a single toddler often do not work with multiples.

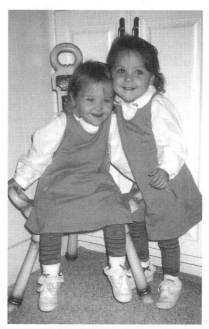

Toddler multiples can be the best of friends and the worst of enemies.

- Because toddlers enjoy receiving praise or approval, single-born toddlers often adjust behaviors that do not please a parent to behaviors that will please them. Toddler multiples also appreciate praise from parents, but they will forgo parental approval when the other multiple(s)' approval impulsively draws them into an activity.

- Active multiples join together and dream up adventures that parents tend to discourage, and multiples' combined abilities mean they actually can–and frequently do–implement ideas that are far beyond a toddler acting alone.

- Multiples cheer each other on. Whether they try something together or only one follows through, the support of another toddler spurs many to try something that would inspire caution in a single toddler.

- Multiples may be playing happily or sharing a treat together. As they mutually enjoy the activity or treat, their behaviors escalate and they get sillier and sillier. Before a mother can say "uh oh," one of two things has probably occurred. In the first, the multiples' laughing banter has led to a poke. Another takes umbrage and follows the poke with a punch or a push. Before long it becomes an all-out boxing match and each is crying.

   With the second scenario the escalating giggles translate into a corresponding escalation of physical activity. Soon something is thrown or knocked over as multiples careen through the room.

- Due to limited verbal ability, many toddlers express pleasure and displeasure physically. A single toddler may pound the floor or throw an object into the air if angry. A multiple is more likely to pound on or throw an object at another multiple when feeling the same way. ("Happy" pounding still hurts the other!)

- When parents impose consequences for inappropriate adventures, whether all participated or one cheered another on, multiples often socialize during

A parent and each multiple will feel much better about any day that includes numerous kisses, cuddles, and an "I love you" for each.

a time-out or calm-down time, or one who is not involved comes over to keep the isolated multiple company.

• When interaction results in one multiple biting, hitting, or kicking another, the "victim" multiple may become more upset with the parent reprimanding the "perpetrator" than he was with the multiple that hurt him.

• A demand for equality by many toddler and preschool multiples can result in interactive behaviors that try parents' patience. Multiples often demonstrate jealous behavior or an apparent struggle or competition for "dominance" in these situations. The following are some common situations arising from the demand for equality.

❑ One multiple seems happily occupied with some activity but every time another asks to be held or breastfed, the busy one is over in a flash demanding to be held and breastfed, too. A few minutes later the situation reverses. The one who first asked to breastfeed is now playing, and the one who was playing now asks for some of mother's attention. Still the one who seems to be enjoying a toy or activity leaves it immediately to demand equal attention from mother.

❑ A parent may have gone to a lot of trouble to locate two (or more) of the same toy in different colors so that each multiple can easily identify his toy, only to find that all the multiples fight over the same toy of a particular color.

❑ No matter what the circumstances every multiple wants the same toy at the same time every time, and nine times out of ten a battle erupts to determine which multiple has first "playing" rights. If a parent diverts the attention of one or more to a different toy, multiples will soon fight over the diversion. Remove the toy in contention and multiples will compete for another available toy.

Imposing corrective measures for toddlers' misbehavior can be challenging for parents of multiples, but often it is laughable as well.

• By 15 to 18 months many multiples have figured out how to respond when a parent asks, "Who did it?" Each simply points to the other in an eloquent, nonverbal, "He did it."

• Knowing that retreat is often a better form of valor, those same 15- to 18-month-olds will run in different directions when they hear a parent coming. They have already figured out that one parent cannot catch two (or more) if they split up.

• If a parent tells each multiple to sit in a specific chair in order to minimize socializing during a time-out, few multiples will actually remain in that chair unless a parent restrains each by using a seat belt or harness, which often is neither feasible nor appropriate. Also, too much time is often lost between the behavior and the consequences for the last multiple placed in a time-out chair. If the point of a time-out is to demonstrate or provide consequences for a behavior, the point often gets lost.

- To eliminate socialization during a time-out, a parent may try to separate and then supervise multiples in different rooms; however, this is not always feasible. Unless each is isolated in a room with a gated or shut door, which often is not appropriate for toddlers, the first multiple will have left the room to rejoin the other member(s) of the set before a parent can settle a second one in a different room. Again, too much time is lost between the behavior and the consequences for the last multiple placed in a separate room, and the toddlers miss the point of the time-out.
- When interaction results in one multiple biting, hitting, or kicking another, parents often do not know whether to first comfort the "victim" or correct the "perpetrator." The victim deserves to be comforted, but the perpetrator is unlikely to make the connection between the action and the corrective measure a minute or two after an incident occurs. (And the victim is likely to forget the incident and soothe or comfort the perpetrator when corrective measures are taken, so the parent now appears as the "bad guy" and the point of correction is lost–again.)

If any of these scenarios sound familiar, what are parents of multiples to do?

There Are No Easy Answers

Although parents may feel tempted to throw up their hands and walk away, each multiple still needs and deserves limits. Parents of multiples must be more vigilant and they have to expend more effort to keep up with two or more same-age toddlers, especially if a trailblazer or two are part of the set. A child's temperament influences how that child responds to the limitations or boundaries parents impose. It also affects how a child responds to the consequences related to his inappropriate behaviors.

Strategies That Work

Fortunately, there are interventions that parents of multiples have found to be helpful.

> **Parents must be ready to get up and physically intervene when toddlers push the limits.**

- A parent and each multiple will feel much better about any day that includes numerous kisses, cuddles, and an "I love you, (toddler's name)" for each.
- At the end of each day, no matter what kind of day everyone had and no matter how many times your

toddlers heard the word "no," positive feelings can be restored by saying "I love you, (toddler's name)" while massaging a toddler's back and head at bedtime, repeating with each multiple.

- Super-childproofing, or multiples-proofing, may be the greatest disciplinary action parents of multiples can take. (See Chapter 29 for specific childproofing ideas.) By making the home and yard a safe place for toddlers and other family members, many incidents that would require parental intervention can be avoided. This also means the word "no" will be heard less often.
- Keep the word "no" to a minimum. Hearing "no" too often might lead some children to eventually lose their wonderful sense of adventure, or worse, lose the confidence to try new things. During childhood, active multiples hear the word "no" many more times than single-born children. Each multiple hears the "no" meant for him alone, the "no" meant for every other multiple alone, the "no" directed at multiples' joint ventures, and the "no" for the activities that only multiples can dream up and implement.

Choices allow each to have a voice and gain some control in various situations.

Sometimes parents limit outings, especially outings to others' homes, if trailblazing or wandering multiples are too difficult to supervise away from their super-multiples-proofed environment. To curious multiples, going to another home may seem like a visit to an exotic foreign land. Their need to investigate by climbing, touching, and tasting may be overwhelming. Keeping track of multiples is crucial to avoid dangerous or seemingly mischievous situations, but parents find they then have little opportunity to talk with the friends or relatives they came to visit. Often it is easier to ask friends and relatives to visit your house for the time being.

Offering each multiple simple choices often reduces misbehavior that may result from toddlers' feelings of frustration and helplessness. Choices allow each to have a voice and gain some control in various situations. Limit the number of options offered (two is usually enough) and do not offer an option that you are not comfortable with. Some of the forms choices may take include:

1. The *either/or* choice–"Would you rather have carrots or peas with supper?" Count on at least one multiple to change her mind once she sees that another multiple made a different choice. Sometimes it takes no effort to accommodate a change of mind and a parent may want to avoid the hassle of insisting each multiple stick with the choice already made, but this may set a precedent for future choices when it may not be as easy to adjust.

2. The *conflict of interest* choice–"Do you want to walk to your room in three minutes when it's time to get ready for bed, or do you want me to

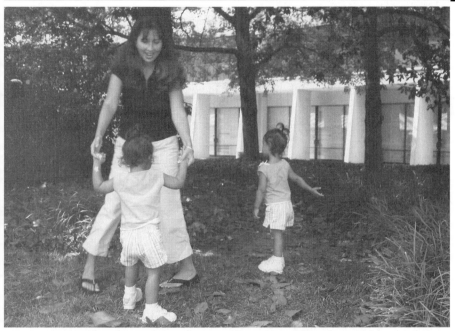

Spending time outdoors releases energy and improves everyone's day.

carry you to your room then?" (Going to bed is not a choice, but each may control some aspects of it.)

3. The *best behavior* choice–"Are you ready to choose a different toy now, or do you need me to take you to your room so you can be alone to calm down?"

4. The *no decision is a decision* choice–"Three minutes are up and it's time for bed. Did you decide whether you want to walk or have me carry you?" (No response from toddler.) "I guess you're telling me you want me to carry you." Pick the child up, being prepared for the child's slippery body movements, and follow through immediately.

Multiples may sometimes act "wound-up" or become frustrated and start fighting when one or more is *overtired or hungry.* Respect each multiple's body clock for food and sleep to avoid many of these situations.

When toddlers are busy interacting or are involved in an activity, they may have difficulty abruptly *switching gears.* Give a several minute warning to help them prepare to move on to the next item on the agenda. Making certain first that they are listening, announce what they will be expected to do next, tell them when they are expected to make the transition, and let them know you are setting a timer for the number of minutes (not more than 5 to 10 minutes for toddlers). When the timer rings, tell them it is now time for the next activity so they must stop whatever they've been doing. Be ready to help them end the current activity and move on if they ignore the timer.

Try interrupting inappropriate behavior by wrapping a toddler in a gentle but firm bear hug. If the child is upset, continue the hug until the child calms down. During the hug, a parent may whisper brief, simple "sweet nothings" to explain why the behavior was not the best choice and other options that might have been better, although a silent hug reassures and calms some children better.

- Jealous behavior can be a drawback to the bear hug. Often the other(s) want to join in the corrective measure. A bear hug may lose its effectiveness as a corrective measure when another one or two are added. However, a group hug can also divert the child's attention from inappropriate behavior and it often demonstrates a positive way to resolve a conflict.

- A variation of the bear hug for older toddlers is to have the multiple being corrected place her hand in a parent's pocket. The hand must stay in the parent's pocket until the child calms and the parent releases it. Until then the child must go wherever the parent goes.

When toddler multiples fight over the same toy and it is unclear who grabbed the toy from whom, place that toy on the time-out shelf until a plan for sharing has been worked out. Three strikes–or three squabbles–over the same toy places that toy in time-out for overnight or longer.

- Return a toy to the multiple initially in possession of it when a toy-grabbing squabble is observed, discussing why one may not take an item that another is playing with.

- Discuss the concept of sharing and taking turns with a toy that more than one wants. Then set a timer and let everyone know that it signals toy trade time.

Although younger toddlers may squabble over the same toy even when two identical toys are available, older toddlers and preschooler multiples often want to play with individual yet identical, toys. When every multiple wants the same small toy, in the same color, and with the same markings, it may be time to respect their collective wishes and buy each the exact toy for the next gift-buying occasion. Consult each multiple before placing an identifying mark on identical toys, so everyone knows which toy belongs to which child. (As they grow older, they will request different toys.)

Biting Toddlers

Most sets of multiples include at least one biter, and most parents quickly learn the cues that one is about to bite. Although multiples usually outgrow this behavior by the time they become preschoolers, the following strategies have helped some parents bring an earlier end to biting behavior.

Some parents find it helps to stop pre-bite jaw action by cupping the toddler's lower jaw in a parent's hand. They do this by placing the thumb of one hand at the temple near one of the toddler's ears and the index finger at the temple near the other ear; the child's jaw rests in the "sling" made by the palm of the parent's hand. The action itself stops the behavior–do *not* apply pressure to the temples.

Another technique is to place a soft, pliable, plastic container lid in the toddler's mouth just when he is about to bite another. The parent then explains that if a child feels a bite coming on he may use a plastic lid instead of the other multiple's body part.

A biter who waits to sink his teeth in another multiple until mother's back is turned is more difficult to deal with, because linking cause with consequence is more difficult if the incident–and visible teeth marks–go undetected for a time and the child who was bitten did not cry out. When a parent hears the victim protest and comforts that child first, the lapse between bite and consequences may be too long for the biter to make the correct connection between action and response. If the parent first deals with the biter, the victim may think his discomfort has been ignored. Sometimes there are no "right" answers. Many parents find it usually works best to comfort the victim while briefly and simply telling the toddler biter how biting hurts.

Strategies That Don't Work

Just as some strategies help, others may hinder parents' long-term goals to teach self-discipline to each multiple.

Corporal punishment imposes "artificial" consequences for misbehavior through the intentional inflicting of an uncomfortable physical sensation as a reprimand. Slapping or spanking sends mixed messages to children. Multiples cannot comprehend the reasoning that makes it all right for a parent to hit them for behavior the parent does not like,

> Corporal punishment, such as slapping or spanking, sends mixed messages to multiples.

yet they are not allowed to hit the other(s) when one does something that another does not like. Corporal punishment teaches toddlers only that it is acceptable for someone bigger and stronger to use physical force.

- It is doubly confusing if any is spanked for hitting another or when a parent bites a multiple that just bit another. How can children's immature thought processes interpret parental actions that "say" to them, "I'm hitting you for hitting your brother" or "I'm biting you because you bit your sister"?

- When a multiple's physical dominance is an issue, corporal punishment only reinforces dominance since someone bigger, stronger, and more powerful is allowed to physically hurt another.

- Some parents believe corporal punishment is encouraged in the writings of ancient religious texts. However, many religious authorities state such long-held beliefs are based on misinterpretations of the original languages the texts were written in. (See Resources for specific resources about discipline with a biblical basis.)

Constant parental intervention for multiples' disagreements or physical fighting may only aggravate the situation. Avoid intervening unless one toddler is in immediate danger from another. Then intercept the punch or push, describe more appropriate ways for resolving differences, separate both/all if necessary, but then stay out of it as much as possible. Avoid passing judgment about who did what unless you actually witnessed the entire squabble from build-up to blow-up.

- When parents stand back, stay out, and simply observe their multiples, they may be surprised to discover the seemingly more mild-mannered toddler often goads the other until the allegedly aggressive toddler finally has had enough and lashes out.
- Many parents are pleasantly surprised to discover that multiples fight less when less parental attention is paid to such fights.
- Multiples deserve to be treated as individuals. Unless a parent witnesses the multiples' misbehavior, consider what multiples may be learning when they are reprimanded collectively but the parent is uncertain whether all actually contributed to the mischief.
- When a parent threatens intervention yet repetition of an inappropriate behavior is followed only by repetition of the threatened intervention, multiples quickly figure out that there is no real consequence for the behavior. They soon tune out the meaningless parental noise.

Labeling children, instead of their behaviors, is hurtful. Avoid labels, such as the "good/easy" twin or the "bad/difficult" quad, which imply that each multiple purposely chooses a positive or negative course of action. Toddlers (and older children) do not choose their temperaments and activity levels. They do not yet possess the cognitive ability to consciously scheme, consider all the implications, or comprehend the consequences of what adults consider as "good" or "bad" behaviors.

Giving up and allowing physically active toddlers to do whatever they want to do may seem the easiest course at times, but long term it is a disastrous solution. When giving in takes the place of loving guidance, parents shortchange themselves, society, and, most especially, their multiples, since these children must someday interact in that much wider society. Parents have a responsibility to provide the individual guidance that each child needs and deserves.

- Providing loving guidance for multiple toddler and preschool trailblazers or wanderers is an around-the-clock task. It involves more than parents' words telling their children what to do; it often involves physically intervening to show them what to do and stopping or diverting inappropriate behavior.
- To maintain the physical and emotional enthusiasm needed for this 24/7 mission, reenergize by taking regular, brief breaks. (See "Brief Separations"

and "Gaining Support" in the sections below.)

- If you gave up today, do not waste time feeling guilty. Reenergize, recommit, and begin again tomorrow.

Multiples' escapades may not seem amusing at the time, but they often sound hilarious in retrospect. Since most multiples are more than ready, willing, and able to provide parents with more humorous material, do not share the details of various incidents with others when there is even a remote possibility that any multiple may overhear–unless you desire repeat performances!

Other Toddler Issues

Language Development

Language ability blossoms during the toddler period. By 15 to 18 months, the increasing receptive language ability of each multiple should be obvious to parents even if multiples were preterm. *Receptive language* is the ability to understand what is said. A child demonstrates this ability when a parent asks a question and the child responds in a way that indicates she understood what was asked. For example, a parent could ask a child if he would like some

> **Some research found delays in expressive language development were more common for multiples.**

juice and the child responds by running to the refrigerator, or a parent might ask a child to get his shoes and immediately the child gets the shoes and brings them to the parent.

Many parents report preverbal toddler multiples seem less frustrated and engage in fewer conflicts after parents teach them some simple signs for objects or certain common actions. A number of books and DVDs or videotapes are available about *infant signing*. (See Resources.)

The timetable for the development of *expressive language*—the ability to actually speak—is broader. Some toddlers have a vocabulary of 50 or more words and are speaking in clear, several-word sentences at 18 months, and others are three years old before they speak in sentences. However, both toddlers may be within the normal range of development. Generally, girls speak somewhat earlier than boys. Still, all toddlers should be able to say a number of words clearly by age two, and all should be forming sentences by age three.

Some research found *delays in expressive language development* were more common for multiples. Preterm birth and its consequences are implicated in some instances. However, the studies also found that multiples tended to receive less individual attention from parents. Compared with parents of single-born children, parents of the studied multiples interacted and spoke less to their infants or toddlers whether as a set or individually. Since multiples have been in each other's company from before birth, they do not always have to rely on words to communicate. In

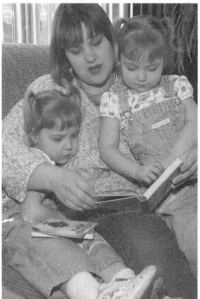

Reading to toddlers helps their speech development.

addition, toddler multiples may reinforce one another's poor speech patterns. Depending on the cause and the degree to which language ability is delayed, speech therapy may be necessary. The following ideas promote speech development in multiples.

• Address each multiple separately and by name even when that means repeating a direction two, three, or more times. "It's time to go to the grocery store. Michael, you need to put your coat on. Lily, you need to put your coat on, too."

• Avoid "baby talk"; pronounce words as you want each to pronounce them.

• Talk to each as you change diapers or give baths. Describe a room as you walk through it with a baby or toddler. Identify everything you see during an outing, such as items on grocery shelves or objects in the park. Describe texture, taste, temperature, color–anything you can think of! You cannot talk to multiples–separately and together–too much.

• Put words in each child's mouth as she attempts to "ask" for something, "Lily, would you like juice? Can you say 'juice'? Watch my mouth say the word"; then repeat the word correctly. (As any child's speech improves, this lesson in how to ask for something should evolve from "Can you say 'juice'?" to "Tell Mommy, 'I want juice,'" to "Ask Mommy, 'May I please have some juice?'")

• Praise attempts at new words and repeat the word correctly, "Very good, Michael! That's right; that's a 'dog'!" Before repeating the word, make eye contact so the child can watch as your mouth forms the word.

• Frequently, one multiple is more verbal than the other(s), and that multiple may take over as the set's spokesperson. Allowing one multiple to be the set's spokesperson may delay the speech of the other(s) since the spokesperson often eliminates another's need to make his wants or needs known. Fortunately, this is easy to halt when parents consistently encourage the verbal ability of each multiple.

• Make a conscious effort to speak to each multiple separately and then wait for a response by the one addressed. If the verbal multiple answers for the one spoken to, gently say something to the effect of, "It is nice that you want to help your brother, Lily, but I'd like Michael to tell me what he wants." Then repeat the request for the multiple originally addressed and again wait for a response.

- Read, read, and then read to multiples some more. Read with lots of expression, which helps them learn patterns of speech and maintain interest in the story.

Early intervention for language-related issues can make a crucial difference in a child's overall development. If any multiple's receptive or expressive language seems to lag behind, parents must act as that child's advocate so the child receives needed help. Discuss questions and concerns with the pediatric care provider. Pursue a hearing examination or a speech evaluation by an accredited speech-language expert if you are uncomfortable with any multiple's language development. (See Resources for "Related Parenting Books.")

Night Waking

Many toddlers still wake during the night, and it is not unusual for two, three, or more individual toddler multiples to be waking at night. Sometimes multiples have been waking since birth, but often they had been sleeping for several consecutive hours and parents had gotten used to a few-hour period of uninterrupted sleep. Then one or more multiples begin waking again during a bout of illness or

> Sleep is not a luxury for parents who must care for active multiples during the day.

prior to teeth erupting, and they continue to wake when the illness is long gone or the teeth are through. Or, after comfortably cosleeping, a couple may find the sleeping arrangement that worked with babies no longer works as multiples grow into larger or more restless toddlers.

Sleep is not a luxury for parents who must care for active multiples during the day. Coping with one or more multiples that wake at night, especially if any wake off and on through the night, can affect a mother's ability to lovingly nurture all of them during the day. When two or more toddlers frequently wake at night and a mother never feels rested, she may not feel able to provide the consistent day-to-day guidance her toddlers need. Mothers report feeling guilty when they quickly become impatient, yell, and react inappropriately to their multiples' normal toddler behaviors due to sleep deprivation. Accidents can happen when a too-tired parent tries to rest her eyes for a few minutes. Also, sleep-deprived mothers of multiples are more likely to experience frequent colds or other physical symptoms.

There are no easy answers. Parents want to meet their toddlers' nighttime needs, yet parents also have a need for adequate rest if they are to be awake, alert, and ready to provide multiple toddlers with loving and safe guidance during the daylight hours. Different solutions have worked better for different families.

- To revise a family cosleeping arrangement, parents sometimes make more space by adding another mattress or two alongside their bed.

❑ Once multiples' receptive language becomes apparent, parents who cosleep part of the night may find that, rather than adding mattresses, they can lay sleeping bags on the floor of their room for any multiple that joins them during night. They tell the toddlers that "big" children may sleep next to, but not in, the parents' bed.

❑ Other parents set up a mattress in the multiples' room and mother or dad joins toddlers in their room if any wakes at night.

- Some parents find toddler multiples sleep with fewer interruptions when they sleep together. Usually these toddlers will be found touching or hugging each other during their sleep. A mattress on the floor of the toddlers' room may be the easiest way to implement this idea. Bed rails can be attached if a mattress is set on a bed frame. (See "Indoor solutions" in Chapter 29.)

- Other multiples sleep more soundly when apart, so parents set up a crib or bed in a separate bedroom or in a room with an older sibling. Creating separate space works well when a home has extra bedrooms, but it can be difficult to implement when space is limited. It often means completely multiples-proofing a second bedroom. If this means altering an older sibling's room or storing the older child's "treasures," this option is unlikely to be well received.

Get into the routine of rubbing each multiple's back and head at bedtime. (Some toddlers may want a full-body massage.) Many parents report their multiples sleep longer when massage regularly precedes the toddlers' nighttime routine. Parents often find they relax as they help their toddlers relax. (See "Resources" for books about infant-toddler massage.)

Some parents find they can talk multiples out of night-waking once the toddlers demonstrate receptive language. These parents first prepare the toddlers for the change.

- To prepare children for any significant change in their routine, begin telling them about it early on the day the plan is to be implemented.

- In brief, simple sentences, explain the anticipated change. An example might be, "You are now big boys (girls), and big boys don't need 'milkies' (insert the multiples' name for breastfeeding here) at night. So if you wake up tonight, Mommy or Daddy will bring you a drink of water and rub your back for a couple of minutes while you stay in your bed."

- Repeat the information about the change numerous times using the same wording. For a change related to night waking, repeat the information at bedtime. You could say, "Remember, if you wake up tonight Mommy or Daddy will bring you a drink of water and rub your back for a couple of minutes while you stay in your bed."

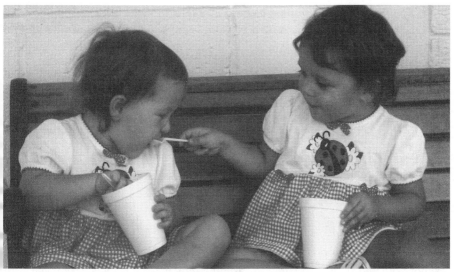

Multiples develop a special bond.

- When the child wakes, the parent reminds the child of the plan they had spoken of throughout the day. "Remember that we said you may have a drink of water if you woke up during the night? Here's your drink of water. When you finish, I'll rub your back when you lie down."

This strategy often works without a hassle or a single tear, but make a "just in case" plan for handling continued requests or cries about coming to the parent's bed.

- Many parents find it helps to initiate a plan such as this when dad has a few days off work, so he can take over the nighttime drink of water duty.
- Some parents choose to keep taking a new drink of water and the offer of a backrub to an awake multiple every 5 to 10 minutes, but they do not take the toddler into their bed.
- Sometimes a mother will go in and offer a brief breastfeeding to a toddler, but she does not take the toddler out of her own bed.
- Other parents take the toddler into their bed if the plan does not work immediately. They are not comfortable with continuing the plan for this particular toddler or they know the disruption is likely to wake the other toddler(s).

The idea behind the "drink of water and backrub" plan is that a parent meets the toddler's need for a parent's presence; it simply is not met in the way the child has come to expect. When it works, the multiple begins to sleep without waking within three to five nights (or less). If any toddler continues to wake beyond this time, consider whether to put a halt to the plan with a particular child. That multiple probably is saying he is not ready; he may be in a "clingy" phase and needs more reassurance. Try again later. A plan that does not work now may work well in a month or two.

There probably is no perfect solution when multiple toddlers continue to wake at night. Parents must weigh each multiple's nighttime parenting needs with their own ability to cope lovingly and consistently with multiple toddlers during the day. Ultimately, the idea is to meet each multiple's overall needs best. (See Resources for Related Parenting Books.)

Brief Separations

Toddler multiples often develop a close bond with the other multiple(s) as well as with their mother and father. Unlike a single-born toddler who lets mother know he prefers to stick by her as she shops, visits a friend, or eats lunch out, many multiples are not bothered by brief separations from mother as long as they can remain with one another. They may become upset, however, if they are separated from the other multiple(s). Since each multiple is an individual, there are exceptions and some multiples have the same difficulty with separations from mother as any singleton toddler.

Because it takes a lot of parental energy to keep up with energetic toddler multiples, parents may need to reenergize–together and separately–by taking regular brief breaks. Go to lunch or a movie with your husband or with friends. Run away from home–literally but briefly–or engage in some other regular exercise. Meditate in a park or a church. Shop or run errands alone for a brief respite. A mother may find she can run errands more efficiently and be back home in half the time it takes to dress multiples for a trip, get them in and out of car seats, grocery carts, or a stroller, push one cart while pulling another when both carts are piled high with items, and mother is also dealing with normal toddler interruptions–multiplied.

When multiples handle brief separations well, it is important that any care provider or sitter clearly understands their individual and interactive activity levels. Daddy can assume more of his multiples' care as they develop into toddlers. When a father is left alone with multiples for several hours on a regular basis, he usually gains a better understanding of the fantastic job you accomplish every day.

When planning a few hours out together, many parents still prefer to have two or more persons watch multiples while they are away. Parents must be very certain of a single sitter's ability to supervise multiples, especially when there is a trailblazer or two in a set. Even an experienced care provider or sitter may have difficulty appreciating multiples' joined capabilities.

Potty/Toilet Learning

After two, three, or more times the usual number of diaper changes, most parents are eager for multiples to learn to use the toilet. Learning to use the toilet usually is easy and does not take long when the child is ready. Most children gain the physical control and mental readiness needed to use a toilet between two and four years of age. Girls generally indicate readiness to use a toilet earlier than boys.

> **Multiples may be ready for potty learning at about the same time or at very different times.**

Multiples may be ready for potty learning at about the same time or at very different times. It is important to respond to the individuals within the multiples set for this developmental issue.

- Identical multiples are more likely to achieve physical readiness at about the same time, but they may not be interested at the same time. However, a spirit of competition may spur a less interested one after the other(s) begins to use the potty.
- Fraternal twins, especially boy-girl sets, may vary widely in physical readiness and in interest.
- When one multiple seems ready but the other(s) is not, go ahead and begin with one. Do not ignore the readiness cues of one in order for all to achieve this milestone at once. It is often easier to deal with this process one at a time, anyway.

Since the basics of how to use the toilet are quickly understood once a child is ready, it probably is best to take a break if it is taking weeks (or months) for a child to learn. Try again later when the child is more ready or interested.

A twins study conducted years ago found there was no benefit in pushing a child who was not yet ready. Parents began "training" one twin to use the toilet between 12 and 18 months. They waited for signs of readiness before the toilet was introduced to the other twin. Readiness varied for those in the "wait" group, but it generally occurred from six to 18 months later. Yet researchers found both twins in a set used the toilet consistently at about the same time, reinforcing the notion that parents train themselves–not the child–when children are placed on a potty chair for weeks or months before they are ready. Most parents of multiples have better things to do!

When any multiple appears to be "toilet ready," mothers have recommended some or all of the following ideas.

- If possible, wait until weather allows multiples to wear fewer clothes, so there is less laundry in case of accidents. (Expect accidents for they will occur!) On the other hand, don't delay when any really wants to learn to use the potty!
- Consider taking any "trainee" out of super-absorbent disposable diapers or "training pants." Replace them with cloth diapers or training pants.

(Training pants are available through some diaper services and there are also disposable brands.)

- Start with only one potty chair for twins, but you may need a second if you have triplets or quads. Multiples rarely need to use the potty at the same time. You can always get another if they do time bathroom breaks close together. A potty seat that fits on an adult toilet may work better for older toddler or preschool trainees.
- Once any begins using the potty, dress that multiple in "potty-friendly" clothes. Elasticized waistbands on pants and easily lifted skirts or dresses work best, because toddlers and preschoolers often do not sound an advance warning when they need to use the toilet. They wait until the urge builds in intensity and requires immediate action.
- Be ready for all to need to use the toilet within moments of buckling the last one into a car seat. Expect to stop–and stop immediately–at every restroom any multiple spots when they are out and about.

A new movement to return to the old idea of beginning toilet training during early infancy has been in the news. This method encourages parents to become sensitive to a baby's elimination cues, which some call *elimination communication.* When a baby cues, a parent places the baby on or over a potty seat. Reports also refer to frequent "accidents" for a number of the babies. It is not clear if a number of children gain earlier control of the muscles used for elimination or whether actual child control of these muscles occurs during the typical two to four years of age.

- A method is valuable if it truly helps a parent become more sensitive to each multiple and his cues while saving parents time and effort.
- A method does not benefit either parents or multiples if it results in rigid scheduling or treatment of babies, causes any parent to feel frustrated or even angry due to babies' accidents, or requires more time and effort to clean those accidents.
- When a method seems to result more in the training of parents than babies yet parents remain calm about accidents, only the parents can determine its worth.
- This method requires diligence for a parent of a singleton. It may be more difficult to monitor or act on the individual elimination cues of two, three, or more young babies when also meeting all of their other needs. If interested in this method, maintain multiples-related realistic expectations.

A Need for Support

Parents coping with multiple toddlers, especially those with trailblazers or wanderers, often think they must be doing something wrong when their toddlers are involved in one disaster after another and they create mess upon mess. Parents of single-born children cannot understand what it is like to try to keep up with multiple toddler explorers. It is difficult or impossible for them to appreciate the interactive effect of multiples and how it affects parental coping day to day. Because many mothers of singletons deal with sibling interactions that occasionally result in similar situations or they have single trailblazers that keep them hopping, they may be able to identify with mothers of active multiples but they just cannot comprehend the around-the-clock constancy of multiples' behaviors and the wearing effect it can have. Parents of sightseer multiples may not need as much support as parents of more physically active multiples, and they may also have difficulty relating to the experiences of mothers of trailblazing multiples.

> **Parents of single-born children cannot understand what it is like to try to keep up with multiple toddler explorers.**

If other mothers do not understand what you are dealing with or you wonder if something is wrong with your parenting, find another mother of multiples to be a *phone friend*. It helps if she shares a similar parenting philosophy, has the same number of multiples, and is dealing with multiples having temperaments similar to your toddlers. Some prefer to talk with a mother whose multiples are slightly older, which can help put multiples' current antics into perspective. In any case it is nice to know that other parents of multiple trailblazers usually feel several messes behind! There are many sources for phone friends.

- A La Leche League Leader or mother may be aware of a potential phone friend.
- Officers of a mothers of multiples organization may be able to provide a link with another mother.
- The Internet has created new opportunities for meeting with other mothers of multiples worldwide.

Multiple toddlers generate unique parenting issues. Parents of multiples may experience both joy and frustration as they care for two or more individuals and the interactive multiples *entity* that forms within many sets. Solutions for guiding one child at a time through toddlerhood do not always work when implemented for toddler multiples. Still each multiple needs and deserves a parent's loving guidance the same as any single toddler.

> **Recognizing and helping each child capitalize on his/her strengths while mastering weaknesses may be the essence of discipline.**

Limits and boundaries for toddlers often focus on their activity levels and a related need to explore, as these behaviors are most likely to result in injury for a toddler or damage to household property. Whether multiples are sightseers that easily go along with the limits parents set or trailblazers that frequently seem oblivious to limits, there are valuable aspects to every activity level and behavioral style–even the more challenging ones for parents! Every style also has its weaker points. Recognizing and helping each child capitalize on his/her strengths while mastering weaknesses may be the essence of discipline.

No wonder many, if not most, mothers (and fathers) of toddler multiples feel overwhelmed at times! When this occurs, call an experienced LLL Leader or another mother of multiples for understanding and support. Since humans were designed to give birth and nurture one offspring at a time, remind yourself as often as necessary, "I am normal. It's the situation that is not normal!" Before you know it, multiples will move into the "easier to watch" preschool years when even trailblazers begin to listen first and act second.

KEY POINTS

❑ Toddler multiples create situations for parents that other parents never face.

❑ Multiples' temperaments affect their actions when alone and together.

- Some toddlers are "naturally" more calm and observant, others are naturally excitable and extremely active, and many fall somewhere in between.

- Parents may worry if a dominant multiple seems to take over in every situation and if one seems more passive and always lets another take over.

❑ Discipline refers to guiding each child to use safe and socially acceptable behaviors.

- Discipline becomes a factor as multiples walk and climb and interact with one another, resulting in unsafe situations.

- Unlike single toddlers who like to please the parent, multiples may be more interested in pleasing each other.

❑ Children understand (receptive) language before they speak (expressive) language.

❑ Although night-waking is common during the second year, sleep is important for parents caring for multiple toddlers during the day. Strategies to encourage toddlers' sleep should be sensitive to everyone's needs.

❑ Because toddler multiples often feel close to one another as well as to their parents, many tolerate brief separations from one or both parents as long as they stay together.

- Any individual multiple may still experience separation anxiety during separations from one or both parents.

- When dealing with this issue, parents will want to be sensitive to the individuals within the set of multiples.

❑ Potty learning usually does not take much time if a particular child is ready—physically and mentally–to use the toilet. Most children will be ready to learn to use the toilet between 2 to 4 years of age.

❑ Parents of two or more active and adventurous same-age toddlers often feel alone and isolated.

- Talk to other parents who are in the midst of, or have been through, toddlerhood with busy multiples. Their understanding, support, and ideas can be life-saving for the toddlers and sanity-saving for parents

RESOURCES

This list is not intended to be inclusive for all organizations, references, products, or product brand names for multiples-related items. Inclusion on this list does not imply author or LLLI endorsement of any organization, reference, product, or brand name.

MULTIPLES-SPECIFIC ORGANIZATIONS AND WEB SITES
Breastfeeding Multiples
La Leche League International (see below); multiples-specific links pages: http://forums.llli.org/forumdisplay.php?f=56

AP Multiples (Attachment Parenting of Multiples; online discussion of breastfeeding, breast-milk-feeding, and attachment parenting by and for parents of multiples) Web site: //groups.yahoo.com/; subscribe (free) with user name and password; insert APMultiples in "Find a Group"

MotheringDotCommune (online forum for discussions of all aspects of parenting multiples, including breastfeeding) Web site: //www.mothering.com/discussions/index.php?; register (free); scroll to Parenting to Parenting Issues; click on Parenting Multiples

Breastfeeding and Attachment Parenting Twins
Web site: //members.tripod.com/~breastfeedingtwins/index.html

France: Allaitement des Jumeaux et Plus ADJ+
11 avenue Lafayette 63120 F Corpiere
Phone: 04.73.53.17.95
Email: questions-espace-allaitement@allaitement-jumeaux.com
Website: www.allaitement-jumeaux.com/

Gromada, Karen; author Web site: www.karengromada.com/

Italian language: Il Mondo dei Gemelli Associazione (see International Associations
for Parents of Multiples: Italy below); breastfeeding multiples-specific page:
//mollar.ilmondodeigemelli.org/MenuAllattSvezzam.htm

Spanish language: www.lalecheleague.org/lang/faqgemelos.html
http://personal.auna.com/gemacarcamo

Photos/illustrations of simultaneous breastfeeding:
www.karengromada.com/photos.htm
www.breastfeeding.com/helpme/helpme_images_twins.html

International Associations for Parents of Multiples
Argentina: Multifamilias
Email: master@multifamilias.com.ar
Web site: www.multifamilias.com.ar/

Australia: Australian Multiple Birth Association (AMBA)
PO Box 105, Coogee, New South Wales 2034
Phone: 1300 88 64 99
Email: secretary@amba.org.au
Web site: www.amba.org.au

Canada: Multiple Births (Naissance Multiples) Canada
PO Box 432, Wasaga Beach, Ontario L9Z 1A4
Phone: 866-228-8824 or 705-429-0901; 705-429-9809
Email: office@multiplebirthscanada.org or francophone@multiplebirthscanada.org
Web site: www.multiplebirthscanada.org/ or
http://www.multiplebirthscanada.org/french/index_f.php

France: La Fédération Nationale Jumeaux et Plus
l'Association, 28 place Saint Georges 75009 Paris
Phone: 01.44.53.06.03; fax : 01.44.53.06.23
Email: infos@jumeaux-et-plus.asso.fr
Web site: www.jumeaux-et-plus.asso.fr/FR/som_site.htm

Germany: Doppelt & Dreifach: Mehrlingselterninitiative Giessen e.V.
Email: info@doppelt-und-dreifach.de or http://www.doppelt-und-
dreifach.de/kontakt/email/email.html
Web site: www.doppelt-und-dreifach.de/

Ireland: Irish Multiple Births Association
Carmichael Centre, North Brunswick St., Dublin 7, Ireland
Phone: 01-874-9056
Email: info@imba.ie
Web site: www.imba.ie

Italy: Il Mondo dei Gemelli Associazione
Strada della Magra, 100, 10156 Torino, Italy
Phone/fax: 178 271 2359
Email: associazione@ilmondodeigemelli.org
Web site: //molar.ilmondodeigemelli.org/

Japan: Japanese Association of Twins' Mothers
Email: info@tmcjapan.org
Web site: www.tmcjapan.org/

Mexico: Asociación de Nacimientos Múltiples, A.C.
Phone: 01-442-2133539; email: presidencia@anmgemelos.com
Web site: www.gemelos.org.mx

New Zealand: New Zealand Multiple Birth Association
PO Box 1258, Wellington, New Zealand
Web site: www.nzmba.info/

South Africa: South African Multiple Birth Association (SAMBA)
Phone: 0861 432 432
Email: sambapresident@mweb.co.za
Web site: www.samultiplebirth.co.za

Spain (Madrid), Amapamu, Centro Cívico Anabel Segura
Avda. de Bruselas, 19; 28108 - Alcobendas (Madrid); email: informacion@amapamu.org
Web site: www.amapamu.org/

Sweden: Svenska Tvillingklubben, Valhallavägen 110, 114 41 Stockholm, Sweden
Phone: 08-662-12 22; email: svenska@tvillingklubben.se
Web site: www.tvillingklubben.se/

United Kingdom: Twins and Multiple Births Association (TAMBA)
2 The Willows, Gardner Road, Guildford, Surrey GU1 4PG England
Phone: 0800 138 0509 (Twinline) or 0870 770 3305; fax: 0870 770 3303
Email: enquiries@tamba.org.uk
Web site: www.tamba.org.uk/

United States: National Organization of Mothers of Twins Clubs (NOMOTC)
PO BOX 700860, Plymouth, Michigan 48170-0955
Phone: 248-231-4480 or 877-540-2200
Email: info@notmotc.org
Web site: http://www.nomotc.org/

Associations for Parents of Higher-Order Multiples

Canada: Higher Order Multiple Support Network (merged with Multiple Births Canada, see above)
Email: homnetwork@multiplebirthscanada.org
Web site: www.tqq.com/

Finland: Association of Finnish Triplet Families
Web site: //tripletti.cjb.net

Germany: ABC-Club Office, Bethlehemstr. 8, D-30451 Hannover
Phone: +49-511-2151945; fax +49-511-2101431
Email: abc-club@t-online.de
Web site: http://www.abc-club.de/

United States: Mothers of SuperTwins (MOST)
PO Box 306, East Islip, NY 11730-0627 Phone: 631-859-1110
Email: info@MOSTonline.org or www.mostonline.org/contact.htm
Web site: www.mostonline.org/

The Triplet Connection, PO Box 429, Spring City, UT 84662
Phone: 435-851-1105; fax: 435-462-746
Email: www.tripletconnection.org/about/contact.php
Web site: www:tripletconnection.org/

Childbirth Preparation for Multiple Birth

Marvelous Multiples, Inc., PO Box 381164, Birmingham, AL 35238
Phone: 205-437-3575; fax: 205-437-3574
Email: marvmult@aol.com
Web site: www.marvelousmultiples.com/; Spanish language page:
www.marvelousmultiples.com/Spanish.htm

Doula: Birth and Postpartum Support

DONA International (Doula information and worldwide referral)
PO Box 626, Jasper, IN 47547
Phone: 888-788-DONA (888-788-3662); fax: 812-634-1491
Email: Info@DONA.org
Web site: www.dona.org/

High-Risk Pregnancy/Bed Rest

Bed rest during Multiple Pregnancy/Pregnancy Bed rest Information and Support for Families and Caregivers (Judith Maloni, PhD, RN, FAAN, Researcher)
Web site: //fpb.cwru.edu/Bedrest/

Sidelines, PO Box 1808, Laguna Beach, CA 92652
Phone: 888-447-4754; fax 949-497-5598
Email: sidelines@sidelines.org
Web site: www.sidelines.org/

Grief Support: Miscarriage, Stillbirth, or Infant Death of a Multiple(s)

Center for Loss in Multiple Birth, Inc. (CLIMB, information in several languages)
PO Box 91377, Anchorage, AK 99509
Phone: 907-222-5321
Email: climb@pobox.alaska.net
Web site: www.climb-support.org/

Multiple Births: Bereavement Support, Ottawa, ONT, Canada
Phone: 613-722-3325; fax; 613-236-7080
Email: haddon@istar.ca
Web site: www.multiplebirthsfamilies.com/bereavement.html

Multiplicity: Multiple Birth Challenges, Loss, Prematurity (Elizabeth A. Pector, MD, mother who experienced perinatal death of one twin)
Email: synspectrum@yahoo.com
Web site: www.synspectrum.com/multiplicity.html or
www.synspectrum.com/articles.html

Twinless Twins International Support Group (for multiples who have experienced the death of a co-multiple), PO Box 980481, Ypsilanti, MI 48198-0481
Phone: 888-205-8962
Email: contact@twinlesstwins.org
Web site: www.twinlesstwins.org/

Twin-to-Twin Transfusion Syndrome

Australia: Twin to Twin Transfusion Syndrome Australia Inc.
PO Box 1343, Carindale, Queensland, Australia 4152
Email: info@twin-twin.org or www.twin-twin.org/contact.htm
Web site: www.twin-twin.org/

United Kingdom: Twin2Twin – UK Twin to Twin Transfusion Syndrome Association, 42 Wentworth Crescent, Harlington, Hayes, Middlesex, England UB3 1NN
Phone: 0208 581 7359 or 01895 846688
Email: correen@twin2twin.org
Web site: www.twin2twin.org/

United States: The Twin–to Twin Transfusion Syndrome Foundation (information, several languages), 411 Longbeach Parkway, Bay Village, OH 44140
Phone: 800-815-9211 or 440-899-8877
Email: info@tttsfoundation.org
Web site: www.tttsfoundation.com/

Zygosity Testing
(At-home sampling cheek swab kit returned for DNA analysis; worldwide mailing)

Affiliated Genetics, Inc., PO Box 58535, Salt Lake City, UT 84158
Phone: 800-362-5559 or 801-582-4200; fax: 801-582-8460
Email: service@affiliatedgenetics.com
Web site: www.affiliatedgenetics.com/

Proactive Genetics, Inc., 525 Blackburn Drive, Martinez, GA 30907
Phone: 866-TWIN-DNA (866-894-6362); fax: 800-701-3109
Email: info@proactivegenetics.com or www,proactivegenetics.com/contact.dna
Web site: www.proactivegenetics.com/

Pro-DNA Diagnostic
5345 boul. de l'Assomption, Bureau 165, Montreal, Quebec Canada H1T 4B3
Phone: 877-236-6444 (Canada & USA), 001-514-253-9998 (outside Canada & USA)
Fax: 514-899-96
Email: info@proadn.com
Web site: www.proadn.com

Hindmilk Feedings for Preterm Infants
Lactation Program and Mother's Own Milk Bank
Texas Children's Hospital, 6621 Fannin Street–West Tower (Room 445), Houston, TX 77030; contact: Nancy M. Hurst, RN, DSN(c), IBCLC (Manager)
Phone: 832-822-3612
Email: nmhurst@texaschildrenshospital.org
Web site: www.texaschildrenshospital.org/CareCenters/Lactation/Default.aspx

Human Milk Banks
Human Milk Banking Association of North America (HMBANA)
1500 Sunday Drive, Suite 102, Raleigh, NC 27607
Phone: (919) 861-4530 ext. 226
Email: aprather@olsonmgmt.com
Web site: www.hmbana.org/
(See Web site for milk bank locations in the USA and Canada; contact HMBANA for locations in other countries.)

Other Organizations for Parents of Multiples
Center for the Study of Multiple Birth
333 E. Superior Street–Suite 464, Chicago, IL 60611
Phone: 312-695-1677
Email: lgk395@northwestern.edu
Web site: www.multiplebirth.com/

Conjoined Twins International (CTI), PO Box 10895, Prescott, AZ 86304-0895
Phone: 928-445-2777
Email: dwdegeraty@myexcel.com or www.conjoinedtwinsint.com/home.htm
Web site: www.conjoinedtwinsint.com/

International Twins Association (ITA)
Email: ITAConvention@aol.com
Web site: www.intltwins.org/

International Society for Twin Studies
Web site: www.ists.qimr.edu.au/

The Multiple Birth Foundation, Hammersmith House Level 4, Queen Charlotte's & Chelsea Hospital, Du Cane Road, London, W12 0HS
Phone: 0208 383 3519; fax: 0208 383 3041
Email: info@multiplebirths.org.uk
Web site: http://www.multiplebirths.org.uk/

The Twins Foundation (twin registry), PO Box 6043, Providence, RI 02940-6043
Phone: 401-751-TWIN (401-751-8946)
Email: tf-inquiry1a@twinsfoundation.com
Web site: www.twinsfoundation.com/

RELATED ORGANIZATIONS
Breastfeeding/Lactation
La Leche League International (referral to local LLL Leaders in United States, Canada, and other countries), PO Box 4079, Schaumburg, IL 60168-4079
Phone: 847-519-7730 or 800-LALECHE; fax: 847-519-0035
In Canada, phone 613-448-1842 or 800-665-4324
Email: llli@llli.org
Web site: http://llli.org/

International Lactation Consultant Association (referral), 1500 Sunday Drive, Suite 102, Raleigh, NC 27607
Phone: 919-861-5577; fax: 919-787-4916
Email: info@ilca.org
Web site: www.ilca.org/

Australian Breastfeeding Association (formerly Nursing Mothers Association of Australia; Breastfeeding Twins and Breastfeeding Triplets, Quads and More booklets available), PO Box 4000, Glen Iris, Victoria 3146 Australia
Phone: 61 3 9885 0855; fax: 61 3 9885 0866
Email: info@breastfeeding.asn.au
Web site: www.breastfeeding.asn.au/

Children/Multiples with Special Needs
Special Child (for parents [of multiples] with special needs)
Email: rfcc-info@specialchild.com
Web site: www.specialchild.com/index.html

Sensory Integration International (general information, local referral), PO Box 5339, Torrance, CA 90510-5339
Phone: 310-787-8805; fax: 310-787-8130
Email: info@sensoryint.com
Web site: www.sensoryint.com/

Infant Care/Infant CPR Classes

American Red Cross (child care classes; local referral),
2025 E Street NW, Washington, DC 20006
Phone: 202-303-4498
Email: www.redcross.org/contactusform/
Web site: www.redcross.org/; local referral: www.redcross.org/where/chapts.asp

Infant Reflux Disease.Com A Guide for Infant Reflux and Pediatric GERD
Email: www.infantrefluxdisease.com/contact.htm
Web site: www.infantrefluxdisease.com/

Infertility Support and Information

American Society for Reproductive Medicine (information, referral),
1209 Montgomery Highway, Birmingham, AL 35216-2809
Phone: 205-978-5000; fax: 205-978-5005
Email: asrm@asrm.org
Web site: www.asrm.org/

Resolve, Inc. (support, local referral),
7910 Woodmont Avenue, Suite 1350, Bethesda, MD 20814
Phone: 888-623-0744 (helpline) or 301-652-8585; fax: 301-652-9375
Email: info@resolve.org
Web site: www.resolve.org/

Postpartum Depression or Anxiety Disorders

Depression after Delivery, Inc. (information, referral, screening tool)
Email: www.charityadvantage.com/depressionafterdelivery/custom/contactus.asp
Web site: ww.depressionafterdelivery.com/Home.asp

Postpartum Support International (PSI) (postpartum mood disorder information,
referral), 927 N. Kellogg Avenue, Santa Barbara, CA 93111
Phone: 805-967-7636; fax: 805-967-0608
Email: PSIOffice@earthlink.net
Web site: http://www.postpartum.net/

Adjunct/Alternative Treatment: Kathleen Kendall-Tackett, PhD, IBCLC; Web site:
www.granitescientific.com/index.htm; Scroll to/click on: Treatment Alternatives for
Postpartum Depression

Postpartum Exercise

Strollercize®, Inc. (classes, workout kit/DVD, book)
309 East 52nd Street 3rd Floor, New York, NY
Phone: 800-Y-STROLL (800-978-7655)
Email: ystroll@strollercize.com
Web site: www.strollercize.com/

Strollercize (Australia): www.strollercize.com/au
Phone: 1 300 78 7655
Email: info@strollercize.com.au

StrollerFit®, Inc. (classes, book), 100 E-Business Way, Suite 290, Cincinnati, OH 45241
Phone: 866- BABY-FIT (866-222-9348 or 513-489-2920; fax: 513-489-2964
Email: service@strollerfit.com
Web site: www.strollerfit.com/

EQUIPMENT

Breast Pumps

Ameda Breastfeeding Products/Hollister Incorporated (hospital-grade, self-cycling
breast pump purchase or rental, double collection kit, etc.), Hollister Incorporated,
2000 Hollister Drive, Libertyville, IL 60048
Phone: 800-323-4060 (USA) or 800-263-7400 (Canada)
Email (USA): www.hollister.com/us/contact/feedback.asp
Web site: www.hollister.com/; distributors worldwide (breastfeeding):
www.hollister.com/us/mbc/breastfeeding/where/international.asp

Medela, Inc. (hospital-grade, self-cycling breast pump purchase or rental, double
collection kit, etc.)
Phone: 800-435-8316
Email: www.medela.com/NewFiles/cust_serv_mail.asp
Web site: www.medela.com/; worldwide index:
www.medela.ch/ISBD/en/breastfeeding/index.php?navid=11

Comparison of breast pump types:
www.lalecheleague.org/llleaderweb/LV/LVJunJul04p52.pdf

Electronic Digital Scales

Medela, Inc. (BabyWeigh™ Scale) (see Medela, Inc., listing with Breast Pumps
above)

At-Breast Feeding-Tube Systems

Lact-Aid International, Inc. (**Lact-Aid® Nursing Trainer System**)
PO Box 1066, Athens TN 37371-1066
Phone: 866-866-1239 or 423-744-9090 (outside USA); fax: 423-744-9116
Email: orders@lact-aid.com
Web site: www.lact-aid.com/

Medela, Inc. (Supplemental Nursing System™) (see Medela, Inc., listing with Breast
Pumps above)

Nursing Bras and Fashions

Bravado! Designs Inc. (nursing bras, including larger sizes)
41 Hollinger Road, Toronto, ON, Canada M4B 3G4
Phone: 800-590-7802 or 416-466-8652; fax: 416-466-8666
Email: customerservice@bravadodesigns.com
Web site: www.bravadodesigns.com/

Breast Is Best (catalog of nursing fashions)
1574 Heathside Crescent, Pickering, ON, Canada L1V 5X1
Phone: 877-837-5439 or 905-837-5439; fax: 905-837-2399
Email: breast-is-best@rogers.com
Web site: www.breast-is-best.com

Decent Exposures (nursing bras), 12554 Lake City Way NE, Seattle, WA 98125
Phone: 800-524-4949 or 206-364-4540
Email: requests@decentexposures.com
Web site: www.decentexposures.com

Expressiva Nursingwear, 1141 Sheridan Road, Atlanta, GA 30324
Phone: 877-933-9773 or 404-315-0692; fax: 206-339-4903
Email: customercare@expressiva.com
Web site: www.expressiva.com/

La Leche League Nursing Bras (available at Nordstroms and other local retailers)
Phone: 888-282-6060
Web site: www.nordstrom.com

Medela, Inc. (nursing bras) (see Medela, Inc. listing with Breast Pumps above)

Motherwear International, Inc. (catalog of fashions for discreet breastfeeding)
320 Riverside Drive, Florence, MA 01062
Phone: 800-950-2500; fax: 413-586-7532
Email: customerservice@motherwear.com
Web site: www.motherwear.com/

One Hot Mama (breastfeeding clothing/swimwear, slings)
6814 Woodrow Wilson Drive, Los Angeles, CA 90068
Phone: 800-217-3750 or 323-969-0790; fax: 323-969-0478
Email: help@onehotmama.com
Web site: www.onehotmama.com/

Special Edition (section for MOT/MOM)
Phone: 888-806-2727; fax: 512-326-8541
Email: customerservice@maternityandnursing.com
Web site: www.maternityandnursing.com/catalog/index2.php?cPath=190

Nursing Pillows

Anna Nursing Pillows (available from La Leche League International, see above)
The Nursing Pillow Company, 260 Osborne Road, Brevard NC 28712
Phone: 888-889-9109; Fax: 704-845-2513
Email: sales@thenursingpillowcompany.com

Double Blessings (EZ-2-Nurse pillow, double strollers, etc.)
Phone: 800-584-TWIN (800-584-8946, USA) (619-441-1873 (Canada), 00-1-619-441-1873 (worldwide)
Email: info@doubleblessings.com
Web site: www.doubleblessing.com/

Pollywog (breastfeeding positioning pillow for babies with reflux/GERD), 5710 NE 56th Street, Seattle, WA 98105
Phone: 866-332-0958 or 206-782-8835
Email: info@pollywogbaby.com
Web site: www.pollywogbaby.com/

OTHER PRODUCTS
Miscellaneous
The Nurturing Mother's Boutique (Twin Connection section; pregnancy/breastfeeding equipment, clothing, support belts, lingerie, etc.)
2050 W 9th Street, Oshkosh, WI 54904
Phone: 888-666-7224 or 920-231-1611
Email: customerservice@momsboutique.com
Web site: http://www.momsboutique.com/shopsite_sc/store/html/

Double to Quadruple Strollers and Prams
Baby Jogger (double and triple models)
8575 Magellan Parkway, Suite 1000, Richmond, VA 23227
Phone: 800-241-1848; fax: 804-262-6277
Email: customerservice@babyjogger.com
Web site: www.babyjogger.com/; worldwide distributors: www.babyjogger.com/intldistributors.htm

Inglesina USA, Inc., 414 Eagle Rock Ave. Suite 308, West Orange, NJ 07052
Phone: 877-486-5112
Email: inglesina-cs@mycomcast.com
Web site: www.inglesina.com/us/index.php; worldwide distributors: www.inglesina.com/en/dealers/index.php

Maclaren USA, Inc, 4 Testa Place, South Norwalk, CT 06854
Phone 877-442-4622 or 203-354-4400; fax: 203-354-4415
Email: info@maclarenbaby.com
Web site: www.maclarenbaby.com/US/index.html (see "About Us/Contact Us"; click on "International Office Info")

Peg-Perego (USA), 3625 Independence Drive, Ft. Wayne, IN 46808
Phone: 800-671-1701 or 260-482-8191
Email: www.perego.com/pages/feedbackcs.html
Web site: www.pegperego.com (worldwide listing)

Runabout™ "Minivan" (double, triple, quadruple, quintuple stroller and "add-a-seat" models), 18770 SW Rigert Road, Aloha, OR 97007
Phone: 800-832-2376 or 503-649-7922; fax: 503-591-9435
Email: runabout@teleport.com
Web site: bergdesign.net/runabout.htm (also see Triplet Connection or MOSTonline about at Associations for Parents of Higher-Order Multiples)

Web site: Review of multiple-seat strollers: //strollers.baby-gaga.com/double-and-triple-strollers.php

Baby Slings/Carriers

Cuddly Wrap, Peapod Creations
PO Box 21 R.P.O. Norwood Grove, Winnipeg, MB R2H 3B8, Canada
Phone: 204.233.5442 or 866-811-8103
Email: info@peapodcreations.ca
Web site: www.peapodcreations.ca

Cuddle Karrier (hip carrier for older baby/babies)
1928 Wildflower Drive, Pickering, ONT L1V 7A7, Canada
Phone: 877-283-3535 or phone/fax: 905-420-1223
Email: cuddlekarrier@canada.com
Web site: cuddlekarrier.com/

MaxiMom (twin or triplet infants carrier) from Tot Tenders
Phone: 800-634-6870; email: info@tottenders.com
Web site: www.tottenders.com/index.html

Maya Wrap, PO Box 44114, Omaha, NE 68144
Phone: 888-629-2972 or 402-614-7340; fax: 402-614-7481
Email: mayawrap@mayawrap.com
Web site: www.mayawrap.com/
worldwide distributor list: www.mayawrap.com/s_distributors.php

New Native Baby Carrier, 135 Aviation Way – Suite 14, Watsonville, CA 95076
Phone: 800-646-1682 or 831-761-2677; fax: 831-761-2677
Email: info@newnativebaby.com
Web site: www.newnativebaby.com/

Over the Shoulder Baby Holder, Post Office Box 5191, San Clemente, CA 92674
Phone: 800-637-9426 or 949-361-1089 (outside USA); fax: 949-361-1336
Email: info@babyholder.com
Web site: www.babyholder.com/
Ride On Carriers™ (hip carrier for older baby/babies), 1932 N Hwy 287, Berthoud, CO 80513
Phone: 866-874-3366; fax: 970-532-4759
Email: info@rideoncarriers.com
Web site: www.rideoncarriers.com/

SlingEZee Sling
571-A Crane St., Lake Elsinore CA 92530
Phone: 951-674-4300 or 800-727-3683; Fax: 951-674-4310
Email: slingezee@yahoo.com
Web site: www.parentingconcepts.com

Double-slinging
(Several sites sell slings/carriers)
www.karengromada.com/photos.htm
www.thebabywearer.com/articles/HowToO/Twins.htm
www.heart2heart.on.ca/sling-twinsposition.html
www.kangarookorner.com/k_how_twins.shtml
www.mamatoto.org/default.aspx?tabid=63
www.onehotmama.com/accessories/twins.htm
www.slingsandmore.com/twin_etc_sling.htm
http://wearyourbaby.com/default.aspx?tabid=63

Infant Cribs/Cots and Hammocks
Amby Baby USA (Amby Baby Motion Bed–hammock-type infant bed), 10285 Yellow
Circle Drive, Minneapolis, MN 55343
Phone: 866-519-BABY or 952-974-5100
Email: info@ambybaby.com
Web site: www.ambybaby.com/; worldwide distributor list: www.babyhammocks.com/

Arm's Reach Concepts, Inc. (Co-Sleeper®)
2081 Oxnard Blvd. PMB 187, Oxnard, CA 93030
Phone: 800-954-9353 or 805-278-2559; fax: 805-604-7982
Email: arc@armsreach.com
Web site: www.armsreach.com/; USA/worldwide distributor list:
www.armsreach.com/stores.asp

Infant Sleep/Relaxation or Infant Reflux/GERD Aids
Baby Slumber/Earth's Magic, LLC (swaddle blankets, white noise CDs, sleep sack),
140 Iowa Lane–Suite 102, Cary, NC 27511
Phone: 888-227-6718
Email: www.babyslumber.com/efeedback/efeedbackV4.php?contact
Web site: www.babyslumber.com/

Miracle Blanket (swaddle blanket), 3951 Southview Terrace, Medford, OR 97504
Phone: 866-286-6386; fax: 805-830-6370
Email: contact form at Web site
Web site: www.miracleblanket.com/index.htm

Slumber Sounds (swaddle blankets, sleep sack, infant massage sets), 321 9th Street,
Leavenworth, WA 98826
Phone: 866-575-2229
Email: custserv@slumbersounds.com
Web site: www.slumbersounds.com/

Pollywog (sleep/diapering wedges or incliners for infant reflux/GERD) (see Pollywog
listing with Nursing Pillows above)

Prenatal Pelvic and Postpartum Diastasis Support

Baby Hugger (prenatal support garments)
Phone: 888-770-0044 or 724-694-0711; fax: 724-694-5081
Email: info@babyhugger.com
Web site: www.babyhugger.com/

Loving Comfort Maternity Support (prenatal and postpartum support garments)
Phone: 800-344-0011
Email: support@cmo-inc.com
Web site: www.maternitysupport.com

Maternal Fitness (TuplerWear™ postpartum splint), 108 East 16th Street 4th Floor,
New York, New York 10003
Phone: 212-353-1947; fax: 212-353-0620
Email: info@maternalfitness.com
Web site: www.maternalfitness.com/

Prenatal Cradle, Inc. (pelvic support garments), PO Box 443, Hamburg, MI 48139-
0443 Phone: 800-607-3572
Email: prenatal@prenatalcradle.com
Web site: www.prenatalcradle.com/

Special Edition (Mom-Ez Maternity Support belt) (see Special Edition listing with
Nursing Bras and Fashionsabove)

GENERAL
Equipment & Childproofing

One Step Ahead (infants)/Leaps and Bounds (children) (childproofing devices,
expandable play yards, etc.), PO Box 517, Lake Bluff, IL 60044
Phone: 800-274-8440/800-477-2189; fax: 847-615-7236/847-615-2478
Email: questions@onestepahead.com
Web site: www.onestepahead.com/

Totsafe.com (childproofing checklist and related devices)
Phone: 586-263-0882; fax: 586-408-6047
Email: support@totsafe.com
Web site: www.totsafe.com/

BOOKS AND VIDEOS (DVDS)
Pregnancy and Birth

**The Doula Book: How a Trained Labor Companion Can Help You Have a
Shorter, Easier, and Healthier Birth** (2002) by Marshall Klaus, John Kennell, and
Phyllis Klaus (available from Perseus Press)

**Having Twins and More: A Parent's Guide to Multiple Pregnancy, Birth and
Early Childhood** (2003, rev. ed.) by Elizabeth Noble with Leo Sorger (available from
Houghton-Mifflin); author Web site: www.elizabethnoble.com/

The Everything Pregnancy Fitness Book (2003) by Robin E. Weiss (mother of twins, includes chapters on multiple pregnancy and bed rest) (available from Adams Media); author Web site: http://robinliseweiss.com

Exceptional Pregnancies: A Survival Guide to Parents Expecting Triplets or More (2000) by Kathleen S. Birch and Janet L. Bleyl (available from The Triplet Connection); author Web site: www.tripletconnection.org/

Maternal Fitness: Preparing for a Healthy Pregnancy, and Easier Labor and a Quick Recovery (1996) by Julie Tupler with Andrea Thompson (available from Simon & Schuster); author Web site: www.maternalfitness.com/

Multiple Pregnancy Sourcebook (2001) by Nancy Bowers (available from Contemporary Books); author Web site: www.marvelousmultiples.com/

When You're Expecting Twins, Triplets or Quads: Proven Guidelines for a Healthy Multiple Pregnancy (2004, rev. ed.) by Barbara Luke and Tamara Eberlein (available from Collins); author Web site: www.drbarbaraluke.com/

DVD or Videotapes

A Natural Delivery of Vertex Twins; available: Ina May Gaskin
Email: inamaygaskin@gmail.com
Web page: http://www.inamay.com/videos.php

Double Duty: The Joys and Challenges of Caring for Newborn Twins (1998) (30 min video) (15 min. edited version avail.);available: The Nurturing Mother's Boutique; see listing with Other Products: Miscellaneous above

Robyn's Births (#B403; 12 min) and **Nancy's Births** (#B107; 13 min) (both of full-term, vaginal twin births); available: INJOY Childbirth Videos: Birth Stories, 1435 Yarmouth Avenue – Suite 102, Boulder, CO 80304
Phone: 800-326-2082 ext. 2 or 303-447-2082; fax: 303-449-8788
Email: custserv@injoyvideos.com
Web page: www.injoyvideos.com/IJBirthLibrary.cfm?id=23

Triplets: Putting the Pieces Together (1997) (17 min); available: INJOY Childbirth Videos (See listing immediately above)
Web page: www.injoyvideos.com/IJOneVolOneVer.cfm?id=168

Postpartum Exercise

Bounce Back into Shape after Baby: The Ultimate Guide to a Fun-Filled, Time and Energy Efficient Workout–With Your Baby (2002) by Caroline C. Creager (available from Executive Physical Therapy, Inc.); author Web site: www.carolinecreager.com/bounceback.html

Lose Your Mummy Tummy (2004) by Julie Tupler with Jodie Gould (available from Da Capo Press); book and video; author Web site: www.maternalfitness.com/

The StrollerFit ExerBook: Bouncing Back (2001) by Lisa Kvietok and Curt Conrad (available from Jasperoo Publishing); author Web site: www.strollerfit.com/

Parenting Multiple-Birth Children

The Art of Parenting Multiples: The Unique Joys and Challenges of Raising Twins and Other Multiples (1999) by Patricia Malmstrom and Janet Poland (available from Ballantine Books); author Web site: www.twinservices.org/

Breastfeeding for One, Two or Three! A Nursing Mother's Survival Guide for One Child, Twins, Triplets or More! (2004) by Maria S. McCarthy (self-published; available from Amazon.com)

Double Duty: The Parents' Guide to Raising Twins, from Pregnancy through the School Years (1998) by Christina Baglivi Tinglof (available from McGraw-Hill); author Web site: www.talk-about-twins.com/

The Everything Twins, Triplets and More Book (2005) by Pamela Fierro (available from Adams Media Corp); author Web site: //multiples.about.com/

The Joy of Twins and Other Multiple Births: Having, Raising, and Loving Babies Who Arrive in Groups (1994, rev. ed.) by Pamela Patrick Novotny (available from Crown Publishing)

Keys to Parenting Multiples (2001, rev. ed.) by Karen Kerkhoff Gromada and Mary Hurlburt (available from Barron's Educational Series); author Web site: www.karengromada.com/

Multiple Blessings: From Pregnancy Through Childhood, a Guide for Parents of Twins, Triplets or More (1994) by Betty Rothbart (available from Harper Perennial)

Raising Multiple Birth Children: A Parents' Survival Guide (1999) by William Laut and Sheila Laut with Kristin Benit (available from Chandler House Press)

Twins: A Practical Guide to Parenting Multiples from Conception to Two Years Old (2005, 2nd ed.) by Katrina Bowman and Louise Ryan (available Allen & Unwin)

Twins to Quints: The Complete Manual for Parents of Multiple Birth Children (2002) compiled by National Organization of Mothers of Twins Clubs, Inc. and edited by Rebecca Moskwinski (available from Harpeth House); author Web site: www.nomotc.org/

Twins, Triplets and More: Their Nature, Development and Care (1992) by Elizabeth M. Bryan (available from St. Martin's Press); author Web site: www.multiplebirths.org.uk/

Social and Cognitive Development

Entwined Lives: Twins and What They Tell Us about Human Behavior (2000) by Nancy L. Segal (available from Plume); author Web site://psych.fullerton.edu/nsegal/

Raising Twins: What Parents Want to Know (and What Twins Want to Tell Them) (2000) by Eileen M. Pearlman and Jill Allison Ganon (available from Collins); author Web site: www.twinsight.com/

Understanding Multiple-Birth Children and How They Learn: A Handbook for Parents, Teachers and Administrators (2004) by John R. Mascazine (available from Authorhouse); author Web page: www.ohiodominicanedu/academics/faculty/mascazine.asp

Postpartum Mood Disorders

Depression in New Mothers: Causes, Consequences, and Treatment Alternatives (2005) by Kathleen Kendall-Tackett, PhD, IBCLC (Available from Haworth Press); Author Web site: www.granitescientific.com/index.htm

Bereavement

Coming to Term: A Father's Story of Birth, Loss and Survival (2001) by William H. Woodwell Jr. (available from University Press of Mississippi); author Web site: www.whwoodwell.com/

A Different Kind of Mother: Surviving the Loss of My Twins (2001) by Christine Howser (available from Authorhouse)

MAGAZINES

Twins Magazine, 111211 E. Arapahoe Road – Suite 101, Centennial, CO 80112-3851
Phone: 888-55-TWINS (888-558-9467) or 303-290-8500
Email: twins.customer.service@businessworld.com
Web site:www.twinsmagazine.com/

RELATED PARENTING BOOKS

Breastfeeding

Breastfeeding Your Hospitalized Baby by Nancy M. Hurst
(pumping for/breastfeeding preterm infants); available online:
www.texaschildrenshospital.org/CareCenters/Lactation/Images/Breastfeeding.pdf)

Defining Your Own Success: Breastfeeding After Breast Reduction Surgery (2001) by Diana West (available LLLI); author Web site: www.bfar.org/

The Ultimate Breastfeeding Book of Answers (2000) by Jack Newman and Teresa Pitman (available from LLLI and Prima Lifestyles/Random House); author Web site: www.drjacknewman.com/

The Womanly Art of Breastfeeding (2003, 7th ed.) by La Leche League International (LLLI) (available in several languages from LLLI); author Web site: www.llli.org /

Infant Growth/Development and Parenting

Attachment Parenting: Instinctive Care for Your Baby and Young Child (1999) by Katie Allison Granju and Betsy Kennedy (available from Pocket Books/Simon & Schuster); author Web site: www.katieallisongranju.com/

The Baby Book: Everything You Need to Know About Your Baby from Birth to Age Two (2003, rev. ed.) by William Sears and Martha Sears with Robert Sears and James Sears (available LLLI and Little Brown); author Web site: www.askdrsears.com/

Biblical Parenting (2002) by Crystal Lutton (pastor and mother of twins) (available from American Book Publishing); author Web site: www.aolff.org/

Bonding: Building the Foundations of Secure Attachment and Independence (1996) by Marshall H. Klaus, John H. Kennell, and Phyllis H. Klaus (available from Addison-Wesley Publishing Co.)

The Complete Book of Christian Parenting & Child Care: A Medical & Moral Guide to Raising Happy, Healthy Children (1997) by William Sears and Martha Sears (available from Broadman & Holman Publishers); author Web site: www.askdrsears.com/

Infant Massage: A Handbook for Loving Parents (2000, rev. ed.) by Vimala McClure (available from Bantam); author Web site: www.iaim.net//index.php

Kangaroo Care: The Best You Can Do to Help Your Preterm Infant (1993) by Susan M. Ludington-Hoe with Susan K. Golant (available from Bantam; author Web page: //fpb.case.edu/Faculty/Ludington.shtm

The Premature Baby Book: Everything You Need to Know about Your Premature Baby From Birth to Age One (2004) by William Sears and Martha Sears (available LLLI and Little Brown); author Web site: www.askdrsears.com/

Your Amazing Newborn (2000) by Marshall H. Klaus and Phyllis H. Klaus (available from Perseus Books)

Fussy or High Need Baby/Children

The Fussy Baby Book: Parenting Your High-Need Child From Birth to Age Five (1996) by William Sears and Martha Sears (available from LLLI and Little Brown); author Web site: www.askdrsears.com/

The Happiest Baby on the Block: The New Way to Calm Crying and Help Your Newborn Baby Sleep Longer (2003) by Harvey Karp (available from Bantam); author Web site: www.thehappiestbaby.com/default.asp

The Out of Sync Child: Recognizing and Coping with Sensory Processing Disorder (2005, rev. ed.) by Carol Stock Kranowitz (available from Perigee Books); author Web site: http://www.out-of-sync-child.com/about_author.html

A Parent's Guide to Living with Infant Acid Reflux (2005) by Annette Cottrell; (available online: www.pollywogbaby.com/refluxandcolic/LivingwithInfantAcid Reflux.pdf); author Web site: http://www.pollywogbaby.com/

Raising Your Spirited Child: A Guide for Parents Whose Child Is More Intense, Sensitive, Perceptive, Persistent, Energetic (1998) by Mary Sheedy Kurcinka (available from Harper Paperbacks); author web site: www.parentchildhelp.com/

The Happiest Baby on the Block: The New Way to Calm Crying and Help Your Newborn Baby Sleep Longer (2003) DVD or videotape by Harvey Karp (available from LLLI)

Night Waking
Good Nights: The Happy Parents' Guide to the Family Bed (And a Peaceful Night's Sleep) (2002) by Jay Gordon and Maria Goodavage (available from LLLI and St. Martin's Press); author web site: www.drjaygordon.com/

Nighttime Parenting: How to Get Your Baby and Child to Sleep (1999, rev. ed.) by William Sears (available from LLLI and Plume/Penguin Putnam); author Web site: www.askdrsears.com

The No-Cry Sleep Solution: Gentle Ways to Help Your Baby Sleep Through the Night (2002) by Elizabeth Pantley (available from McGraw-Hill); author Web site: www.pantley.com/elizabeth/

The No-Cry Sleep Solution for Toddlers and Preschoolers (2005) by Elizabeth Pantley (available from McGraw-Hill); author Web site: www.pantley.com/elizabeth/

Toddlers: Breastfeeding, Development, Gentle Discipline
Adventures in Gentle Discipline: A Parent-to-Parent Guide (2005) by Hilary Flower (available from LLLI); author email: hilary@nursingtwo.com

Adventures in Tandem Nursing (1999) by Hilary Flower (available from LLLI); author email: hilary@nursingtwo.com

The Discipline Book: How to Have a Better-Behaved Child from Birth to Age Ten (1995) by William Sears and Martha Sears (available from LLLI and Little Brown); author Web site: www.askdrsears.com/

The Happiest Toddler on the Block: The New Way to Stop the Daily Battle of Wills and Raise a Secure and Well-Behaved One- to Four-Year-Old (2004) by Harvey Karp (available from Bantam); author Web site: www.thehappiestbaby.com/default.asp

How to Talk So Kids Will Listen & Listen So Kids Will Talk (1999) by Adele Faber and Elaine Mazlish (available from LLLI and Harper Collins); authors' Web site: www.fabermazlish.com/index.htm

How Weaning Happens (2000) by Diane Bengson (available from LLLI)

Kids, Parents and Power Struggles: Winning for a Lifetime (2001) by Mary Sheedy Kurcinka (available from Harper Paperbacks); author Web site: www.parentchildhelp.com/

Mothering Your Nursing Toddler (2000, rev. ed.) by Norma Jane Bumgarner (available from LLLI); author Web site: www.myntoddler.com/

The Nursing Mother's Guide to Weaning (1994) by Kathleen Huggins and Linda Ziedrich (available from Harvard Common Press)

RELATED WEB SITES
Lactational Amenorrhea (LAM) Web Site
http://www.fhi.org/en/RH/FAQs/lamfaq.htm

Twins and Language Development
www.mom2many.com/documents/first_words_on_twin_language.pdf
//members.tripod.com/Caroline_Bowen/mbc.htm

Infant signing
//signwithme.com/002_browse_signs.asp

APPENDIX

Storage and Handling of Human Milk

Each medical institution has its own milk storage and handling guidelines for babies who are hospitalized. The following guidelines apply to home use of expressed milk for full-term, healthy babies. Human milk has properties that protect it from bacterial contamination.

Term Colostrum
(milk expressed within 6 days of delivery)
At 80.6 to 89.6 degrees F (27 to 32 degrees C)—12 hours

Mature milk
At room temperature

At 60 degrees F (15 degrees C)—24 hours

At 66 to 72 degrees F (19-22 degrees C)—10 hours

At 79 degrees F (25 degrees C)—4 to 6 hours

At 86 to 100 degrees F (30 to 38 degrees C)—4 hours

In a refrigerator

At 32 to 39 degrees F (0 to 4 degrees C)—8 days

In a freezer

In a freezer compartment located inside a refrigerator—2 weeks

In a self-contained freezer unit of a refrigerator—3 or 4 months (temperature varies because the door opens and closes frequently).

In a separate deep freezer at a constant 0 degrees F (-19 degrees C)—6 months or longer.

Choice and Use of a Storage Container

• All storage containers, bottles, nipples, cups, spoons, or any other feeding utensils need to be clean.

• To clean a hard-sided milk storage container, use hot, soapy water, rinse well, and allow to air dry.

• Label each container with the month, date, and year so that it can be used in the order in which it was expressed.

For freezing, there are several choices

• Glass is the first choice because it is the least porous, so it offers the best protection for frozen milk.

• The second choice is clear, hard plastic (polycarbonate).

• The third choice is cloudy, hard plastic (polypropylene).

Whichever container material is chosen, when milk is frozen

• The storage container should be sealed with a solid, single-piece cap,

• An inch (2.5 cm) should be left at the top to allow for expansion,

• The caps should be tightened after the milk is frozen.

Milk storage bags, a type of plastic storage container, are popular and convenient.

• Milk bags take up less storage space than hard-sided storage containers.

• Milk thaws more quickly in bags, due to more surface area in contact with the milk.

• Bags can be attached directly to a breast pump, cutting down on time spent transferring milk, reducing the number of pump parts that need to be cleaned after each pumping, and decreasing the risk of contamination that can occur when pouring milk from one container to another.

• Some recommend against their use, particularly for hospitalized babies, because there is more risk of leakage than with hard-sided containers and they are not as airtight, increasing the possibility of contamination.

• Although some consider milk bags more difficult to pour milk from, some brands have built-in tear spouts.

• Some thicker milk storage bags are pre-sterilized, include self-sealers, and have areas for labeling.

Bottle-liner bags for infant feeding bottles are not recommended. Freezing milk in this less-durable type of plastic liner can be risky, because

• They are designed for feeding not storage,

• Removing air from the bag can be tricky,

• The seams may burst during freezing, and

• The bag may leak during thawing.

If the mother chooses to freeze her milk in disposable bottle liners, suggest she follow this procedure for extra protection

• Put the bag of milk inside another empty bag to avoid tearing,

• Squeeze out the air at the top,

• Roll down the bag to about an inch (2.5 cm) above the milk,

• Close the bag and seal it,

• Place the sealed bag upright in a heavy, plastic container with a lid, and then seal the lid before putting it in the freezer.

Handling and Thawing Human Milk

The color of human milk can vary from bluish, yellowish, or even brownish in color.

• Some foods or dyes consumed by the mother may change the color of mother's milk.

• Frozen milk may take on a yellowish color, but this does not mean it is spoiled, unless it smells sour or tastes bad.

Human milk separates into milk and cream, because it is not homogenized like cow's milk from the store. Swirl milk gently to mix it before a feeding.

A mother can combine batches of milk that were expressed at different times during the day, provided she follows the storage guidelines for the older milk.

Fresh milk can be added to frozen milk provided it is first cooled for about 30 minutes and there is less fresh milk than frozen milk. (Human milk should not be thawed and refrozen.)

To thaw frozen milk

• Hold the container under cool running water and gradually add warmer water until the milk is thawed and heated to room temperature.

• If more than one container is being thawed, both can be combined for a feeding.

• After the milk is thawed, the milk should be gently shaken before testing the temperature.

Human milk should not be heated in a microwave oven, because

• Valuable components of the milk will be destroyed if it is heated over 130 degrees F (55 degrees C),

• Microwave ovens heat liquids unevenly, causing "hot spots" in the milk that could burn the baby.

Marmet Technique of Manual Expression

The Marmet Technique of manual expression and assisting the milk ejection reflex (MER) has worked for thousands of mothers—in a way that nothing has before. Even experienced breastfeeding mothers who have been able to hand express will find that this method produces more milk. Mothers who have previously been able to express only a small amount, or none at all, get excellent results with this technique.

Technique Is Important

When watching manual expression the correct milking motion is difficult to see. In this case the hand is quicker than the eye. Consequently, many mothers have found manual expression difficult—even after watching a demonstration or reading a brief description. Milk can be expressed when using less effective methods of hand expression. However, when used on a frequent and regular basis, other methods can easily lead to damaged breast tissue, bruised breasts, and even skin burns.

The Marmet Technique of Manual Expression was developed by a mother who needed to express her milk over an extended period of time for medical reasons. She found that her milk ejection reflex did not work as well as when her baby breastfed, so she also developed a method of massage and stimulation to assist this reflex. The key to the success of this technique is the combination of the method of expression and this massage.

This technique is effective and should not cause problems. It can easily be learned by following this step by step guide. As with any manual skill, practice is important.

Advantages

There are many advantages to manual expression over mechanical methods of milking the breasts:

- Some mechanical pumps cause discomfort and are ineffective.
- Many mothers are more comfortable with manual expression because it is more natural.
- Skin-to-skin contact is more stimulating than the feel of a plastic shield, so manual expression usually allows for an easier milk ejection reflex.
- It's convenient.
- It's ecologically superior.
- It's portable. How can a mother forget her hands?
- Best of all it's free.

How the Breast Works

The milk is produced in milk-producing cells (alveoli). When the milk-producing cells are stimulated, they expel milk into the duct system (milk ejection reflex).

A small portion of the milk may flow down the ducts and collect in the milk ducts under the areola known as terminal ducts (distal portion of lactiferous ducts).

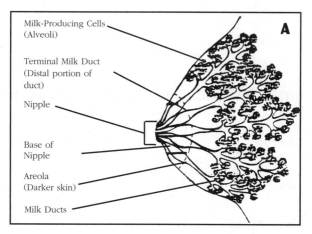

Milk-Producing Cells (Alveoli)

Terminal Milk Duct (Distal portion of duct)

Nipple

Base of Nipple

Areola (Darker skin)

Milk Ducts

A

Expressing the Milk

Draining the Terminal Milk Ducts

1. Position the thumb and first two fingers on the breast about 1" to 1 1/4" (2.5 to 3.125 cm) behind the base of the nipple.

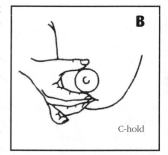

C-hold

B

   - Use this measurement, which is not necessarily the outer edge of the areola, as a guide. The areola varies in size from one woman to another.
   - Place the thumb pad above the nipple at the 12 o'clock position and the finger pads below the nipple at the 6 o'clock position forming the letter "C" with the hand, as shown. This is a resting position.
   - Note that the thumb and fingers are positioned so they are in line with the nipple.
   - Avoid cupping the breast.

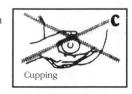

Cupping

C

2. Push straight into the chest wall.

   - Avoid spreading the fingers apart.
   - For large breasts, first lift and then push into the chest wall.

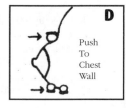

Push To Chest Wall

D

3. Roll thumb forward as if taking a thumbprint. Change finger pressure from middle finger to index finger as the thumb rolls forward.

- **Finish Roll.** The rolling motion of the thumb simulates the wave-like motion of the baby's tongue and the counter pressure of the fingers simulates the baby's palate. The milking motion imitates the baby's suck by compressing and draining the terminal milk ducts without hurting sensitive breast tissue.
- Note the moving position of the thumbnail and fingernails in illustrations D, E, and F.

4. Repeat Rhythmically to drain the terminal milk ducts.

- Position, push, roll; position, push, roll…

5. Rotate the thumb and finger position to reach other terminal milk ducts. Use both hands on each breast. Illustration G shows hand positions on the right breast.

- Note clock positions of fingers in illustration G: 12:00 and 6:00, 11:00 and 5:00, 1:00 and 7:00, 3:00 and 9:00

Avoid These Motions
- Squeezing the breast. This can cause bruising.
- Pulling out the nipple and breast. This can cause tissue damage.
- Sliding on the breast. This can cause skin burns.

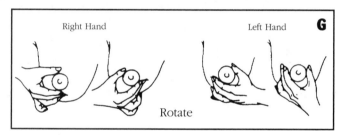

Assisting the Milk Ejection Reflex (MER)
Stimulating the flow of milk.

1. Massage the milk producing cells and ducts.

- Start at the top of the breast. Press firmly into the chest wall. Move fingers slowly, pressing firmly in a small circular motion on one spot on the skin.
- After a few seconds, pick fingers up and move to the next area on the breast. Do not slide on breast tissue.
- Spiral around the breast toward the areola using this massage.

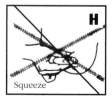
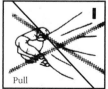
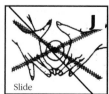

- The pressure and motion are similar to that used in a breast examination.
2. Stroke the breast from the chest wall to the nipple with a light tickle-like stroke.

- Continue this stroking motion from the chest wall to the nipple around the whole breast.
- This will help with relaxation and encourage the milk ejection reflex.

3. Shake the breast gently while leaning forward so that gravity will help the milk eject.

Procedure

This procedure should be followed by mothers who are expressing in place of a full feeding and those who need to establish, increase, or maintain their milk supply when the baby cannot breastfeed.

- Express each breast until the flow of milk slows down.
- Assist the milk ejection reflex (massage, stroke, shake) on both breasts. This can be done simultaneously, and only takes about a minute.
- Repeat the whole process of expressing each breast and assisting the milk ejection reflex twice more. The flow of milk usually slows down sooner the second and third time as the ducts are drained.

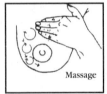
Massage

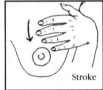
Stroke

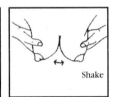
Shake

Timing

The entire procedure should take approximately 20 to 30 minutes when manual expression is replacing a feeding.

- Express each breast 5 to 7 minutes.
- Massage, stroke, shake for about one minute.
- Express each breast 3 to 5 minutes.
- Massage, stroke, shake for about one minute
- Express each breast 2 to 3 minutes.

Note: If the milk supply is established, use the times given only as a guide. Watch the flow of milk and change breasts when the flow gets small. If little or no milk is present yet, follow these suggested times closely. Any portion of the procedure or timing may be used or repeated as necessary.

Reverse Pressure Softening
By K. Jean Cotterman, RNC, IBCLC

More health care providers are observing that mothers receiving multiple intrapartum IVs experience delay in expected postpartum fluid shift. Increased edema during the puerperium complicates engorgement, increases sub-areolar tissue resistance, distorts the nipple, and interferes with comfortable, efficient latching on. Edema may appear early, or later, within 48 to 96 hours, often lasting 10 to 14 days. (This may depend on both the quantity of IV fluid given and the time of infusion in relation to placental delivery, the stimulus for lactogenesis II.)

Reverse pressure softening (RPS) is a simple intervention that has proven very helpful in the first 14 days postpartum. RPS uses gentle positive pressure to soften a 1 to 2 inch area of the areola surrounding the base of the nipple, temporarily moving some swelling slightly backward and upward into the breast. RPS may be applied by the health care provider and/or taught to the mother/significant other, if necessary, over the telephone.

Interstitial fluid volume increases 30% above normal before edema becomes visible (Guyton 1977). To contain edema, areolar tissues must expand, limiting their ability to extend the nipple well into the baby's mouth. Early proactive use of RPS causes no harm and may facilitate increased milk transfer, reduce risk of nipple trauma, and help resolve engorgement.

Conversely, pumping may attract edema into the flange area, especially at maximum vacuum settings. Areolar tissue may then appear "thickened," seeming to "bury" the subareolar ducts. Then, neither infant tongue action, fingertip expression, nor the pump itself removes milk very successfully.

RPS is best performed immediately before each attempt to latch the baby on, for as many feedings as needed.

- The mother may prefer to apply RPS herself, or the HCP, with her permission, may apply RPS
  - facing the mother, or
  - from slightly behind the mother, reaching over her shoulders, or
  - placing her fingers over those of the mother, to reinforce pressure.
- The firmer or more swollen the areola, the more time is needed to achieve pliability.
  - RPS often forms temporary "dimples" or "pits," but edema soon re-enters the pits after pressure is released.
  - Positioning the mother with severe edema flat on her back during RPS delays re-

entry of swelling, allowing a longer window of time for latching the baby on.

– Firmly but gently, press steadily on the areola, right at the nipple base.

– Pressure should not be firm enough to cause pain. Avoid discomfort with less pressure for longer intervals.

– Press inward toward the chest wall for a full 60 seconds or longer. (10 to 20 minutes or more may be needed; this is a good time for instructions.)

• Any finger combination may be used. (See diagrams.)

– Mothers may find short nails with curved fingertips of both hands the most effective method.

– One-handed methods are convenient if the other hand is busy.

– HCPs may find straight-fingers or two-thumb methods more convenient.

– Use the flats of two thumbs or the first several fingers on each hand lengthwise above and below the nipple, creating a 1 to 2 inch long depression.

– Continue to alternate in opposite quadrants, with repeated 2 minute periods of pressure, partially overlapping the first set of pits, to keep edema displaced from the entire area at the base of the nipple.

• After RPS, additional fingertip expression to further soften the areola is much easier, more comfortable, and more productive. Creating a special niche for the chin often permits deeper latch-on.

Benefits of RPS include:

• Steady stimulation of nerves under the areola automatically triggers the milk ejection reflex, propelling milk forward in the breast, nearly always within 1 to 2 minutes or less.

• Excess interstitial fluid is temporarily moved in the direction of natural lymphatic drainage.

• Displacing milk slightly backward into deeper ducts relieves over-distention of sub-areolar ducts, reducing latch discomfort and facilitating milk transfer.

• Areolar elasticity is freed for

– extending the nipple more deeply into baby's mouth.

– responding to the rippling of the tongue.

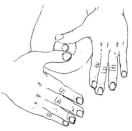

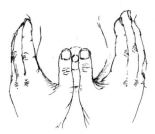

Two-step, two-handed.
Using straight thumbs, press at base of nipple.
Move 1/4 turn, repeat with thumbs above and
below nipple.

Alternate position of hands.

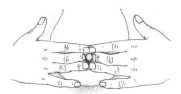

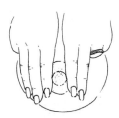

Two-handed, one-step method. Press into areola at
base of nipple with 3 fingers from each hand.
Fingernails are trimmed short; fingertips are
curved inward.

Two-step method using two hands.
Use two or three straight fingers on each side,
with first knuckles touching nipple. Move 1/4 turn,
repeat with fingers above and below nipple.

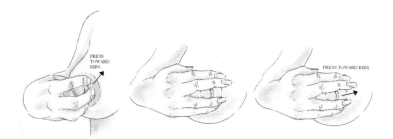

PRESS
TOWARD
RIBS

PRESS TOWARD RIBS

One-handed "Flower Hold."

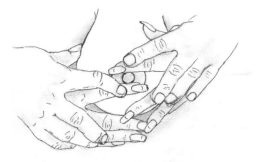

Health care provider places fingers over mother's fingers to
help apply firm pressure.

Illustrations by Kyle Cotterman.

Guyton, AC, *Basic Human Physiology:*
Normal Function and Mechanisms of
Disease, 2nd Ed., W. B. Saunders Co.
Philadelphia, 1977, p. 321.

Updated April 2005

Breastfeeding Log

Day of Week:

Date:

For: (Insert multiple A's name – print using large letters for easier use when sleep deprived!)

Time	12	1am	2am	3am	4am	5am	6am	7am	8am	9am	10am	11am	12	1pm	2pm	3pm	4pm	5pm	6pm	7pm	8pm	9pm	10pm	11p	Daily Total
Breastfeed																									
Wet/Urine																									
B.M./stool																									

For: (Insert multiple B's name)

Time	12	1am	2am	3am	4am	5am	6am	7am	8am	9am	10am	11am	12	1pm	2pm	3pm	4pm	5pm	6pm	7pm	8pm	9pm	10pm	11pm	Daily Total
Breastfeed																									
Wet/Urine																									
B.M./stool																									

For: (Insert multiple C's name)

Time	12	1am	2am	3am	4am	5am	6am	7am	8am	9am	10am	11am	12	1pm	2pm	3pm	4pm	5pm	6pm	7pm	8pm	9pm	10pm	11pm	Daily Total
Breastfeed																									
Wet/Urine																									
B.M./stool																									

Two or more multiples could be monitored for a single day on this chart, or adapt so that one multiple is monitored for several days on one page – using a several-day sheet for each. For individual charts consider printing on a different color of paper for each baby.

A checkmark could be placed in the appropriate spot for each row; some parents also create "codes" to track how long a feeding took, how wet a diaper was, or how large or what color a stool was, etc.

One or more columns could be added to any baby's log for: pumping sessions, alternative/supplementary feedings, etc.

PHOTO CREDITS

Dave Arendt, pages 1, 3, 9, 16, 47, 73, 80, 129, 133, 139, 141, 144, 145, 153, 161, 167, 169, 197, 211, 212, 220, 223, 226, 230, 231, 232, 241, 246, 252, 256, 268, 273, 276, 289, 291, 298, 301, 302, 307, 325, 331, 335, 369, 374

Lindy Stoll, 7, 23, 115, 131, 209, 305, 313, 357

Betsy Liotus, 11, 191, 219, 270

Colleen Karotkin, 26, 66, 185, 253, 267, 314

Karen Jordan, 35, 59, 142

Jennie Dagerath, 38

Colleen White, 43

Andrea Szabo, 51, 63, 76, 137, 151, 249

Unnur Fridriksdottir, 55

John Roleson, 85

Catherine Schroeder, 87

Carolyn Miller, 90

Medela, 97, 103, 124

David Wernick, 121 (top, middle)

Elaine Caper, 121 (bottom)

Mary Kornick, 122, 297

Nancy VanderKlok, 146, 157

Genevieve Raymond, 147, 215, 265

Laura Johnson, 147 (top)

Paul Torgus (illustrations), 162

Beth Morgan, 237, 255, 317, 365, 377

Cheryl Gallagher, 240

Arms Reach, 242

Jenne, 245

Kim Cavaliero, 261, 294

Joanna Satterfield, 310

Mary Kornick, 337, 339

Jennifer Upton, 343

INDEX

About La Leche League

La Leche League International is a nonprofit organization founded in 1956 by seven women who wanted to help other mothers learn about breastfeeding. Currently, there are La Leche League Leaders and Groups in countries all over the world.

La Leche League offers information and encouragement primarily through personal help to those women who want to breastfeed their babies. A Health Advisory Council comprised of medical consultants from all over the world offers advice and assistance when necessary.

La Leche League is the world's largest resource for breastfeeding and related information, distributing more than three million publications each year. THE WOMANLY ART OF BREASTFEEDING, a basic how-to-book, has helped countless mothers through almost any nursing crisis. Other books published by La Leche League are sold in bookstores and through the LLLI online store at www.llli.org.

For further information, we urge you to locate a La Leche League Group in your area by checking your local telephone book or by calling 1-800-LA-LECHE in the USA (800-665-4324 in Canada) or by writing to LLLI, P. O. 4079, Schaumburg, IL 60168-4079 USA (LLLC, 18C Industrial Drive, Box 29, Chesterville, Ontario, Canada).

Visit our Web site at www.llli.org.